D1195526

Electronic Spatial Sensing
for the Blind

NATO ASI Series

Advanced Science Institutes Series

A Series presenting the results of activities sponsored by the NATO Science Committee, which aims at the dissemination of advanced scientific and technological knowledge, with a view to strengthening links between scientific communities.

The Series is published by an international board of publishers in conjunction with the NATO Scientific Affairs Division

A	Life Sciences	Plenum Publishing Corporation
B	Physics	London and New York
C	Mathematical and Physical Sciences	D. Reidel Publishing Company Dordrecht and Boston
D	Behavioural and Social Sciences	Martinus Nijhoff Publishers Dordrecht/Boston/Lancaster
E	Applied Sciences	
F	Computer and Systems Sciences	Springer-Verlag Berlin/Heidelberg/New York
G	Ecological Sciences	

Series E: Applied Sciences – No. 99

Electronic Spatial Sensing for the Blind

Contributions from Perception, Rehabilitation, and Computer Vision

edited by

David H. Warren
Edward R. Strelow

Department of Psychology
University of California
Riverside, California 92521
USA

1985 **Martinus Nijhoff Publishers**
Dordrecht / Boston / Lancaster
Published in cooperation with NATO Scientific Affairs Division

Proceedings of the NATO Advanced Research Workshop on Visual Spatial Prosthesis for the Blind, Lake Arrowhead, California, USA, September 10-13, 1984

Library of Congress Cataloging in Publication Data

```
NATO Advanced Research Workshop on Visual Spatial
   Prostheses for the Blind (1984 : Lake Arrowhead,
   Calif.)
   Electronic spatial sensing for the blind.

   (NATO ASI series.  Series E, Applied sciences ;
no. 99)
   "Proceedings of the NATO Advanced Research Workshop
on Visual Spatial Prostheses for the Blind, Lake
Arrowhead, California, USA, September 10-13, 1984"--T.p.
verso.
   Bibliography: p.
   Includes index.
   1. Eyes, Artificial--Congresses.  2. Blind, Appara-
tus for the--Congresses.  3. Blind--Orientation and
mobility--Congresses.  4. Spatial systems--Congresses.
5. Electronic systems--Congresses.  I. Warren, David H.
II. Strelow, Edward R.  III. North Atlantic Treaty
Organization.  Scientific Affairs Division.  IV. Title.
V. Series.
RE986.N38  1984         617.7'9        85-21453
ISBN 90-247-3238-7
```

ISBN 90-247-3238-7 (this volume)
ISBN 90-247-2689-1 (series)

Distributors for the United States and Canada: Kluwer Academic Publishers, 190 Old Derby Street, Hingham, MA 02043, USA

Distributors for the UK and Ireland: Kluwer Academic Publishers, MTP Press Ltd, Falcon House, Queen Square, Lancaster LA1 1RN, UK

Distributors for all other countries: Kluwer Academic Publishers Group, Distribution Center, P.O. Box 322, 3300 AH Dordrecht, The Netherlands

Printed in The Netherlands

PREFACE

During September 10-14, 1984, we held a Research Workshop at the Lake Arrowhead Conference Center, California, bringing together leaders in the field of electronic spatial sensors for the blind from the psychology, engineering, and rehabilitation areas. Our goal was to engage these groups in discussion with one another about prospects for the future of electronic spatial sensing, in the light of emerging technologies and the increasing sophistication of behavioral research related to this field. The papers in this book give an update on several of the key research traditions in this field. Broader overviews are provided in the paper by Brabyn, and in our Historical Overview, Final Commentary and the Introductions to each section. In a field as complex as this, some overlap of discussion is desirable and the reader with a serious interest in this field is advised to sample several opinions.

This volume, and the conference on which it is based, received assistance from many people and organizations. The Scientific Affairs Division of the North Atlantic Treaty Organization supported the conference as part of their program of Advanced Research Workshops, and the Science and Technology to Aid the Handicapped Program of the National Science Foundation provided additional major financial support. The Center for Social and Behavioral Sciences Research of the University of California, Riverside provided financial as well as major logistical support. Ande Deaver was particularly helpful in this latter respect, seeing flawlessly to the myriad administrative details necessary to have the conference proceed smoothly. We are grateful to the Department of Psychology for help at various stages of the conference preparation and particularly for the services of Fanto Garro who provided excellent technical support.

We are indebted to Robert Mann, William Gallagher, Larry Scadden, and Paul Bertelson for their advice in the early stages of planning, and to many others, including the participants, for help in refining the concept and organization of the conference.

Finally, we wish to thank Marilyn Dick, Nancy Rettig, and Gail Lee for their many hours of work typing and retyping draft after draft, and for their excellent work in producing the final copy of the manuscript.

David H. Warren & Edward R. Strelow

TABLE OF CONTENTS

x

PARTICIPANTS - CONFERENCE ON VISUAL SPATIAL PROSTHESES
FOR THE BLIND: September, 1984

University of California Conference Center
Lake Arrowhead, California, USA,

Bach-y-Rita, P. (Prof.)
The Medical School,
University of Wisconsin
Madison, Wisconsin, USA

Easton, R. D. (Prof.)
Boston College
Chestnut Hill, Massachusetts, USA

Brabyn, J. A. (Dr.)
Smith-Kettlewell
   Institute of Visual Sciences
San Francisco, California, USA

Epstein, W. (Prof.)
University of Wisconsin
Madison, Wisconsin, USA

Brambring, M. (Prof.)
Universität Bielefeld
West Germany

Foulke, E. (Prof.)
University of Louisville
Louisville, Kentucky, USA

Carterette, E. C. (Prof.)
University of California,
Los Angeles, California, USA

Freedman, S. (Dr.)
American Foundation for the Blind
New York, New York, USA

Collins, C. C. (Prof.)
Smith-Kettlewell
   Institute of Visual Sciences
San Franciso, California, USA

Gallagher, W. F. (Exec. Director)
American Foundation for the Blind
New York, New York, USA

Davidson, I. F. W. K. (Dr.)
O.I.S.E.
Toronto, Ontario, Canada

Giannini, M. (Dr.)
Veterans Administration
Washington, D.C., USA

Deering, M. F. (Dr.)
Fairchild Research Center
Palo Alto, California, USA

Haber, L. (Prof.)
University of Illinois, Chicago
Chicago, Illinois, USA

Dodds, A. G. (Dr.)
The University of Nottingham
Nottingham, United Kingdom

Haber, R. N. (Prof.)
University of Illinois, Chicago
Chicago, Illinois, USA

Dodwell, P. C. (Prof.)
Queen's University
Kingston, Ontario, Canada

Harris, C. S. (Dr.)
AT & T Bell Laboratories
Murray Hill, New Jersey, USA

Heyes, A. D. (Dr.)
The University of Nottingham
Nottingham, United Kingdom

Hornby, G. (Mr.)
Auckland Teachers College
Auckland, New Zealand

Hughes, B. (Mr.)
University of Wisconsin
Madison, Wisconsin, USA

Humphrey, G. K. (Prof.)
The University of Lethbridge
Lethbridge, Alberta, Canada

Jansson, G. (Prof.)
University of Uppsala
Uppsala, Sweden

Kay, L. (Prof.)
University of Canterbury
Christchurch, New Zealand

Kay, N. (Mrs.)
University of Canterbury
CHristchurch, New Zealand

Larrimer, J. (Dr.)
National Science Foundation
Washington, D. C., USA

Lie, I. (Prof.)
University of Oslo
Blindern, Oslo, Norway

Mackay, R. S. (Prof.)
California State University
San Francisco, CA
        and
Boston University
Boston, Massachusetts, USA

Pollack, I. (Prof.)
University of Michigan
Ann Arbor, MI, USA

Redden, M. (Dr.)
American Association for
  Advancement of Science
Washington, D. C., USA

Scadden, L. A. (Dr.)
National Science Foundation
Washington, D. C. USA

Sonnier, B. J. (Dr.)
University of California,
Riverside, California, USA

Spungin, S. (Dr.)
American Foundation for the Blind
New York, New York, USA

Strelow, E. R. (Dr.)
University of California,
Riverside, California, USA

Tobin, M. J. (Dr.)
Research Center for the Education
  of the Visually Handicapped
Birmingham, England

Todd, S. (Mr.)
Veteran's Administration
New York, New York, USA

Tou, J. (Prof.)
University of Florida,
Gainesville, Florida, USA

Veraart, C. (Dr.)
Universite Catholique de Louvain
Brussels, Belgium

Wanet, M.-C. (Mlle.)
Universite Catholique de Louvain
Brussels, Belgium

Warren, D. H. (Prof.)
University of California
Riverside, California, USA

ADDRESSES OF THE AUTHORS

Adjouadi, M. (Dr.)
Department of Computer Science,
University of Florida
Gainsville, Florida, 32611, USA

Bach-y-Rita, P. (Prof.)
Department of Rehabilitative Medicine,
The Medical School,
University of Wisconsin
Madison, Wisconsin, 53141, USA

Brabyn, J. A. (Dr.)
Rehabilitation Engineering Center
Smith-Kettlewell Institute of Visual Sciences
San Francisco, California, 94115, USA

Brambring, M. (Prof.)
Fakultät für Psychologie
Universität Bielefeld
West Germany

Collins, C. C. (Prof.)
Smith-Kettlewell Institute of Visual Sciences
220 Webster Street
San Franciso, California, 94115, USA

Deering, M. F. (Dr.)
Fairchild Research Center
4001 Miranda Avenue
Mail Stop 30-888
Palo Alto, California, 94304, USA

Dodds, A. G. (Dr.)
Blind Mobility Research Unit
The University of Nottingham
Nottingham, NG7 2RD, United Kingdom

Dodwell, P. C. (Prof.)
Department of Psychology
Queen's University
Kingston, Ontario, Canada, K7L 3N6

Easton, R. D. (Prof.)
Department of Psychology
Boston College
Chestnut Hill, Massachusetts, 02167, USA

Epstein, W. (Prof.)
Department of Psychology
University of Wisconsin
W.J. Brogden Psychology Building
1202 W. Johnston Street
Madison, Wisconsin, 53706, USA

Foulke, E. (Prof.)
Perceptual Alternatives Laboratory
University of Louisville
Louisville, Kentucky, 40208, USA

Freedman, S. (Dr.)
American Foundation for the Blind
15 West 16th Street
New York, New York, 10011, USA

Haber, R. N. (Prof.)
Department of Psychology
University of Illinois, Chicago
P.O. Box 4348
Chicago, Illinois, 60680, USA

Heyes, A. D. (Dr.)
Blind Mobility Research Unit
The University of Nottingham
Nottingham, NG7 2RD, United Kingdom

Hornby, G. (Mr.)
Auckland Teachers College
74 Epsom Avenue
Auckland, New Zealand

Hughes, B. (Mr.)
Department of Rehabilitative Medicine
The Medical School
University of Wisconsin
Madison, Wisconsin, 53141, USA

Humphrey, D. E. (Dr.)
The University of Lethbridge
4401 University Drive
Lethbridge, Alberta, T1K 3M4, Canada

Humphrey, G. K. (Dr.)
Department of Psychology
The University of Lethbridge
4401 University Drive
Lethbridge, Alberta, T1K 3M4, Canada

Jansson, G. (Prof.)
Department of Psychology
Uppsala University
Uppsala, Sweden

Kay, L. (Prof.)
Department of Electrical Engineering
University of Canterbury
Christchurch, New Zealand

Kay, L. (Mrs.)
Department of Electrical Engineering
University of Canterbury
Christchurch, New Zealand

Lie, I. (Prof.)
Institute of Psychology
University of Oslo
Box 1094
Blindern, Oslo 3, Norway

Mackay, R. S. (Prof.)
2083 16th Avenue
San Francisco, California, 94116, USA

Muir, D. W. (Prof.)
Department of Psychology
Queen's University
Kingston, Ontario, Canada, K7L 3N6

Pollack, I. (Prof.)
Mental Health Research Institute
University of Michigan
Ann Arbor, MI, 48109, USA

Riesen, A. H. (Prof.)
Department of Psychology
University of California
Riverside, California, 92521, USA

Satherley, M. (Ms.)
New Zealand Psychological Service
Auckland, New Zealand

Sonnier, B. J. (Dr.)
Department of Psychology
University of California
Riverside, California, 92521, USA

Spungin, S. J. (Dr.)
American Foundation for the Blind
15 West 16th Street
New York, New York, 10011, USA

Strelow, E. R. (Dr.)
Department of Psychology
University of California
Riverside, California, 92521, USA

Tou, J. T. (Prof.)
Department of Computer Science
University of Florida
Gainesville, Florida, 32611, USA

Veraart, C. (Dr.)
Lab. de Neurophysiologie
Faculte de Medecine
Universite Catholique de Louvain
Ave. Hippocrate, 54, UCL 5449
B-1200 Brussels, Belgium

Wanet, M.-C. (Mlle.)
Lab. de Neurophysiologie
Faculte de Medecine
Universite Catholique de Louvain
Ave. Hippocrate, 54, UCL 5449
B-1200 Brussels, Belgium

Warren, D. H. (Prof.)
Department of Psychology
University of California
Riverside, California, 92521, USA

HISTORICAL OVERVIEW

The Nature of the Problem

Providing electronic replacement for human visual functions is a complex problem with unanswered questions in many areas of science and technology as well as rehabilitation. The general problem and tentative lines of solution have been studied since the beginning of the century: an electronic spatial sensor was developed by 1897 (14) and technology for both a spatial sensor and a reading machine was developed by Fournier d'Albe between 1912 and 1920 (10,22).

While these early devices were primitive, they nevertheless defined the general steps in providing visual prostheses which have been followed to the present time. First, a sensing problem is identified, for example, the reading of print from normal books. Second, a machine is built to handle the sensing problem, in Fournier d'Albe's case by an optical sensor. Finally, the information sensed by the machine is presented to a blind user in a form with which he or she is capable of dealing, typically by an auditory or tactile display.

At none of these stages are the problems simple, although providing the blind with access to print has proved easier than giving pictorial or environmental information. The basic stimulus information for reading, print on a page, presents a comparatively well-constrained sensing problem in that the mechanical device for registering print can operate from fixed distances under controlled viewing conditions. In dealing with the perception of objects in space, on the other hand, a spatial sensor must process stimuli presented under extremes of illumination and at a variety of viewing angles and distances.

A more subtle and serious problem in space perception has been selecting the spatial information to present to the blind person. All devices used to the present time reduce visual information considerably over what would be provided by the eyes.

However, this selection has been governed more by the idiosyncrasies of particular device technologies than by informed selection
on the part of their designers about the most relevant aspects of
stimulation (25).   The problem of identifying the environmental
stimulus features which are used by the sighted for common sensing
tasks, such as the control of mobility, falls within the realm of
experimental psychology, but few researchers in this field have
been concerned with the study of real-world perception. Recently,
the Direct/Ecological Perception movement (e.g., 12,20) has made
the understanding of such real-world problems part of its agenda,
particularly the mobility problem. Insights to such problems may
also come from the areas of computer vision and robotics, such as
the design of self-guided robots (3,21), where the problems of
guided travel have parallels with blind mobility.

By comparison with reading, with its natural speech code,
there is no natural code for spatial representation, and no
modality that is equipped to receive the full richness of spatial
layout contained in a visual scene.   Scenes can, of course, be
described verbally, but only to a superficial level without extreme length, as is acknowledged by the adage that "a picture is
worth a thousand words."   The problem of presenting artificial
spatial information to a non-visual sense thus involves (a)
selecting key aspects of spatial information for the blind person,
(b) selecting an appropriate remaining sense modality to receive
the display, and (c) coding the critical information for presentation to that modality in such a manner that it can be readily
used and interpreted.

Coded spatial information has been presented to the blind
principally by auditory and tactile displays, although attempts
have been made to use vestibular stimulation as well as direct
cortical stimulation. The latter would seem to offer great potential in the long term for prostheses, although it seems unlikely
that any major progress will be made in direct brain stimulation
until there is much better understanding of neural processes than
is now the case. By comparison, the use of an intact sensory
system, such as hearing or touch, has the advantage of allowing
signals to be presented using the body's own natural transducers
(i.e., receptor surfaces) which are in direct communication with
the brain.

In summary, while the provision of artificial visual experience for the blind involves the registering and display of environmental information by technological means, subsumed in the
problem is the need to understand what information is useful for
common sensing tasks and to understand the manner in which this
information should be coded and displayed so that it may be
readily interpreted.

Current Devices

To the present time, most work on the design of spatial sensors has dealt with the provision of spatial information to assist mobility in the blind. Mobility is an important aspect of research with spatial sensors but is not the only rationale for their use; the emphasis on electronic travel aids (ETAs) as opposed, for example, to devices aimed at providing recognition of scenes, reflects the more difficult technological and behavioral aspects of the latter problem. A variety of devices have been produced to sense the presence of objects in the "middle distance" from arm's reach to 20 or 30 feet. These devices have generally been called obstacle detectors since the philosophy behind their use has been to allow the user to avoid collision with obstacles in the travel path. The term also reflects the fact that the operation of most of these devices does not allow any substantial differentiation among, or recognition of, the number or types of objects encountered.

One of the earliest such devices was the Pathsounder (24), originally designed to be worn on the chest. This device uses ultrasonic sensing to provide distance information of the nearest obstacle in front of the user via audible or tactile signals. The Mowat Sensor (23) is a hand-held sonar device with a similar vibratory display in which vibratory rate codes distance. The Single-Object-Sensor (18) is a head-worn device similar to the Mowat Sensor except that it employs an audible clicking display to provide distance and direction information. A somewhat similar ultrasonic device has been made available commercially by the Siemens corporation. The Nottingham Obstacle Detector (1) is another sonar device which uses an audible code in which pitch rises step-wise with the distance of an object. As well, there have been attempts to employ the commercially available sonar unit from Polaroid as an experimental mobility aid with variable sensing characteristics (19).

A long line of research with optical triangulation principles led to the Laser Cane, a sensor incorporated into a walking cane (11). This device is capable of indicating the presence of objects ahead, above, or below the cane, and providing a warning of the presence of objects in a collision zone by audible or tactile signals.

These devices have neither attempted to nor generally been capable of portraying the complexities of the spatial environment to the blind user but instead indicate the presence of obstacles in the travel path and in some cases provide limited distance or directional information.

A number of sonar devices of Kay have employed a frequency-modulation principle of operation which has allowed the collection of substantially more spatial information than has been generally true of the obstacle detectors. Kay has called his approach "environmental sensing". The first of his devices was the Sonic Torch (15), a hand-held device with an audible display presented through a single hearing aid-type earphone. The sound of this device is a pulsed tonal complex in which pitch rises linearly with distance. The Torch gives no indication of direction but its narrow sensing beam can be physically scanned across space to indicate the location of objects. Object recognition is based on tonal quality in which the echoes from complex surfaces give a complex tonal pattern. This device was the first spatial sensor for the blind to become commercially available, with over one thousand units produced. The successor to the Sonic Torch was the Binaural Sensory Aid (16), known now primarily by its trade-name Sonicguide. This is essentially a Sonic Torch with an extra receiving channel. The difference in signal strength between the two receiving channels gives a direction code based on binaural, interaural amplitude cues. It is worn on the head as a pair of spectacles, or in various headband arrangements (27). A more recent version of this form of device is the Trisensor (9,17) which employs a third receiving channel in the center 10-15 degrees of the field of view in order to allow the user to resolve objects in complex settings. The several display codes in this device (inter-aural amplitude, pitch, tone quality, and center-field intensity) represent the maximal effort to date to provide environmental information to a blind user through audible means.

Outside of the mobility tradition, the other major attempt to provide visual-type spatial experience to the blind has been by the Tactile Vision Substitution System (TVSS) (2), which presents the tactile projection of a video image to the back or to the abdomen. Initial models used a display of vibrating points although later electrocutaneous displays were tried. Work with this device has centered on the general question of whether tactile projections of visual images could be interpreted. Several reports showed that recognition of objects was possible, at least in conditions of restricted viewing (33), and that some understanding of the visual concept of objects was possible by a blind user (13). As well, the TVSS was shown to allow improvement in walking performance in an indoor setting (7) based on the "productive walking index" of Armstrong (1), although the mobility aspect of this aid has not been emphasized.

Features of the TVSS have been combined with an ultrasonic environmental sensor to give a spatial sensor which detects the distance and direction of objects and presents information via a plan-position display on the chest, rather than the characteristic visual-type frontal image of the TVSS (5). Some success has been reported in the mobility setting.

Possibily the most impressive aspect of research in electronic spatial prostheses is the diversity of devices used. There has been great variation in the principles of registering environmental information, in the spatial information selected, and in the coding and display of information. While some devices have been more successful than others, no one device has been overwhelmingly successful. All the devices cited have shown at least some limited capability to represent space, and several have shown usefulness in applied settings. However, rather than stressing the success or weakness of particular devices we feel that each different device should be considered an experiment in providing artificial vision, each providing a lead on a different aspect of the general problem.

Evaluation Techniques and Behavioral Research Issues

Because of the interest in the design of Electronic Travel Aids (ETAs) a major research question has been how to assess their usefulness to assist the mobility of the blind (1, see also Brabyn, and Dodds, this volume). This apparently simple question has not proved easy to answer in an unambiguous fashion. Many questions can be raised about what are the appropriate tasks to examine, and how to measure performance. Mobility involves a collection of perceptual, motor, and cognitive factors, and the overall skill is not easy to measure or even analyze, with or without the use of sensory aids (26). The procedures generally followed employ a range of measures of performance of mobility in the field, such as speed, collisions, and stride length to determine if travel is helped by the sensor.

An alternative approach to field evaluation of mobility devices has been proposed by Brabyn (4), who argued that the effectiveness of the information in various kinds of sensors could be assessed by breaking down the mobility task into its perceptual-motor components. A sensitive computer-mechanical link was developed, capable of measuring the loss of control of the body path caused by reduced spatial information, which has been applied to a number of problems in prosthesis research (4,6,28,29,30; see also Brabyn, this volume). Vision allows considerable accuracy of setting a travel path, and the accuracy of guidance provided by a sensor should be one measure of its usefulness of a spatial sensor. Improvements in guidance performance by the provision of a sensor, up to the point where a visual level of skill is reached, would also represent a quantifiable goal for sensor design. In fact, measurements of this sort have shown that visual levels of performance have been achieved on some tasks with simulations of devices (4, see Brabyn, this volume).

There are many other factors both in the realm of psychology and technology which have been largely neglected in the evaluation process to the present time. Seemingly obvious technological factors such as reliability are frequently overlooked. More seriously, there has been no general attempt to define criteria of performance of sensors to provide electronically unambiguous information about objects in space. All of the devices under consideration as electronic spatial sensors have idiosyncrasies of operation which affect, in some cases seriously, their ability to deliver information about environmental objects. For example, both optical and ultrasonic environmental sensing systems require a wide dynamic range in order to deal with signals with widely varying levels of physical energy. The human visual system, by comparison, deals with the wide range of light energy by a combination of mechanical adjustments of the aperture (the iris), photochemical adaptation, and neural processes, which allow it to identify objects in varying conditions of illumination ranging from starlight to the brightness of snowfields and deserts. Electronic and mechanical sensors generally operate far below this level of performance with results ranging from a loss of informational detail about objects to the complete failure to detect objects in the environment.

It should also be realized that the ultimate criterion of a device such as an ETA is its acceptance on the market as a viable commercial product and that even positive reports from behavioral assessors cannot guarantee this result. A device may not be accepted because it is too expensive, technically unreliable, or because it may not be easily used. Even the inclusion of user satisfaction questions will not necessarily predict the use of such aids by the blind (see Kay's discussion of the market aspect of sensory aids and Spungin and Freedman in the rehabilitation section of this volume). Alternatively, negative results, i.e., no advantage to the use of the sensor, have to be treated with the skepticism reserved for negative results in other areas of research. The failure to find a result may reflect as much on the adequacy of the evaluator's conceptualization of what to measure and how to conduct such a study as on the properties of the device itself.

We are not in a good position to evaluate the man-machine interaction involved in sensory aid use when we understand so little of the nature of the psychological processes involved in the use of these devices; the complexity of this problem is such that we should probably not expect a complete analysis of the human factors of performance within the foreseeable future. One major problem which should be given more priority in research is the development of training programs. These have a direct bearing on the evaluation issue, since any evaluation is as much a test of the training program employed as it is of the sensor itself. There is considerable variablity in the underlying spatial understanding of blind persons, which itself could have a bearing on the level of performance achieved. Many of the presumptions about training do not appear valid in light of research (see Warren & Strelow, this volume) and it is doubtful that any training programs to date represent more than sophisticated guesses about how this should be done.

For the most part, training approaches are not well-developed even for spatial sensors used for mobility. The approach to training, typically, has been to give the user an explanation and demonstration of the typical signals of the device and what they mean, and then to accompany the user on a series of naturalistic trials in which the user's encounters with the normal enviornment or a training environment such as configurations of poles are the primary instructional material, with the guide providing some commentary and additional interpretation. For the most part, the user learns to use the device through a trial and error process.

It seems likely that this process can be improved upon. Psychologists have, both in the laboratory and in the educational setting, learned a great deal about more and less effective ways of arranging experience and tailoring instructional strategies, and this knowledge and methodology should be developed to fruition and brought to bear in the area of spatial sensors. To be sure, a great deal of additional research may need to be done on the interpretability of the codes used by a sensor, and on the nature of learning of the correspondence between those codes and the physical dimensions which they are designed to represent. Such research should be able to provide the basis for designing effective training strategies for bringing the new user to an early useful level of expertise.

The second kind of psychological problem falls in the area of rehabilitation. It is not necessarily the case that the visually impaired person, particularly the one who has recently lost sight, will automatically accept a device to replace some of his visual function. This may be particularly true if the device is an obvious one which has the effect of "branding" its user as blind or otherwise "different." The psychological problems that have been reported in studies of the visual restoration phenomenon (31) should serve as evidence enough that a dramatic change in a person's perceptual capabilities, as with the provision of a new kind of sensory aid, may not be eagerly accepted or easily adopted. Habits, including habits of perception, are long in developing and can be slow to change, particularly if emotional issues complicate the picture.

Technological Developments in the Future

Improvements on currently available visual prostheses could come from general developments in many areas of technology which could improve the design of existing devices. For example, most devices have suffered problems of reliability, limited portability, and limited battery life. The cameras used in some applications have had limited ability to deal with the contrast of normal illumination, while limitations in the performance of the ultrasonic transducers set basic limitations on the performance of FM sonars. The TVSS and tactile sonar projects have drawn attention to the need to improve the mechanical characteristics of tactile displays.

While the improvement of existing devices is not an unimportant consideration, we are also concerned that newer areas of technology be brought to bear on the general problem. Virtually all of the devices discussed above have their origins in the technologies of two or three decades ago, and it is imperative that efforts be made to examine what the more contemporary approaches can add to this field. Of particular significance, we feel, are the fields of artificial sensing.

We use the term artificial sensing to refer generally to research in the use of artificial devices to detect and identify objects at a distance, from information or images collected by various sensing devices such as video or photographic cameras, charge-coupled devices, and ultrasonic sensors. This field includes such areas as computer vision, pattern recognition, and image enhancement (3). These areas have developed independently of research with visual prostheses, and have been accelerated by the increasing use of computers and robots for industrial purposes. Nevertheless, they deal with similar problems to those of prosthetic designers.

We have been struck by the progress in image processing, classification of characters, scene analysis, and certain aspects of robotics, particularly the navigation of machines through the environment, and the potential relationship of these areas to the visual prosthesis problem. For example, the design of a sensing system to allow a robot machine to travel among environmental objects (21) has a considerable parallel with the problem of mobility for a blind person. The spatial information which is effective for machine purposes could also serve a blind user, if an appropriate coding strategy could be identified.

Image enhancement techniques offer a potential means of improving the performance of the video sensors in devices such as the TVSS under conditions of degraded viewing or illumination. Principles of scene analysis can be applied to the extraction of significant environmental information from optical sensors. Preliminary attempts have been made at applying this work to prostheses for the blind (see 8; Tou & Adjouadi, and Deering, this volume).

Purpose of the Volume

With the emergence of a roster of ETAs for blind mobility over the past two decades, and particularly with the prospects that new engineering advances may provide the capabilities for breakthroughs that will permit new generations of other spatial sensors to be designed and developed, our view is that a great deal of communication among experts in several areas is needed to ensure that future developments provide the greatest benefit for the blind and visually impaired user. Close communication among engineers, psychologists, and rehabilitation personnel will be needed for optimal progress.

Accordingly, we held an Advanced Research Workshop involving representatives of all of these areas in September 1984. A series of formal papers was presented, and much discussion occurred between and among these groups of experts. This volume contains the edited papers from that conference, as well as several integrating, commentary, and summarizing pieces that were developed after the conference. We hope that the volume will serve as a report of the "state of the art" of the field of electronic spatial sensors, as well as a guideline for the identification of problem areas that must be addressed by those in the field as we look forward to the developments of the future.

The Editors

REFERENCES

1.   Armstrong, J. (1973). Summary report of the research pro-
     grams on electronic mobility aids. Report, Psychology De-
     partment, University of Nottingham.

2.   Bach-y-Rita, P., Collins, C. C., Saunders, F., White, B., &
     Scadden, L. (1969). Vision substitution by tactile image
     projection. Nature, 221, 963-964.

3.   Ballard, D. H. & Brown, C. M. (1972). Computer Vision. New
     Jersey: Prentice-Hall.

4.   Brabyn, J. A. (1978). Laboratory Studies of Aided Blind
     Mobility. Ph.D. Thesis: University of Canterbury.

5.   Brabyn, J. A., Collins, C. C., & Kay, L. (1981). A wide-
     band CTFM scanning sonar with tactile and acoustic display
     for persons with impaired vision (blind, diver, etc.).
     Proceedings of the Ultrasonic International Conference,
     Brighton, England.

6.   Brabyn, J. A. & Strelow, E. R. (1977). Computer-analyzed
     measures of characteristics of human locomotion and mobility.
     Behavior Research Methods and Instrumentation, 9, 456-462.

7.   Collins, C. C., Scadden, L. A., & Alden, A. B. (1977).
     Mobility studies with a tactile imaging device. Conference
     on Systems and Devices for the Disabled, Seattle.

8.   Deering, M. F. (1982). Real time natural scene analysis
     for a blind prosthesis. Fairchild Technical Report #622.

9.   Easton, R. D. & Jackson, R. M. (1983). Pilot test of the
     trisensor, a new generation sonar sensory aid. Journal of
     Visual Impairment & Blindness, 77, 446-449.

10. Fournier d'Albe, E. E. F. (1920). The optophone: An instru-
     ment for reading by ear. Nature, 105, 295-297.

11. Freiburger, A. M. (1967). Fabrication of obstacle detectors
     for the blind. Bulletin of Prosthetics Research, 10, 8.

12. Gibson, J. J. (1979). The Ecological Approach to Visual
     Perception. Boston: Houghton-Mifflin.

13. Guarniero, G. (1974). Experience of tactile vision. Per-
     ception, 3, 101-104.

14. Jansson, G. (1978). Human locomotion guided by a matrix of tactile point stimuli. In G. Gordon (Ed.), Active Touch. Oxford: Pergamon Press.

15. Kay, L. (1964). An ultrasonic sensing probe as a mobility aid for the blind. Ultrasonics, April-June, 106-114.

16. Kay, L. (1974). A sonar aid to enhance spatial perception of the blind: Engineering design and evaluation. The Radio and Electronic Engineer.

17. Kay, L. (1982). Spatial perception through an acoustic sensor. Report, University of Canterbury.

18. Kay, L., Bui, S. T., Brabyn, J. A., & Strelow, E. R. (1976). Single object sensor: A simplified binaural mobility aid. Journal of Visual Impairment & Blindness, 70, 22-24.

19. Maure, D. R., Mellor, C. M., & Uslan, M. (1979). AFB's computerized travel aid: Experimenters wanted. Journal of Impairment & Blindness, 73, 380-381.

20. Michaels, C. F. & Carello, C. A. (1982). Direct Perception. New York: Appleton Century Crofts.

21. Moravec, H. P. (1982). Robot Rover: Visual Navigation. Ann Arbor: UMI Research Press.

22. Nye, P. W. & Bliss, J. C. (1970). Sensory aids for the blind: A challenging problem with lessons for the future. Proceedings, Institute of Electrical and Electronic Engineers, V58, 12, 1878-1898.

23. Pressey, N. (1977). Mowat Sensor. Focus, 11, 35-39.

24. Russell, L. (1965). Travel path sounder. Proceedings, Rotterdam Mobility Research Conference. New York: American Foundation for the Blind.

25. Strelow, E. R. (1982). Sensory aids: Commercial versus research interests. Journal of Visual Impairment & Blindness, 76, 241-243.

26. Strelow, E. R. (1985). What is needed for a theory of mobility: Direct perception and cognitive maps: Some lessons from the blind. Psychological Review, 92, 226-248.

27. Strelow, E. R. & Boys, J. T. (1979). The Canterbury child's aid: A binaural spatial sensor for research with blind children. Journal of Visual Impairment & Blindness, 73, 179-184.

28. Strelow, E. R. & Brabyn, J. A. (1981). Use of foreground and background information in visually guided locomotion. Perception, 10, 191-198.

29. Strelow, E. R. & Brabyn, J. A. (1982). Use of natural sound cues by the blind to control locomotion. Perception, 11, 635-640.

30. Strelow, E. R. & Brabyn, J. A., & Clark, G. R. S. (1976). Apparatus for measuring and recording path velocity and direction characteristics of human locomotion. Behavior Research Methods and Instrumentation, 8, 442-446.

31. Valvo, A. (1971). Sight Restoration After Long-term Blindness: The Problems and Behavior Patterns of Visual Rehabilitation. New York: American Foundation for the Blind.

32. Warren, D. H. & Strelow, E. R. (1984). Learning spatial dimensions with a visual sensory aid: Molyneux revisited. Perception, 13, 331-350.

33. White, B., Saunders, F. A., Scadden, L. A., Bach-y-Rita, P., & Collins, C. C. (1970). Seeing with the skin. Perception & Psychophysics, 7, 23-27.

A REVIEW OF MOBILITY AIDS AND MEANS OF ASSESSMENT

John Brabyn

Smith-Kettlewell Institute of Visual Sciences

Mobility has been defined by Foulke (22) as "the ability to travel safely, comfortably, gracefully, and independently through the environment." The most popular mobility aid is, of course, the long cane, but whether or not this solves the problems of "grace" and "independence" is questionable at best. The long cane, introduced in its present form by Hoover (27) in the late 1940s, effectively allows detection of obstacles within a 3-foot range, and tends to warn other pedestrians to get out of the way. The former feature requires fast stopping reaction when an obstacle is encountered, while the latter does not add to the grace and independence of travel.

Consequently, during the 1960s, a host of electronic aids appeared (11,12,23,28,29,39,43,45,47) concentrating on the mobility problems of blind people. The proliferation of such aids slowed down somewhat in the 1970s, and a few aids reached commercial production. By the early 1980s, the flow of significant new developments in the area of mobility aids had slowed to a trickle, and no aid yet developed has achieved any significant degree of penetration of the potential market.

Evidently, we have been doing something wrong. Hence the need to step back and assess the situation, review the fundamental problems of mobility, and devise strategies for future progress.

ELECTRONIC MOBILITY AIDS: HISTORY

Following the development of radar and sonar technologies for remote sensing during World War II, and the introduction of transistor technology which made portable electronic devices practical, inventors began to see the potential for various obstacle-detection devices to aid blind people. Devices utilized the transmission of an energy wave (usually ultrasonic) and the reception of echoes from objects in or near the traveler's path. The choice of ultrasound for the transmission medium, as opposed to light or radio waves, was dictated by the convenience with which echo ranging could be performed in this medium due to the relatively slow speed of propagation. Optical sensing was used in some cases where the operation of the system was passive, or where range measurement was not a design goal (e.g., in the Laser Cane).

Sonar technology, as it existed by 1960, was well-developed for underwater purposes, but its use above water was complicated by much-increased signal attenuation and difficulty of coupling a transducer effectively to the air. These problems were overcome, and ultrasound became the most popular sensing medium for mobility aids. The main limitations of the technology were limited useful range and difficulties experienced with refections from smooth surfaces (which act like mirrors to ultrasound).

Clear-Path Indicators vs. Environmental Sensors

Once the technical problems had been solved, the principal arguments among developers revolved around the amount and type of information that is desirable to present to the user, and the manner in which it should be presented. Development followed two schools of thought. One class of aids, known as obstacle detectors or clear-path indicators (22), warned only of the presence and sometimes the approximate range of obstacles directly in the travel path, while generally not being concerned with identification of the obstacles detected. Such devices generally had the advantage of relatively lower cost.

Included in this category is the Russell Pathsounder (43), which uses a 30-degree ultrasonic beam transmitted from a chest-level unit suspended from the user's neck. It can provide tactile and auditory warning of objects up to six feet ahead and allows some range estimation. The Mowat Sensor (41) is a hand-held, pulsed sonar system with tactile output. The narrow-beam, flashlight-sized device vibrates with a period proportional to target range. The Nottingham Obstacle Detector (2) is similar in operation and shape to the Mowat Sensor, except that it provides an auditory readout of range with eight notes corresponding to the musical scale. The Laser Cane (40) is a conventionally shaped long cane with laser emitters and receivers aimed to detect over-hangs, down-curbs, and targets straight ahead within a selectable range of six to 12 feet, giving auditory and tactile warnings.

A second category of aids, known as environmental sensors (22), attempts more than mere detection of obstacles. The first of these to be developed (and one of the most well-known) was the Kay Sonic Torch (28). One of the few devices designed to replace rather than merely supplement the long cane or guide dog, the Sonic Torch (no longer in production) was a handheld, narrow-beam ultrasonic device with an auditory output presented via an ear-phone. The Sonic Torch, in contrast to those ultrasonic travel aids of the obstacle-detector class (which normally use simple single-frequency pulse transmission), transmitted a wide-band-width (40-80 kHz), frequency-modulated, ultrasonic energy wave. Reflected signals from the Sonic Torch were converted to the audible region by multiplication with the transmitted signal. The result was an audible signal extremely rich in information, the pitch corresponding to range and timbre corresponding to variation in target surface texture, the latter enabling a degree of target identification.

Later developments in this concept led to the Binaural Sen-sory Aid (29), known commercially as the Sonicguide. Employing the same methods of transmission and reception, this device looks like a pair of spectacle frames worn on the head with a wide-beam (60-90 degree) transmitter. The two receiving transducers are splayed a few degrees to the left and right, and their signals are presented separately to the left and right ears, giving a built-in direction cue. The Sonicguide is typically used in conjunction with the long cane or guide dog, like most other electronic mobility aids.

RECENT DEVELOPMENTS IN MOBILITY AIDS

Most of the aids used as examples above are now commercially available, but have not achieved broad penetration of the market. All are relatively expensive, costing anywhere from $300 to $3,000. Most are designed to supplement (rather than replace) the long cane, and there is disagreement over whether the additional information that they provide is worth the very considerable extra cost and the effort of training. A skilled user of the long cane can use the sounds emitted by the cane tip for natural echolocation, providing him with a surprising amount of informa-tion about large objects in the immediate environment (51). This category of user, although not typical of the general population, would require substantial additional input from an electronic aid before its use became worthwhile. The sophisticated auditory display of such an aid may tend, however, to mask the subtle echolocation cues mentioned above. For those individuals who do not possess refined echolocation skills, this argument is not valid. Automatic level controllers, which adjust the loudness of the display in accordance with background noise levels, may also reduce such interference (49). Other reasons must be sought for the apparent lack of general acceptance of existing electronic mobility aids.

In the late 1970s and early 1980s, device developers came up with some new solutions and refinements to address these problems. Criticism of the amount of information presented by the Kay Sonicguide was partly answered by the development of a prototype single-channel system with a narrow beamwidth, eliminating the constant signals returned by objects in the periphery, while retaining the object-identification advantages of the binaural version.

To shed light on the controversy regarding the optimal form of range cue for an obstacle detector, the American Foundation for the Blind developed a microprocessor-assisted ultrasonic ranging device (36) using the sonar electronics from the Polaroid camera focusing mechanism. The microprocessor can be programmed to present the output in any one of a variety of auditory codes, including the spoken voice. Other Polaroid-based ranging systems have also been developed (25). In the Federal Republic of Germany, the Siemens Company produced its own spectacle-worn and hand-held obstacle-detector systems, while in England the developers of the Nottingham Obstacle Detector devised a modified head-worn version, the Sonic Pathfinder (26, see also Heyes, and Dodds, this volume) designed to allow discrimination of target direction while remaining basically an "obstacle detection" system.

Investigations were made of the feasibility of tactile information presentation for a mobility aid, in order to overcome the criticized masking effects of auditory displays (and also for use by the deaf-blind). Earlier research in this field, at the Smith-Kettlewell Institute of Visual Sciences and elsewhere (13, 14), had centered on the direct presentation of television camera images on the skin, on a point-for-point basis using large (32 x 32- or 20 x 20-point) tactile arrays worn on the abdomen (See Collins, and Bach-y-Rita & Hughes, this volume). It was concluded that this concept has educational value when confined to simple images and shapes, but the complex scenes encountered outdoors cannot be readily interpreted through the skin for use in mobility.

Two alternative approaches were then investigated for pre-processing the tactile information in order to simplify the display. The first approach used a scanning sonar system (6) to present a plan-type view of the environment on the skin, displaying range and azimuth information in the same manner as a PPI radar display. This approach was successfully tested, but the expense of the large tactile arrays mitigated against successful commercialization. An alternative approach using computer processing of video images to extract only the features thought to be vital to mobility (such as curbs, poles, fences) was then tested. Range and direction were coded on a one-dimensional tactile array, and supplemental synthetic speech information was used in the system output (15, see also Collins, and Deering, this volume).

In order to overcome the difficulties experienced with ultrasonic obstacle sensors when attempting to detect smooth surfaces at oblique angles, an infrared ranging system was designed at the Smith-Kettlewell Institute. The prototype device uses a disparity technique which does not require complex electronics for propagation delay measurements. The initial version uses an auditory output, with an inverse relationship between pitch and range. The beam is extremely narrow (approximately 5 degrees), and smooth surfaces such as linoleum can be detected at angles up to approximately 60 degrees from the perpendicular.

Orientation Aids

A further limitation of electronic travel aid development up to 1980 was that all the aids developed up to that time addressed only the problem of successfully negotiating a safe path through the environment (although some aids, such as the Sonic-guide, can assist materially in the identification of landmarks).

Orientation can be defined simply as knowing where one is in absolute terms of reference. In particular, the blind pedestrian suffers from a lack of access to sign information (imagine the difficulty of a sighted person attempting to find his way around a strange city with no written signs). Recently, researchers have made the first steps toward applying technology to this global navigation problem. The "Talking Signs" system (35), developed at the Smith-Kettlewell Institute, utilizes a network of low-cost infrared transmitter modules placed on normal navigational signs in the environment, such as street corners, bus stops, corridors, room and building numbers. A voice output corresponding to the wording of the sign is produced by a hand-held receiver which receives the infrared transmissions and converts them into a spoken message. Each transmitter contains a computer memory chip on which its message is stored. This system is now in commercial production.

A similar idea is being pursued by the Georgia Institute of Technology in the development of its SONA (Sonic Orientation Navigation Aid) system (32). This orientation aid uses radio-activated auditory beacons to accomplish the task. If, for example, a user is searching for an elevator, he enters a corresponding numerical code on a keypad mounted on his hand-carried transmitter. The transmitter then interrogates any receivers in the vicinity. If a receiver is present on an elevator nearby, it will accept the code and produce an auditory beep.

Obviously, successful dissemination of such orientation and navigation systems is problematical, due to installation costs. Even though substantial and expensive modifications to the environment have been made for the benefit of wheelchair users, it does not currently appear likely that the same expense will be lavished upon the blind.

MOBILITY AID ASSESSMENT

Early Efforts

Until now, the development of electronic mobility aids for the blind has been largely conducted by engineers with their own theories about what information should be used by the blind pedestrian, and how it should be presented. Relatively little knowledge exists regarding the basic mechanisms of human mobility. The mechanical process of locomotion has been studied by those interested in limb prostheses, but that research does not address the more complex sensory and cognitive-related aspects of the problem. As a result, researchers have little basic knowledge to use as a starting point when designing and evaluating mobility aids for the blind. What are the essential components of information needed for mobility? What spatial cues does a sighted person rely on for maintaining a safe course through the environment? Once these cues are identified how can they best be coded and displayed to the user? (See 48, and Foulke, and Jansson, this volume.)

If we do not really understand mobility, how can we measure it to ascertain whether an artificial aid is actually improving a blind person's performance? This problem has dogged the evaluation of mobility aids since their inception.

Early evaluations of mobility aids such as the Sonic Torch (17,21,33,42,46), the Russell Pathsounder (18,44,), the Sonic-guide (1,38,55,56), and the Laser Cane (40) revolved around largely subjective rating systems scored by observers. Some attempts were made to utilize indoor obstacle courses. In some cases, user performance with the aid was judged inferior to unaided performance, and in most cases the results were inconclusive. Certainly, the production and marketing of the various aids went ahead regardless.

Theories of mobility were put forward by Foulke (22), Kay (31), and recently by Strelow (48). Subsequently, other researchers attempted to refine mobility assessment techniques, relating their methods to these theories. The Blind Mobility Research Unit at the University of Nottingham (2,3,33) used sophisticated videobased recording and rerecording techniques for measuring mobility performance outdoors. They developed indices of safety, efficiency, and stress as operational criteria of good mobility (See Dodds, this volume).

The "Locomotor Control" Approach

In contrast to these and other approaches using obstacle courses and grading systems which are subjective to a greater or lesser degree, investigators at the University of Canterbury (4,7,8,52) proposed breaking down the mobility task into the two components of orientation and locomotor control. Locomotor control was defined as the ability to control the bodily path, during mobility, with respect to the immediate environment. This subset of the overall mobility task is one which can, at least in theory, be measured in a quantifiable manner in the laboratory by obtaining continuous records of subject position and associated derivative measures (velocity, acceleration, etc.). This approach to mobility assessment dovetailed the theory of mobility put forward by Kay (31), and allowed mobility studies to be put within that framework.

Instrumentation was developed for continuous measurement of a subject's position in the large mobility laboratory (4,8,9,52). Performance measures were derived which related to the accuracy with which bodily path was controlled in certain tasks such as shorelining, approaching an object from a distance, and traveling around a square or a circle. After experimentation, the measure found to be most relevant and sensitive was the RMS deviation from a straight line (for the shorelining and object-approaching tasks) and the RMS deviation from these ideal paths (the "ideal path" was specified by the experimenter). In certain cases, variations in velocity and acceleration were also useful.

The locomotor control assessment system was utilized to compare the locomotor control performance of subjects utilizing various sonar-based mobility aids, especially in the shorelining task. It was also utilized to explore performance of blind subjects utilizing auditory cues only (51), as well as studying the relative importance of foreground and background information in mobility (50).

A further extension of the technique was modification of the instrumentation to allow dynamic simulation of mobility aid displays in real locomotor control tasks (4,8). The system's computer, which monitored the subject's position, the position of obstacles or "targets," and the subject's head orientation, was utilized to generate appropriate auditory and tactile display parameters which were fed back to the subject. In this manner, range and direction code variations for ultrasonic mobility aids were investigated with a view to optimizing locomotor control performance, and the feasibility of navigating through a maze of poles utilizing a tactile display was established (4).

Using this locomotor control instrumentation as a tool for investigating subcomponents of mobility, it was possible to compile a table (Table 1) showing a continuous quantifiable variation in performance levels from "unaided" performance through to "sighted" peformance. It should be stressed here that this approach investigates only an important subset of the overall mobility task, but one which can be exactly quantified and which therefore lends itself to experimental rigor.

Recent Work

Similar approaches to monitoring and simulating the locomotor control portion of mobility have since been undertaken by other investigators (10,16,54). Dr. Gunnar Jansson of the University of Uppsala, Sweden and Susanna Millar at Oxford University in the U.K. have replicated the Canterbury monitoring system for their own studies.

Recent progress in assessing mobility through the more traditional techniques of time and significant event measurement through a specified indoor or outdoor mobility course have included the application of this method by several investigators (24,37) to assess the mobility skills of the low vision population, with and without various low vision aids. These traditional techniques have been further refined by the Nottingham group in assessing the mobility of the totally blind (20, see also Dodds, this volume). In the latter field, and with a view to the establishment of parameters for blind mobility aids, Shingledecker (53) and others have investigated the use of "secondary task" performance as one approach to the problem of mobility assessment. Total elapsed time of travel was found to be a sufficient criterion to discriminate differences between aided and unaided performances of blind subjects using the Talking Signs Orientation System (5).

Table 1. Shorelining task: hierarchy of performance (from 4).

Condition	Number of subjects tested	Performance (RMS deviation from a straight line) (cm)
Simulated Sonicguide, experienced user, enhanced direction cue	1	3
Sighted	12	3.5
Experienced Sonicguide user	2	7
Reduced vision - no background	6	8
Naive subjects and Sonicguide (real or simulated)	15	12
Natural obstacle sense - blind subjects shorelining a wall	6	13
Veering - 0° start	12	14
Natural obstacle sense - naive subjects shorelining a wall	5	20
Natural obstacle sense - blind subjects shorelining row of poles	6	22
"Random" - veering, 180° start	6	36

In summary, the traditional techniques of mobility measurement, when carefully applied, can give a useful indication of overall skill in goal-oriented mobility, navigation, and orientation, and for the evaluation of orientation aids which allow the user to recognize landmarks, read street signs, etc. However, due to the large number of variables involved in such studies, the more systematic laboratory techniques which examine the interrelationships between perception and locomotor control may well hold more promise for the establishment of perceptual needs in mobility, the refinement and comparison of prototype aids, and enhancement of our understanding of the process through which a sighted individual is able to guide his body in a smooth path with respect to objects in the immediate environment.

CONCLUSION

To date, development of electronic travel aids for the blind has largely preceded our understanding of the needs of the mobile blind pedestrian in terms of the exact nature of any desirable additional information and the way in which it should be presented. Initial and faltering steps have, however, been made in the enhancement of our understanding of the mobility process, and in techniques whereby the value of electronic travel aids may be assessed.

In terms of market acceptance, all mobility aids developed to this point have been relatively unsuccessful. The market evidently considers any useful incremental information obtainable from an electronic mobility aid to be too expensive, too difficult to learn, or too inconvenient to justify the use of the aid.

Consequently, a fresh look at the problem is desirable. Greater understanding of the information input needed for the locomotor control aspects as well as the orientation aspects of the mobility task is needed. New technologies which can address the global orientation needs of the blind (such as lack of access to sign information) as well as improvements in existing technology are needed. Closer cooperation between those who attempt to understand the mobility process, blind mobility practitioners, and those who design mobility aids should result in a steady improvement in the future prospects for electronic travel aids.

REFERENCES

1.   Airasian, P. W. (1973). Evaluation of the binaural sensory
      aid.   American Foundation for the Blind Research Bulletin,
      26, 51-71.

2.   Armstrong, J. D. (1973). Summary report of the research
      programme on electronic mobility aids.   Department of Psy-
      chology, University of Nottingham, Nottingham, England.

3.   Armstrong, J. D. & Worsey, R. C. (1972).   The adding of
      visual information to previously recorded video-tapes: A
      functioning system.   Quarterly Journal of Experimental
      Psychology, 24, 351-353.

4.   Brabyn, J. A. (1978).   Laboratory studies of aided blind
      mobility. University of Canterbury, Ph.D. thesis.

5.   Brabyn, L. A. & Brabyn, J. A. (1983).   An evaluation of
      'Talking Signs' for the blind. Human Factors, 25, 49-53.

6.   Brabyn, J. A., Collins, C. C., & Kay, L. (1981).   A wide
      bandwidth CTFM scanning sonar with tactile and acoustic dis-
      play for persons with impaired vision (blind, diver, etc.).
      Proceedings of the Ultrasonic International Conference 1981,
      Brighton, England.

7.   Brabyn, J. A., Kay, L., & Strelow, E. R. (1977). Effects of
      simulated cue variations on an experienced Sonicguide user.
      Paper presented at Experimental Psychology Society Meeting,
      Oxford, U.K., May.

8.   Brabyn, J. A., Sirisena, H. R., & Clark, G. R. (1978). In-
      strumentation system for blind mobility aid simulation and
      evaluation. IEEE Transactions, BME-25, 6, 556-559.

9.   Brabyn, J. A. & Strelow, E. R. (1977).   Computer-analyzed
      measures of characteristics of human locomotion and mobility.
      Behavior Research Methods and Instrumentation, 9, 456-462.

10.   Brown, B., Brabyn, L.A., Welch, L., Haegerstrom-Portnoy, G.,
      & Colenbrander, A., (In preparation).   The contribution of
      vision variables to mobility in SMD patients.

11.   Charden, G. (1965). A mobility aid for the blind. In Pro-
      ceedings of the Rotterdam Mobility Research Conference. New
      York: American Foundation for the Blind.

12. Clark, L. (Ed.) (1983). Proceedings of the International Conference on Technology and Blindness. New York: American Foundation for the Blind.

13. Collins, C. C. (1967). Tactile image projection. National Symposium on Information Display, Abstract, 8, 290.

14. Collins, C. C. & Madey, J. M. J. (1974). Tactile sensory replacement. Proceedings of the San Diego Biomedical Symposium, 15-26.

15. Collins, C. C. & Deering, M. F. (In press). A microcomputer-based blind mobility aid.

16. Collins, C. C. & O'Connor, W. (1978). Blind mobility studies with a microcomputer. Proceedings of the San Jose Computer Conference.

17. Cranmer, T. V. (1967). Evaluation of the sonic mobility aid in Kentucky. R. Dufton (Ed.), Proceedings of the International Conference on Sensory Devices for the Blind. London: St. Dunstans.

18. Curtis, W. R. (1971). Pathsounder travel aid evaluation. In P. W. Nye (Ed.), Proceedings of the Conference on Evaluation of Mobility Aids for the Blind. Washington, D. C.: National Academy of Engineering.

19. Deering, M. F. & Collings, C. C. (1981). Real-time natural scene analysis for a blind prosthesis. Proceedings of the International Conference on Artificial Intelligence, IJCAI-81, Vancouver, B. C., Canada, 704-709.

20. Dodds, A. G., Carter, D. D. & Howarth, C. I. (1983). Improving objective measures of mobility. Journal of Visual Impairment & Blindness, 77, 438-442.

21. Elliot, E. (1967). Evaluating a sonic aid for blind guidance. Proceedings of the International Conference on Sensory Devices for the Blind. R. Dufton (Ed.), London: St.Dunstans.

22. Foulke, E. (1971). The perceptual basis for mobility. American Foundation for the Blind Research Bulletin, 23,1-8.

23. Freiberger, H. M. (1967). Fabrication of obstacle detectors for the blind. Bulletin of Prosthetics Research, 8.

24. Guenst, D. J. (1980). A study of the relation between clin-
     ically measured visual loss and orientation and mobility
     performance. Unpublished master's thesis, Department of
     Optometry, University of Melbourne, Melbourne, Australia.

25. Heyes, A. D. (1982). A 'Polaroid' ultrasonic travel aid for
     the blind? Journal of Visual Impairment & Blindness, 76,
     199-201.

26. Heyes, A. D. (1984). The sonic pathfinder: A new electronic
     travel aid. Journal of Visual Impairment & Blindness, 78,
     200-202.

27. Hoover, R. E. (1950). The cane as a travel aid. In P. A.
     Zahl (Ed), Blindness. Princeton: Princeton University Press,
     353-365.

28. Kay, L. (1964). An ultrasonic sensing probe as a mobility
     aid for the blind. Ultrasonics, 2, 53.

29. Kay, L. (1964). Ultrasonic spectacles for the blind. Sen-
     sory Devices for the Blind. R. Dufton (Ed.). London: St.
     Dunstans.

30. Kay, L. (1973). The design and evaluation of a sensory aid
     to enhance spatial perception of the blind. Report No. 21,
     Department of Electrical Engineering, University of Canter-
     bury, New Zealand.

31. Kay, L. (1974). Towards Objective Mobility Evaluation:
     Some Thoughts About a Theory. New York: American Foundation
     for the Blind.

32. Kelly, G. W. (1981). Sonic orientation and navigational
     aid (SONA). Bulletin of Prosthetics Research, 1, 189.

33   Leonard, J. A. (1973). The evaluation of blind mobility.
     American Foundation for the Blind Research Bulletin, 26,
     73-76.

34. Leonard, J. A. & Carpenter, A. (1964). Trial of an acoustic
     blind aid. American Foundation for the Blind Research Bul-
     letin, 26, 73-76.

35. Loughborough, W. (1979). Talking lights. Journal of Visual
     Impairment & Blindness, 73, 243.

36. Maure, D. R., Mellor, C. M., & Uslan, M. (1979). AFB's com-
     puterized travel aid: Experimenters wanted. Journal of
     Visual Impairment & Blindness, 73, 380-381.

37.   Morrissette, D. L. & Goodrich, G. L. (1983). The night vision aid for legally blind people with night blindness: An evaluation. Journal of Visual Impairment & Blindness, 77, 67-70.

38.   Murphy, T. J., Johnson, N. C., Stealey, S. E., & Kenji, I. (1973). Evaluation of the binaural sensor in the rehabilitation of the blind. Report from the Illinois Visually Handicapped Institute.

39.   Nelkin, A. (1965). Ultrasonic aid for the blind. In Proceedings of the Rotterdam Mobility Research Conference. New York: American Foundation for the Blind.

40.   Nye, P. W. (Ed.) (1973). A preliminary evaluation of the Bionic Instruments--Veterans Administration C-4 laser cane. National Academy of Sciences Final Report.

41.   Pressey, N. (1977). Mowat Sensor. Focus, 3, 35-39.

42.   Riley, L. H., Weil, G. M., & Cohen, A. Y. (1968). Evaluation of the sonic mobility aid. American Foundation for the Blind Research Bulletin, 17, 181-120.

43.   Russell, L. (1965). Travel path sounder. Proceedings of the Rotterdam Mobility Research Conference. New York: American Foundation for the Blind.

44.   Russell, L. (1971). Pathsounder travel aid evaluation. In P. W. Nye (Ed.), Proceedings of the Conference on Evaluation of Mobility Aids for the Blind. Washington, D. C.: National Academy of Engineering.

45.   Sekroder, P. & Susskind, C. (1964). Electronics and the blind. Advances in Electronics and Electron Physics, 20, 261-301.

46.   Sharpe, R. (1968). The evaluation of the St. Dunstans manual of instruction for the Kay sonic aid. Report, University of Nottingham, Psychology Department.

47.   Starkiewica, W. & Kuliszewski, I. (1965). Progress report on the electropalm mobility aid. In Proceedings of the Rotterdam Mobility Research Conference. New York: American Foundation for the Blind.

48.   Strelow, E. R. (1985). What is needed for a theory of mobility: Direct perception and cognitive maps--Lessons from the blind. Psychological Review, 92, 226-248.

49. Strelow, E. R. & Boys, J. T. (1979). The Canterbury Child's Aid: A binaural spatial sensor for research with blind children. Journal of Visual Impairment & Blindness, 73, 179-184.

50. Strelow, E. R. & Brabyn, J. A. (1981). Use of foreground and background in locomotor control. Perception, 10, 191-198.

51. Strelow, E. R. & Brabyn, J. A. (1982). Locomotion of the blind controlled by natural sound cues. Perception, 11, 635-640.

52. Strelow, E. R., Brabyn, J. A., & Clark, G. R. (1976). Apparatus for measuring and recording path, velocity, and direction characteristics of human locomotion. Behavior Research Methods and Instrumentation, 8, 422, 446.

53. Shingledecker, C. (1983). Measuring the mental effort of blind mobility. Journal of Visual Impairment & Blindness, 77, 7, 334-339.

54. Tachi, S., Mann, R. W., & Rowell, D. (1983). Quantitative comparison of alternative sensory displays for mobility aids for the blind. IEEE Transactions, BME-30, 571-576.

55. Thornton, W. (1973). Evaluation of the binaural sensor or sonic glasses. Research report. London: St. Dunstans.

56. Ward, A. L. (1973). An evaluation of the ultrasonic binaural sensor in rehabilitation of the blind. Final Report. Little Rock: Arkansas Enterprises for the Blind.

ACKNOWLEDGEMENT

This research was supported in part by NIHR Grant #G008005054 and by the Smith-Kettlewell Eye Research Foundation and conducted at the Smith-Kettlewell Institute of Visual Sciences, Medical Research Institute, San Francisco, California.

TECHNOLOGIES OF SPATIAL SENSING

INTRODUCTION

Researchers from many disciplines, both basic and applied, are concerned with the issues raised by electronic spatial sensing. Foremost are those, generally engineers, who have designed the actual devices used as spatial sensors. This section will deal primarily with the technology of such sensors.

Sensory Substitution and Environmental Sensing

This volume includes papers by a number of researchers in this field whose work goes back several decades, and who have provided some of the original concepts of device design and use, notably Paul Bach-y-Rita, Carter Collins and Leslie Kay. Bach-y-Rita and Collins collaborated on devices which presented spatial images in tactile form on the skin in a directly presented form, or in what a Gestalt psychologist would call an "isomorphic form." Kay's systems, on the other hand, provide audible, coded pictures of the environment; his designs draw upon his experience with underwater naval sonar and the airborn sonars of bats. While these technologies have many points of difference, they have in common the presentation of complex information about the environment to a blind user, with a minimum of processing, to bring out specific environmental features. The clearest alternative to this approach is seen in the philosophy of the obstacle detector, which attempts to reduce the complexity of the environment to one piece of goal-related information, that there is or is not an unobstructed passage in front of the traveler.

There is some risk in simplifying issues to this extent. No obstacle detector gives only such clear-path indication; all provide additional environmental information such as range information, if only by the operation of the range limitation of the device acting to define an outer limit to the distance of an obstacle. As well, in both the Kay and the early Bach-y-Rita/

Collins devices, considerable processing of information takes place inherently in the operation of these devices, so that the user is not in any real sense given "raw" environmental information. Still, in both cases, the emphasis is on the user's extracting useful information in these displays after some period of interaction, rather than the designer's deciding what should be emphasized. In this respect their approach resembles some current theories of perception which stress that attention shifts to behaviorally significant features of the environment through processes of perceptual learning (e.g. 2,3). Whatever the theoretical leanings of these groups, this approach also had the virtue of practicality, given that there were and still are limited technological alternatives for spatial sensing and that there is a paucity of knowledge of the stimulus information controlling many of the tasks of spatial perception.

Both Collins and Bach-y-Rita were interested in the projection of visual information to the skin prior to their period of collaboration. Collins has a background in several areas of engineering and physics and has also been involved with attempts to provide surrogate sensory experience via other modalities. Bach-y-Rita came to the tactile projection concept from a theoretical interest in long-term changes in the nervous system. It took several years from their first discussions to get the working model into operation, and several more years to get regular research funding.

In the papers by Collins, and Bach-y-Rita and Hughes, this early work is reviewed, although each paper is more concerned with current work. Collins addresses the need for more sophisticated computer vision-type processing of optically derived spatial information prior to tactile or audible display. His more recent research interests are also represented in the paper of his ex-student Deering (see below). Bach-y-Rita and Hughes consider the problems of the TVSS-type device, less from the perspective of the informational analysis of the scene than from the need for more effective presentation of information in the tactile display. Their paper presents a first report of a novel system which attempts to get around the limitations of conventional tactile displays by a technique of "Time Division Multiplexing." The latter part of their article addresses a number of the more purely psychological issues of seeing with the skin," concerning the conditions under which it may be possible to obtain similar perceptual experience from information presented to different modalities. This issue is dealt with again by Epstein in a later section.

Kay's paper gives little review of his many years work in this field, and the reader is referred to the introduction at the beginning of this volume and to Brabyn's review paper. Kay's research has centered primarily on the use of continuous-wave, frequency-modulated sonars, and grew out of his experience as a naval sonar engineer in Britain. His binaural sensory aid provides continuous distance and direction information in terms of pitch and stereophonic directions cues, and a degree of object recognition based on timbre. He has, as well, one tactile device to his credit, built in collaboration with Collins and Brabyn, and a pulse sonar system somewhat like the systems of Heyes. He has had two of his sensors for the blind in commerical production, the Sonic Torch and the Binaural Sensory Aid, now generally known by the tradename Sonicguide. His research includes several other applications of sonar technology such as devices for monitoring heart movements, materials testings, and underwater sonars for military and commercial purposes. This latter application, in the form of a spatial sensor for use by scuba divers, has led to his latest design for the blind, the Trisensor. This device is not, as yet, widely available, but research versions have been used in different laboratories. Their use is discussed in the papers by Easton; Hornby, Kay, Satherley & Kay; Muir, Humphreys, Dodwell & Humphreys; Strelow & Warren; and Warren & Strelow in the next section. Kay's paper also discusses the relationships between ultrasonic and optical imaging and an issue which is a feature of several other papers, the relationship between robotics and sensory aids research.

Obstacle Detectors

The concept behind an obstacle detector is the provision of comparatively simple but significant information about the environment, and is best illustrated in this volume by the Sonic Pathfinder described in the paper by Heyes. This device provides three channels of direction information, straight ahead and left or right; step-wise range information is provided in the form of a tonal display. However, in an attempt to simplify the display, the side channels are turned off if there are objects in the center of the field of the device. The detection of objects in the environment is accomplished by a pulse sonar with priority of encoding of the first returning impulse. Thus this system primarily registers the nearest object in the field, again simplifying the display.

The attempt to make a simple display does not always lead to simple perceptions, but can instead, as Heyes notes, give rise to ambiguity in situations where several objects are present simultaneously at similar distances. A large part of Heyes' paper deals with programming the microprocessor which controls this system to provide a more interpretable auditory display in these difficult situations. Evaluation of this technology is discussed by Dodds in the next section.

Information Selection and the Physics of Spatial Sensing

The selection of the information to present to a blind user may be achieved by the processing of signals after they are provided by a spatial sensor such as a sonar or camera; however, just as importantly selection may also be accomplished inherently or deliberately by the operation of the sensor itself. The importance of the first stage of physical spatial sensing is often overlooked, especially by non-technologists who may assume that later stages of processing can bring out whatever feature of the environment one desires. However, the first stage of environmental sensing limits what is available for an electronic spatial prosthesis, and subsequent processing cannot provide information about what is not already there. The paper by Mackay discusses a range of physical principles involved in the extraction of information from the environment, which set the fundamental performance of such devices. Mackay shows how differing physical parameters of the spatial sensors bring out different aspects of the environment. He discusses the implications of these principles, with primary application to ultrasonic sensors. This paper and its companion short comment provide examples of what might be gained from alternative physical principles for guidance devices.

Computer Vision and Robotics

The extraction of information from a variety of sensing systems such as x-rays, light cameras, or ultrasonic systems constitutes a major part of contemporary research in electrical engineering and computer science. Of particular interest to the problem of electronic spatial sensors for the blind is research on the development of sensors capable of object recognition or with the capability of representing spatial layout. This research has been motivated by a variety of applications in robotics. One general goal is providing factory robots with some ability to "see what they are doing"; another is the development of self-guided, land-based military hardware (See 1 for a general review).

If a conspicuously successful artificial sensing system were to emerge for military or industrial purposes, then clearly lessons would be sought for application to spatial sensing by the blind. In the current volume, the papers by Deering and Tou and Adjouadi best embody this perspective. Both papers describe systems which employ computer-based artificial intelligence to analyze optical information. Tou and Adjouadi describe their algorithms for analyzing spatial scenes and presenting this information to the user in the form of verbal descriptions of synthetic speech. They describe the implementation of a preliminary but not yet portable version of this technology. Deering's goals are similar, but he does not commit himself to a fully verbal description of the environment; rather he combines verbal descriptions with a tactile display which presents coded information about the distance and direction of objects. His system, while bulky, has nevertheless been partly tested in the street mobility situation. He notes the problem of the slowness of computer-based spatial analysis, and proposes that the advent of Very-Large-Scale-Integrated Circuits (VLSI) for spatial processing in robotics systems will relieve much of the burden on computer systems and make real-time processing of scenes feasible in aids for the blind.

Technology and Behavioral Research with Spatial Sensors

To the present time, technological developments have been the driving force behind the development of artificial spatial sensors for the blind. The availability of technologies for the performance of some of the tasks of visual perception has allowed research into several aspects of the problems of use of artificial sensors for the blind. In a number of instances, these technologies have seen application as workaday aids to the mobility of the blind.

It may be debated just how far along we are to effective replacement of visual functions of the blind. As later sections will make clear, the problems of the use of such sensors are by no means easy or straightforward, and our inability to deal with them may ultimately set as severe limitations as problems with the technology itself. However, while we may have to accept many of the limitations of the human being, technological devices are inherently more amenable to modification. Much of the excitement of this field in fact comes from the sense of the possibilities of technological developments, now and in the future.

The Editors

REFERENCES

1. Ballard, D. H. & Brown, C. M.   (1972).   Computer Vision.
    New Jersey: Prentice-Hall.

2. Gibson, E. J. (1969). Principles of Perceptual Learning
    and Development. New York: Appleton-Century-Crofts.

3. Gibson, J. J. (1979). The Ecological Approach to Visual
    Perception. Boston, MA: Houghton, Mifflin.

4. Strelow, E. R. (1982).   Sensory aids: Commercial versus
    research interests.   Journal of Visual Impairment & Blind-
    ness, 76, 241-243.

ON MOBILITY AIDS FOR THE BLIND

Carter Compton Collins

Smith-Kettlewell Institute of Visual Sciences

I will briefly summarize the results of some 20 years of
research at the Smith-Kettlewell Institute of Visual Sciences
which I have directed toward the development of mobility aids for
the blind. I will attempt to point out what we can learn from
these investigations that may prove valuable in directing the
thrust of future developments.

Our work in this field has evolved in three stages utilizing
successively tactile television, tactile sonar, and yet more
sophisticated image processing with synthetic speech as well as
tactile outputs.

Tactile Television

Although the skin normally plays a limited perceptual role,
in 1964 Bach-y-Rita and I started working on a tactile television
system which projects a point-for-point vibratory mechanical
analog image of the environment into the skin (5). We have used
the back, but more recently the abdomen, in presenting an elevation view of the world, that is, as a photograph normally appears
(6). With such an apparatus the tactile sensory system is capable
of learning to mediate certain perceptual phenomena previously
considered to be uniquely visual, such as size constancy and
space perception (1). Subjects learned size constancy to the extent that they involuntarily ducked their heads when the tactile
image was suddenly magnified by a turn of the zoom lever on the
camera (26). In the information selecting process that results
from continued use of this device we apparently learn to eliminate
a great amount of information such as modality of the cutaneous

stimulation and the body locus of the man-machine interface. With the elimination of the tactile component, the information entering the central nervous system is effectively processed like "visual" information about objects in three dimensional space (11, see also Bach-y-Rita and Hughes, this volume).

In preparation for the development of a portable, lightweight stimulator array which could be utilized in a mobility aid, in 1968 Saunders and I started investigating the characteristics of electrotactile stimulation. We found the two-point limen of the

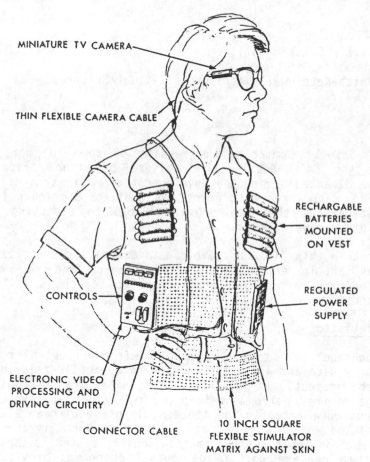

MINIATURE TV CAMERA

THIN FLEXIBLE CAMERA CABLE

RECHARGABLE BATTERIES MOUNTED ON VEST

CONTROLS

REGULATED POWER SUPPLY

ELECTRONIC VIDEO PROCESSING AND DRIVING CIRCUITRY

CONNECTOR CABLE

10 INCH SQUARE FLEXIBLE STIMULATOR MATRIX AGAINST SKIN

Figure 1. Schematic drawing of the 1024-point portable (wearable) electrotactile seeing aid. The miniature TV camera mounted on a pair of glasses permits the object at which the wearer points his head to be imaged on the skin of his abdomen. The image is converted point-to-point to a pattern of electronic pulses applied to the skin by an array of small, concentric electrodes in a flexible undergarment.

skin for electrocutaneous stimulation is about six mm on the abdomen and three mm on the forehead. Ten levels of relative stimulus intensity can be discriminated in a large array which would permit tactile images with 10% differences in shades of gray to be perceived (14).

In general, a recognition device (which identifies a feature of the environment, such as an obstacle or landmark) requires a high resolution, narrow field of view analogous to foveal vision for discovering the salient details of objects in a complex travel path. For recognition of details, a resolution of two tactile display lines per degree of visual field has been found to be necessary. We have determined that performance increases linearly (with tactile display resolution) up to 1000 points without saturation. However, large electrode arrays must conform perfectly to the surface of the skin or the stimuli can become unpleasant (13).

An avoidance device which finds a clear path for the user to follow requires a wide field of view analogous to peripheral vision for orientation and locomotion. Scadden, Alden, and I have studied a 1000 point wearable electrotactile television system with a 90° field of view as a mobility aid as shown in Figures 1 and 2 (15). Blind subjects were able to perceive large discrete objects such as tables and chairs as coherent but nebulous masses of tactile stimulation. They could locate and avoid these obstacles, steering a clear path by manipulating the flow pattern of these obstacles over their skin. They safely avoided 95% of indoor obstacles (100% in half of the cases) and their travel efficiency (percent time spent walking) increased to 86% with less than two hours of experience with the system. These tests have demonstrated the feasibility of the concept that optical information alone presented on the skin can contain sufficient information to permit the blind to avoid obstacles and steer a clear path for successful indoor mobility.

However, on testing this system outdoors in the real world sidewalk environment, it was found that there was simply too much information which overloaded the tactile system. Perhaps 90% was the wrong kind of information, that is, comprised of interfering tactile detail in the background surrounding the objects of regard, which appeared to mask the primary mobility information. The bandwidth of the skin as an information-carrying medium is limited and apparently cannot handle the vast amount of data in a raw television image as complex as a sidewalk scene. Consequently, even when the blind user has learned to recognize some objects within a simple scene presented via a tactile array, the amount of user concentration necessary is too great to be sustained for long periods of time, let alone allow the user to perform other

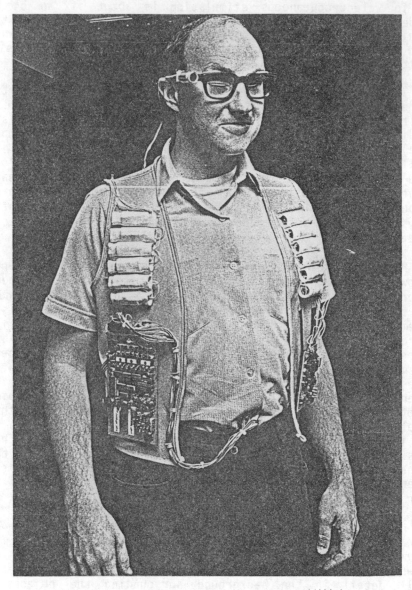

Figure 2. The 1024-point portable seeing aid as worn by a blind individual. The rechargeable batteries and electronics are shown attached to a convenient vest. The electrotactile stimulator matrix is bound to his abdomen by an elastic bandage under his shirt.

tasks at the same time such as carrying on a conversation. The brain apparently does not do well in selectively attending to some parts of the tactile picture while simultaneously ignoring activity in other parts. A "frame" of stimulation around the object of interest masks perception of the object. So far, we have found that adults are not able to learn to use an unprocessed analog tactile image display for real-time sidewalk mobility. More processing appears necessary to produce a readily assimilable display. It appears that we must eliminate some 99% of the detailed clutter but retain the essential mobility information. This might be considered similar to a signal-to-noise enhancement process. We should offload the brain of these visual pre-processing steps. Such pre-processing should be done automatically, and then be presented to the blind pedestrian in a simplified, natural, and reduced form to permit him to move more quickly and effortlessly through his environment.

The success of a two dimensional tactile display for communicating real-time mobility information can be enhanced by avoiding masking of desired information by background stimuli. We have found that to be quickly and clearly interpreted by the tactile system, an image should optimally be of very simple configuration and be composed of only a few discrete points or lines of stimulation. Further study will be required to determine whether subjects can learn to usefully handle more than three simultaneous targets. We have learned that superior results are achieved by simplification of the display rather than by expanding the resolution of the image presented through the skin.

A Tactile Sonar

In 1976, Kay, Brabyn and I started collaboration on the development of an ultrasonic phased-array scanning sonar system with a 20 x 20 mechanical stimulator array to be utilized for outdoor mobility studies (4). Ultrasound automatically filters high spatial frequency noise by virtue of its longer wavelength (0.5 cm) compared with light (0.5 micrometers). It reflects only from normal (perpendicular) surfaces so only a few points are returned. Fortunately, most of the salient obstacles are selectively detected. This is nearly ideal for tactile input which apparently requires an oversimplified image containing a single point or very few points in order to be rapidly, simply and correctly interpreted.

The resulting image, which was encoded after the fashion of a radar plan-position indication (PPI) display, is uncluttered by detail and yet is rich in necessary mobility information (i.e., obstacle ranges and bearings). These images are easily interpreted by blind users when presented on the skin by the electromechanical image projector (Figure 3). When asked to locate

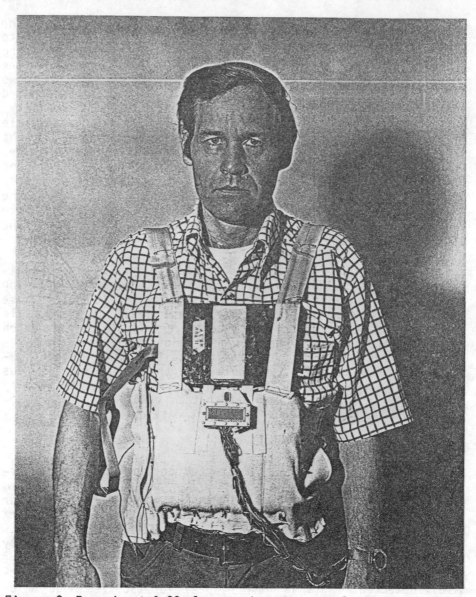

Figure 3. Experimental 20 element phased-array ultrasonic scanning sonar blind mobility aid system with a lightweight, 400 point two-dimensional electromechanical stimulator array serving as a tactile image projector displaying an uncluttered and easily interpreted plan-view of the environment on the abdomen of the wearer.

objects in an obstacle course, subjects were 87% successful, the
same percentage obtained when they attempted the task using their
canes (with which they had had many years of experience). The
productive walking index averaged about 88% in both cases.
However, the lack of step-down detection capability with this
system would prove to be an unacceptable flaw for blind mobility
without the use of a cane or guide dog. In addition, large two-
dimensional arrays of mechanical stimulators are in themselves
heavy, require large, rather than heavy, batteries for operation,
and will probably also cause a system to be more expensive than
the blind can afford.

An Image Processing Approach

       For the ideal mobility system of the future, I strongly be-
lieve that we should take a more sophisticated approach, utilizing
the power of artificial intelligence for processing large amounts
of detailed visual information in order to substitute for the
missing functions of the eye and much of the visual pre-processing
performed by the brain. We should off-load the blind traveler's
brain of these otherwise slow and arduous tasks which are normally
performed effortlessly by the sighted visual system. Object
recognition should be automatically performed by a computer, re-
lieving the need for a difficult, time-consuming, and attention
absorbing task. To process the large amount of information (and
noise) in a natural scene in real-time with currently available
microprocessors, we must use some strategy of simplification. We
should extract features in the scene which are essential for
mobility.

       In 1976, I proposed that one such set of important features
for sidewalk mobility might be the many straight lines of manmade
objects (poles, curbs, and the sidewalk) and the angles they form
due to perspective. Fortunately, by far the greatest number of
obstacles encountered in sidewalk mobility consist of very simple
geometric configurations. Consequently, a quite simplistic obstacle detection algorithm may provide profound assistance to the
blind.

       By 1977, I had recruited Mike Deering to collaborate in de-
velopment of a computer vision system to execute these algorithms
and to compile optimized real-time programs for operating the
experimental apparatus. We chose the just-then available MC 68000
microprocessor for the job. In the resulting system input is
obtained from a miniature, solid state TV camera worn by the
user. The description and location of obstacles and navigational
landmarks are presented to a blind pedestrian through a combination of simple tactile codes and machine-generated speech which
permit the blind person to acquire desired landmark goals as well
as to avoid obstacles (Collins, 1978).

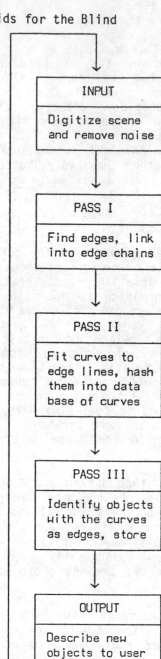

Figure 4. Simplified overall software flowchart for the computer-based blind mobility aid system showing the three-pass obstacle recognition process.

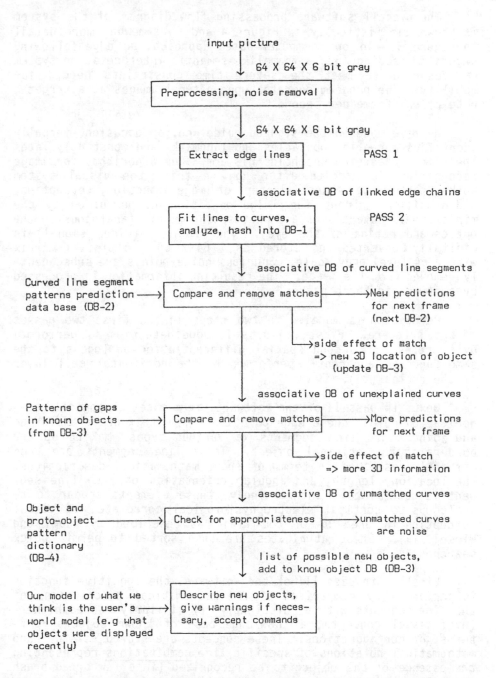

input picture

64 X 64 X 6 bit gray

Preprocessing, noise removal

64 X 64 X 6 bit gray

Extract edge lines   PASS 1

associative DB of linked edge chains

Fit lines to curves,   PASS 2
analyze, hash into DB-1

associative DB of curved line segments

Curved line segment
patterns prediction ———→ Compare and remove matches ———→New predictions
data base (DB-2)   for next frame
                                                        (next DB-2)

                    ———→side effect of match
                        => new 3D location of object
                           (update DB-3)

associative DB of unexplained curves

Patterns of gaps
in known objects ———→ Compare and remove matches ———→More predictions
(from DB-3)   for next frame

                    ———→side effect of match
                        => more 3D information

associative DB of unmatched curves

Object and
proto-object ———→ Check for appropriateness ———→unmatched curves
pattern   are noise
dictionary
(DB-4)
                    list of possible new objects,
                    add to know object DB (DB-3)

Our model of what we   Describe new objects,
think is the user's ———→ give warnings if neces-
world model (e.g what   sary, accept commands
objects were displayed
recently)

Figure 5. Detailed flowchart of the single frame processing loop.
Pass 1 and pass 2 are clearly marked. Pass 3 comprises the remainder of the processing steps indicated in the flowchart.

The overall software processing flow diagram of the system is shown simplistically in Figure 4 and in somewhat more detail in Figure 5. In our computer-based approach, an edge-following algorithm feeding into a framelike semantic interpretation system was designed to meet the severe time constraints needed for mobility. The program operates upon natural images at a targeted rate of one frame per second.

We have modeled the sighted guide who, on occasion, verbally identifies potential obstacles and landmarks and constantly leads the blind pedestrian who holds his arm. Our algorithms for image recognition are modeled after how we think the visual system works, performing sequential steps of image detection, perception, and cognition. Input for image detection is performed by the miniature TV camera lens and photosensor matrix (analogous to the optics and retina of the eye). The TV image (video signal) is digitally converted and stored as a 64 x 64 x 6 digital matrix with a 64 level gray scale. Spurious noise points are subsequently removed from the image. The resulting information is processed by software in three passes.

Perception is modeled in two steps in the first two passes of the software. First, in pass I, edge detection is performed by a process of second spatial differentiation analogous to the same function apparently performed by the horizontal cell layer of the retina (25).

Next, in pass II of the software, from a set of logical categorization rules, these edge-points of the matrix are transformed and joined into line segments of various types, making up the borders of the original object. These line segments are then compactly described in terms of short mathematical descriptions. The location, length, and angular orientation of each line segment is determined. Interestingly, these elements appear to be analogous to cortical electrophysiological correlates of visual perception in area 17 of the brain as described by Hubel and Wiesel (19). These attributes are then sorted to permit quick searches.

Finally, in pass III of the software, the cognitive function is performed by comparison of the mathematical descriptions of the line segments with a "dictionary" of similarly stored higher-level visual concepts, a knowledge base of known objects, patterns, or configurations. These concepts are stored as shorthand mathematical notations of specific line combinations representing the essence of the object to be recognized (in a few broad brush strokes as a cartoonist would represent objects).

In the comparison process, the linked-list of line segments (representing the outlines of an object just found in the environment) is analyzed to find instances of matching with the stored abstract patterns representing features in the environment such as a step, edge of a path, pole, box, or other obstacle. The program is able to conceptualize from many detected edges to instances of higher-level abstractions (concepts) of patterns (i.e., obstacles, etc.) by matching patterns which are stored in memory (12,16).

For example, a horizontal line low in the visual field may represent a curb or stepdown. A vertical line may represent the edge of a post, doorway, or object. Two inclined lines converging upwards toward the horizon may represent the edges of the path or sidewalk.

When instances of stored patterns are encountered and subsequently verified, the patterns are then converted into a user-interface language and output to the (blind) user. The computer can verbally describe these high-level abstractions to the user, indicate where they are located (preferably by tactile stimulation), and how they have changed since the last pictorial information frame.

Object location information is presented once per second by touching the forehead in the direction of the object using a single line of 16 small, lightweight tactile stimulators mounted on a spectacle frame or band on the forehead. Range is coded as number of frequency of taps. Objects are recognized by the AI software of the computer in about one second and are identified by machine-generated stereophonic speech which appears to be coming from the direction of the object. In a verbose mode, the system might say "pole, one o'clock, eight feet." However, we can argue that verbal output should be utilized only for object identification and then be coded as short, monosyllabic words with a small duty cycle so as to interfere minimally with sound shadow navigation and echo location techniques frequently employed by blind travelers.

A surrogate vestibular system (angular accelerometer or compass) stabilizes and locks the computer's model of the world (its cognitive map) to the real world for its own computations regardless of rapid rotations of the wearer's head and body, which can present a completely new scene to the computer, thus requiring extra time for new reorientation calculations. However, to the user, the world appears to move past appropriately as he moves through it. The system identifies many obstacles in real-time, including curbs, poles, posts, overhangs, fences, boxes, trash cans, vehicles, etc., and warns the pedestrian before he walks off the edge of the sidewalk or into an obstacle.

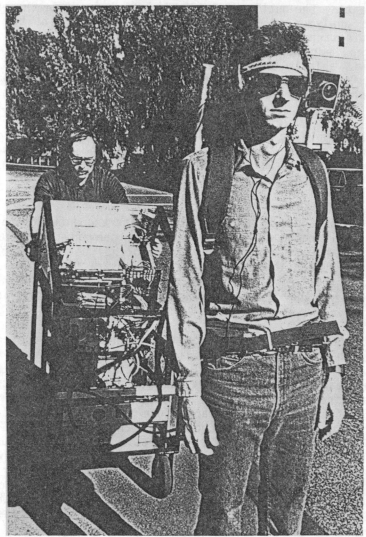

Figure 6.   Photograph of the feasibility testing prototype "Seeing Eye Computer" system in operation.   The wide-angle TV camera is seen behind the left ear of the subject.   The band of 16 miniature solenoid tactile stimulators worn on his forehead indicate object location (azimuth and range) to the blind subject.   The miniature earphones convey stereo synthesized object identification.   The hardware cart which contains the battery operated computer and associated equipment is pushed along behind the subject by the experimenter so he can monitor the system's operation and the subject's performance by wire on a CRT.   The final user's system will be miniaturized to a wearable configuration.

In preliminary tests the prototype system shown in Figure 6 guided a blind user on the sidewalk, identified poles, parked autos, trash cans, and low objects across his path in time for them to be avoided. A feasibility evaluation in comparison with other mobility aids is planned in field tests with blind subjects to determine how much improvement in mobility can be provided. If the tests prove feasibility, engineering design has shown that Complementary Metal Oxide Semiconductor (CMOS) and Very Large Scale Integrated Circuit (VLSI) technology should permit the system to be miniaturized into shoulder bag size or a belt-mounted configuration to be worn by blind pedestrians. The eventual success of this project could extend the horizon of the blind beyond the reach of the long cane.

DIRECTIONS OF FUTURE RESEARCH

Now, what have we learned and where should we go from here? What other visual features and cues are required for mobility and what is the relative importance of each?

Processors. We have learned that higher speed and more powerful processors will be required to perform more complete analyses of the visual scene. Our prototype microcomputer mobility system has provided much insight into the sort of user interaction that a vision-based blind guidance device requires, as well as experience with real-time processing of images from real-world sidewalks. But a robust system for blind guidance will have to incorporate more complex scene analysis than the present one. We have investigated a number of proposed enhancements, including fast hardware for motion disparity analysis, texture gradient clustering, and other techniques for obtaining surface description information.

Texture and slope. In addition to the features recognized by our prototype system we will need to determine the texture and slope of the ground ahead. Our blind colleagues state that these are very important for orientation and mobility even without electronic aids. Texture permits discrimination of a concrete sidewalk from an asphalt street or grassy border. Variations of slope of the sidewalk indicate potential hazard areas such as a driveway, intersection, street, parking lot, nonrecessed doorway ramp, and so forth. In crossing the street, the crown of the road tells blind pedestrians that they have reached the middle of the street and the change of slope of the gutter warns of an upcoming curb on the other side. It is actually the derivatives of the roll, pitch, and yaw of the walking surface that convey this type of information about the safety of forward mobility. The 90 degree downward variation of slope is perhaps most impor-

tant, representing a curb, hole, trench or step-down. So, both
real physical texture and slope can provide important orientation
and mobility cues.

The next major improvement of our system will take spatial
frequency into account in order to extract surface description
information. This will allow us to handle a greater range of
sidewalk scenes, such as those with complex surface texture
noise, e.g., leaves, water, and shadows on the sidewalk.

Visual input. To perform analyses such as these and to
improve recognition of obstacles and desired landmarks, we will
need a higher resolution TV camera than our initial 64 x 64 x 6
array which was chosen to permit processing in the required
real-time interval of one second by an available microprocessor.

Aside from binocular vision requiring two eyes, cameras or
optical paths, each separate eye of the human visual system
actually comprises two separate, concentric visual systems--peri-
pheral and foveal. We could achieve similar functions in a
machine vision system by utilizing two cameras per eye (or channel), one with a wide (peripheral) field and the other a narrow
(foveal) field, that is four cameras or, alternatively, four
time-shared optical systems using a single camera.

A retinal analog with peripheral and foveal retinal equiva-
lents (separate, concentric visual systems) could be utilized to
good advantage. On the one hand we would like higher resolution
in order to achieve a wider field of view, as much as 180° if we
emulate human peripheral vision. We need a wider field of view
for orientation, in order to utilize the complete optical flow
pattern of information which appears to be extremely helpful for
mobility (17,18,21) to quickly detect potential threats from all
angles, and to detect and locate objects which we want to examine
subsequently in more detail.

On the other hand, we require higher resolution for recognition which involves processing features with high spatial frequency content. This high resolution may usefully be limited to
a narrow field of view, perhaps a few degrees, as with the fovea
of the eye.

Reading signs. An important addition to blind orientation
and mobility aids will be the means permitting a blind traveler
to read street signs, shop names, etc. With the appropriate
combination of existing technology this capability could become
available in the near future. Our next generation of intelligent
vision system will have a head-fixed peripheral, wide angle
(180°) TV camera and a pair of narrow angle (2°) horizontally and

vertically steerable, servo controlled miniature foveal cameras.
When a sign has been pointed out in its wide angle peripheral
image field, the computer vision system would direct the center
of the narrow angle foveal camera fields onto the sign to fill
the frame. With contrast enhancement and existing optical
character recognition technology, signs should be able to read
letter-by-letter in machine generated speech. With speech-by-rule
software, many sign names might be read directly to the blind
traveler in synthetic speech.

It would be desirable to employ an interactive means for
directing the attention of the computer system to a particular
sign or other chosen target for user initiated inquiry. We could
utilize eye movements for rapid and frequent searches of the

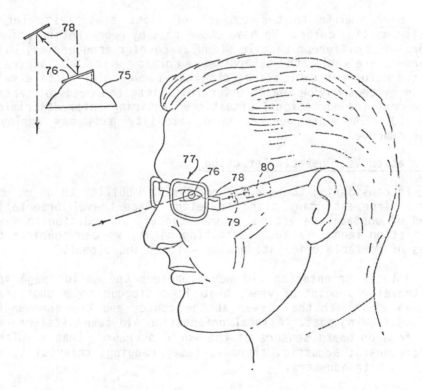

Figure 7. A scleral contact lens fitted with a mirror may permit
the wearer to direct a computer pointer or the angle of view of a
small television system by his own eye movements. An angled mirror
on the spectacle frame relays the contact mirror image to the
objective lens of the TV camera. Development of very small imaging
devices would eventually allow the camera to be mounted in the
earpiece of the spectacles.

visual scene if desired. For this I have designed a scleral contact lens and mirror system as shown in Figure 7, to permit natural eye movements of the recent blind to aim the television camera or a fiducial point at any selected object of regard (7).

Photosensors. A photo-sensor camera array with a larger dynamic range would also be extremely useful. At present a computer-controlled iris diaphragm or camera frame sampling time is required with two separate exposures to simultaneously capture information in both a shadowed area and a brightly sunlit region. In addition, the light sensitivity of cameras should be improved some one hundred fold to match the lower end of the photopic (daylight) sensitivity of the eye. Scotopic (night) vision is at least 10,000 times more sensitive than present solid-state cameras.

Color. While on the subject of light sensitivity let us briefly mention color. We have shown that by representing primary colors with different tactile stimulus carrier frequencies, blind observers are able to determinate colors with 90% accuracy. Tactile color perception suggests that three color tactile tele- vision systems may be feasible for fulfilling the needs of certain employment and educational situations requiring color discrimina- tion (8). The next generation of mobility aids may employ a color computer.

Orientation Vs. Obstacle Detection

In considering the general problem of mobility in an unfami- liar environment, many blind travelers place travel orientation ahead of obstacle detection in importance. In addition to fixed orientation landmarks such as talking signs, we can consider two types of portable orientation aids - local and global.

A local orientation aid would present the world image from the traveler's point-of-view, that is analogous to a photograph or plan view with the viewer at the center and the surrounding objects flowing past. A local orientation aid takes its informa- tion from on-board sensors of the world surround, that is ultra- sonic (sonar), acoustic, thermal, laser ranging, television, and other such transducers.

A global orientation aid would present a traveler's position on a local map with respect to the absolute world coordinates, such as latitude and longitude, or street intersections, as well as the topography and structures defined by the coordinates (i.e., a section of a city map with street names, addresses, bus stops, crosswalks (particularly the unmarked ones), names of business establishments, etc.). A global orientation aid could take coordinate information from existing navigational systems such as LORAN, a satellite navigational system such as Transit or Navstar-GPS, doppler radar, or by utilizing inertial navigation principles. The paramount problem with any of these techniques is that they must be capable of being implemented with adequate performance in a sufficiently economical and lightweight package, but this may prove feasible in the near future. We have recently designed such a package which incorporates a detailed three-dimensional city street map, including street names and addresses in read only memory (ROM). The user may inquire his location and directions for getting to his stated goal from the CMOS computer system.

Mobility aid requirements.   A mobility aid may usefully acquire and process information from a large surrounding region of the environment, but in keeping with the most widely used and successful mobility device, the long cane, should present only those obstacles within the narrow, immediate foreward sector with a restricted range of six to ten feet, which the user can readily keep in mind and process rapidly and comfortably. An exception to this rule might be a mobility aid which could identify objects well enough and sufficiently in advance to lead a traveler to a requested landmark.

The major function of a mobility aid should be to detect a clear path and then direct the user on that course, particularly in the clutter and noise encountered in a crowd on the sidewalk.

The questions a blind traveler asks of a mobility aid are context dependent, that is depend on where he is. Although there are few hard facts which relate to what is required for mobility, our sophisticated blind colleagues, Bill Gerrey, Tom Fowle, and Jay Williams, have assigned their personal priorities for a side-walk mobility aid, requesting the following: 1) make a noise (such as a cane tapping on the ground) for echo-location and sound-shadow navigation; 2) determine the texture of the ground ahead; 3) determine the slope of the ground ahead, including a 90° falloff indicating a curb or trench; 4) detect obstacles (note that this was placed last on their list of priorities).

In my considered opinion, the attributes of an obstacle detector should be to tell the traveler: (1) where the clear paths are, and to answer the questions: (2) is something in my path?; (3) where? (a) direction, (b) distance; (4) identify (what is it?); (5) what velocity, fixed or moving? (a) in what direction? (b) how fast? (both of these are used to determine if the traveler is on or will remain on a collision path with the obsta-cle); (6) what size is it? (should I avoid it or step over it?).

In the process of addressing such questions, we have found that we need more processing of the visual information available from a television camera and, just as important, we need further knowledge of how best to interface the processed information to the remaining sensory modalities of the blind. We must at least satisfactorily communicate this visual information to a blind user.

Interactive control. In general, sophisticated microcomputer pre-processing may be expected to increase the potential speed, path width, and volume of information flow to the brain; however, the brain must be allowed to participate in each state and operation of the data acquisition and analysis process in order to be able to usefully interpret the information. The user should be able to select from a flexible inventory of stored programs and be able to control all processes with some form of undetectable (cosmetically acceptable) interactive control terminal (13).

I speculate that such a control terminal might take its inputs from a miniature pocket-sized key pad, or from imperceptible combinations of finger movements detected by finger joint strain gauges or EMG electrodes. With such a bionic interface the user would essentially be able to communicate with the computer in a form of sign language almost by only thinking of the finger movements. If necessary, other muscle groups could be utilized such as the arm, neck, or even facial expressions involving the lips, nose, or, as mentioned, furling the brow. There would also have to be a means for disabling such controls when we wished to use the hands or facial expressions otherwise.

Use of the Non-Visual Modalities

Now let us discuss the utilization of the remaining modalities for supplying information for blind mobility. First, the blind already employ each of the remaining senses in a natural manner for acquiring mobility information from the environment. They use their natural passive auditory capability for recognizing sounds characteristic of certain activities. These include traffic noises, determining when it is safe to cross the street, when the bus or subway has arrived, and locating entrance gates, escalators, and ticket machines. Other characteristic sounds come from shops, restaurants, garages, playgrounds, etc. The presence and identity of an individual can be detected not only from his voice but from his walking pattern and the fast or slow character of his activity which can be heard as the rustling of clothing, etc.

One of the most important adaptations of our natural auditory capability is acoustic echo-location and sound-shadow navigation,

sometimes improperly called "facial vision." This ability permits
a large number of blind people to detect many obstacles larger
than a foot in diameter, and particularly at elevations near the
head level; however, it is often possible to detect a rising curb
on the ground by means of the noise emitted by tapping a cane or
other noises, although whether location can be detected is unclear. (See 24 for a discussion of limitations of this skill.)
Of course, perhaps the most valuable application of natural
hearing is the naturalized verbal communication code of speech
which is rich, compact, and efficient.

The natural tactile sense is very important for mobility
particularly when used with the long cane. The mechanical texture
of the ground ahead can be determined by the character of the
tactile output from the handle of the cane. Concrete, asphalt,
earth, grass, and other textures each have a different "feel".
One can differentiate sidewalk from roadway or the edge of the
path. Also, very important information about surface roughness
and slope of the ground are discriminated by tactile and kinesthetic cues through the soles of the feet. The importance of
slope changes have already been discussed in detecting curbs,
holes, stairs, ramps, and the blind pedestrian's location when
crossing the street.

The tactile and thermal senses are also used naturally in
detecting air movements, for example, of a breeze, which can be
employed as a cue for the location of an upcoming intersection.
The natural thermal sense permits orientation with respect to the
sun, although this ability can be blocked by clouds. To some
extent the presence of a wall warmed by the sun can be detected
(on the skin of the face) and used as a landmark in contrast to
an adjacent open space.

The olfactory sense is naturally utilized, not continuously
but on an interrupt basis, providing supporting data for navigation and orientation, that is, confirming a traveler's location.
For example, many shops produce characteristic odors such as the
bakery, candy shop, restaurant, a shop grinding coffee beans, a
garage, paint shop, and the shoemaker's, etc.

Electronic Sensing in Relation to the Non-Visual Modalities

Let us now consider how the remaining modalities might best
be interfaced and utilized to convey the processed information
from a visual spatial prosthesis to a blind user without pre-
empting the natural uses of the remaining modalities just discussed, primarily auditory and tactile.

We must convey two types of mobility information, location (direction and distance) on the one hand, and identity of obstacles and desired landmarks on the other.

The auditory modality. We can utilize the natural auditory localization capability to communicate the direction of the target by creating a delay and/or amplitude difference between the stimuli generated for the two ears. Artificial codes can utilize discrete or swept frequencies, pulse modulation, or manipulation of the sound character such as chirping, heterodyning, etc.

Utilization of verbal coding for mobility is probably best done in intermittent, short, information intensive utterances, and then only for object identification. However, verbal input is probably not ideal for continuous feedback of position information which may be better displayed through the tactile modality. The channel capacity for verbal communication is limited in bandwidth and throughput. For instance, in guiding a blind pedestrian we can only talk so fast in describing the environment ahead and to the sides. But there are also other limitations when using the speech modality for communicating mobility information. As mentioned, many blind individuals gainfully utilize their hearing for echo-location and sound-shadow navigation which provide valuable, rapidly assimilated cues for the location of multiple objects in the environment. Therefore, in order not to interfere with these abilities, efficient acoustic coding is required which should probably utilize a small duty cycle and allow for recovery of auditory sensitivity for echo location. This indicates a need to present short duration output information pulses (words) to the subject with longer interpulse intervals, although input information processing should proceed continuously so as not to lose information. An auditory level controller (e.g. 3,23) can also reduce some interference with normal listening.

Hearing carries more information than the other remaining modalities and I believe should be reserved for communicating the most important, information intensive, and difficult concepts such as target identity. But, again, we don't want to overload hearing since it is used for echo ranging. Auditory coding for object identification should utilize a reduced vocabulary comprising single, monosyllabic word descriptions to minimize interference with echo location. These words can be presented binaurally to further convey direction information, in which case an object can be made to sound as if it is the source of its own sound cue. This has proved to be a great aid in object localization.

The tactile modality. Let us now discuss the tactile modality as a means for communicating mobility information by artificially generated stimuli. As previously discussed, the cutaneous sense is utilized in a natural manner by the feet and hands (with a cane) but the haptic sense of the rest of the body is not used for much else. The skin is naturally a two dimensional receptor surface and we have found it well-suited for presenting position information comprising the direction, range, or height of a target. However, the skin works best in the single dimensional input mode. Although the tactile sense may have a smaller bandwidth than the auditory, the tactile modality is quite fast with a flicker fusion frequency of perhaps 400 Hz, which is faster than that of the eye. However, as previously mentioned, we have found that mobility information should be simplified to the presentation of only a few discrete stimulus points, preferably one or two if presented simultaneously. The confusion of masking appears to become too great with a third simultaneously presented point. However, we do not have data on how much improvement might be appreciated through extensive learning. All in all, the tactile modality can relieve the ears remarkably well and the two modalities can be utilized in a complementary fashion, with location best presented through the tactile modality and identification by means of the auditory modality. They could make an excellent team.

As mentioned, we have successfully utilized a tactile coding scheme comprising a single-dimensional, linear array of mechanical tactile stimulators. The stimulator array can be worn on a belt around the waist or in a small band worn on the forehead as shown in Figure 6. For cosmetic acceptance, it could also be concealed in the frame of a pair of glasses. This arrangement is well-suited for presenting directional information in a natural analog manner as angular location of the stimulation. Distance is coded as the rate or number of taps in the indicated direction. This scheme leaves hearing free for echo-location and object identification information.

More complex alternative schemes have utilized a two-dimensional array of tactile stimulators. This has permitted either an elevation projection (resembling a photograph or moving picture) or a plan projection (like a map) to be displayed directly on the skin. The third dimension could be coded, for example, as frequency of stimulation. With an elevation projection, range could be coded; and with a plan projection, target height could be coded as frequency.

Electrotactile stimulation meets most all of the engineering requirements, being flexible, lightweight, and efficient, it uses little power and, therefore, smaller, lighter batteries, it displays higher tactile resolution, and the stimuli are more punctate. However, electrotactile stimulation has not met favorable acceptance by about 25% of our subjects because there are times when it may not seem comfortable. For two dimensional displays in particular, smaller, lighter, more efficient mechanical stimulators should be developed. I have built a few promising prototypes whose details of fabrication will be published elsewhere.

I speculate that perhaps a two dimensional thermal display (slow) or two dimensional frictional display might be employed in the future. In a frictional display the tactile slip of each horizontally vibrating stimulator could be modulated. The background would be slippery and the images would appear as frictionally coupled horizontal vibratory displacement of the skin. This technique might be conceived as electrophoretically modulating the lubricity of the individual elements of a horizontally vibrating mechanical tactile stimulator array. A suggested alternative has been a raised two dimensional display to be scanned with the fingers.

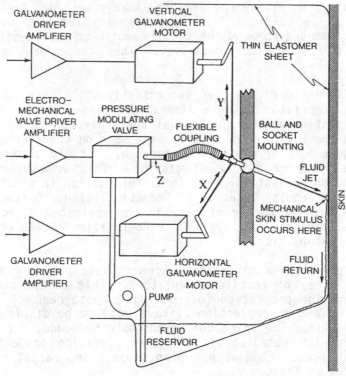

Figure 8. Diagram of prototype fluid jet tactile stimulator system. The jet is raster scanned over the surface of the skin in synchrony with the TV camera scan and fluid pressure is modulated with variations of light intensity to produce a hydromechanical image on the skin. Alternatively, the jet may be steered to trace outlines of pictures or characters cursively onto the skin, a preferred and natural method of communicating images through the skin.

The man-machine interface (skin stimulator matrix) utilizing discrete stimulator arrays constitutes the greatest single expense in a two dimensional tactile display system. However, a continuously scanned rather than discrete stimulator array could be much less expensive since it would utilize only one element instead of many moderately priced units, which can otherwise rapidly add up to thousands of dollars. To address this question I have developed the mechanical analog of an oscilloscope, a raster scanned and intensity modulated miniature fluid jet tactile image projector (9,13) shown in Figures 8 and 9. The preferred mode of operation with a fluid jet stimulator is cursively tracing patterns onto the skin. Cursive tracing is apparently a natural mode of communication through the skin since even without training most people display fast and more accurate performance in image recognition with cursive tracing (2). Our subjects have correctly identified fairly intricate two-dimensional patterns impressed onto their skin by the X-Y deflected fluid jet stimulator. Cursive stimulation is effective up to a velocity of two meters per second on the skin of the abdomen (13). With fluid jet

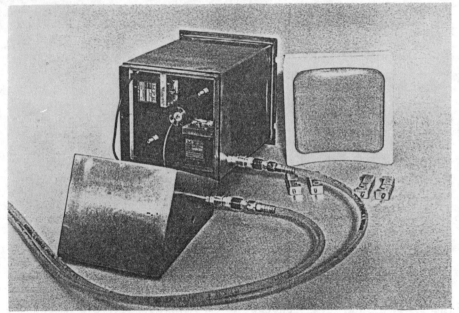

Figure 9. The experimental fluid jet tactile stimulator system showing the components: a) horizontal and vertical galvanometer motors driving b) fluid nozzle mounted in c) ball and socket support and fed high pressure fluid through d) small flexible tubing with e) fluid supply and return hoses. The thin rubber membrane front projection screen, f) through which two-dimensional tactile-images are scanned or preferably cursively traced onto the skin is shown detached from the front of the apparatus.

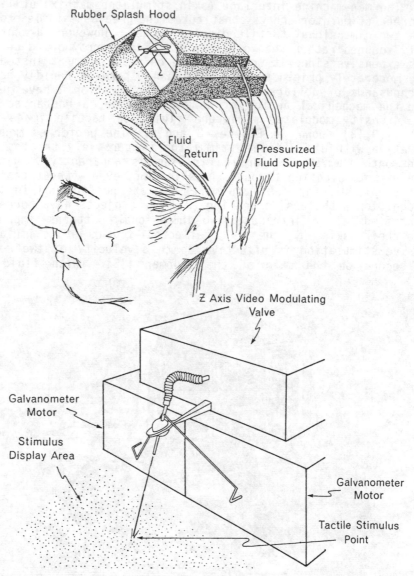

Figure 10.   Artist's concept of a miniature fluid mechanical oscilloscope utilized as a tactile TV monitor which can be worn under a cap. An X-Y pen-motor deflected water jet, with Z-axis modulation by means of a fast-acting electromagnetic valve, cursively traces two-dimensional tactile information onto a 10 cm square area of the forehead (which demonstrates much finer resolving power and better subject performance than the abdomen). The skin is kept dry by an interposed sheet of thin rubber which also returns the flow of warmed water to a small recirculating pump.

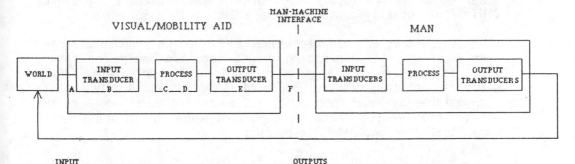

INPUT

OPTICS
Wide Angle and Foveal
Oculomotor Control
TV CAMERA
Small, Lightweight
High Resolution
Large Dynamic Range

OUTPUTS

VOICE
Machine Generated
Stereo

TACTILE STIMULATOR ARRAY
One or Two Dimensional
Small, Lightweight, Efficient

Figure 11.

A Optics: (1) wide angle and foveal--two systems, and two cameras utilizing non-linear scan, foveal, and peripheral presentations; (2) Camera panning or position pointing (a) head mount, (b) small oculomotor contact mirrors.

B TV cameras (binocular): (3) small, lightweight; (4) high resolution; (5) large dynamic range of intensity - iris control; (6) non-overloading (non-blooming, etc.).

C Input pre-processing - VLSI

D Processing - program including the required artificial intelligence.

E Output: (7) voice (stereo), machine-generated; (8) tactile stimulators - small, lightweight, efficient - one or two dimensional arrays.

F Interface - parameters: (9) sensitivity, ergs of mechanical or electrical energy; (10) spatial resolving power--two-point limen, static and dynamic; (11) temporal frequency response-- low for energy conservation and battery life; (12) coding-- for direction, range, and height (three dimensional); (13) color; (14) body locus--effective, powerconservative, cosmetic.

stimulation in our laboratory, subjects have been able to discriminate movements of as little as 1 mm on the abdomen and 0.1 mm on the fingertip (20), which is considerably smaller than the two-point discrimination (or resolving power) measured by any other technique previously used. A thin rubber diaphragm prevents fluid from actually contacting the skin.

The success of this technique has led me to propose a miniature fluid jet for impressing images onto the scalp for future applications. The scalp and forehead have fine resolving power. A two-dimensional pressure modulated fluid jet would only have to scan a three by four inch area, and operating at an angle to the skin, such a device could be concealed under a cap and thus be cosmetically acceptable (Figure 10).

CONCLUSION

We have attempted to determine pragmatically the extent to which a missing sensory modality may be replaced by other remaining modalities. When vision is lost, the most similar remaining modality organized as a two dimensional array of fast-responding receptors is the tactile sense. Our experiments (as described in many of the references) have demonstrated the feasibility of utilizing the skin to transmit visual images to the brain; however, as impressive as it is, the extent of this cross-modality transfer is limited in bandwidth and fundamental visual processing capability. Its forte appears to lie in instantaneous one or two-dimensional spatial localization. Although it is possible to recognize objects when projected onto the skin, the process requires considerable image dissection and conscious analysis by the subject.

Tactile object recognition for mobility application has so far proved too time and attention consuming, too tedious, and too exhausting for continuous use. However, although the spatial localization of a few clearly defined and simultaneously presented objects can be naturally, effortlessly, and reasonably accurately determined, we appear to require further high power, real-time processing of the wide field of view, moving analog images encountered in mobility in order to reliably identify them. Although our early efforts in this direction have shown considerable promise, we have found that the identity of objects appears to be much faster, more reliable, and more easily communicated verbally.

Since the CNS is so exquisitely adaptable, it had been our contention in the past that the brain could adequately learn to process and interpret tactile TV images. Our work has shown that this is true, given sufficient time and effort. However, the real-time, large throughput (wide angle of view) processing operation required by the mobility task has proved to be more than our most experienced and capable blind subjects, using the highest resolution tactile TV system ever built, were capable of successfully performing on the sidewalk.

We have addressed this problem by providing sophisticated, state of the art, real-time computer image processing of the visual information in order to offload the overloaded human tactile image interpretation system (10,12,16). This approach appears to be promising and in my opinion is the method of choice for future research and development of mobility aids for the blind.

ACKNOWLEDGEMENTS

This work was supported by NSF grant #PFR 7906299 from the Science and Technology to Aid the Handicapped Program, NIH Research Grant No. RO1 EY-00686, EY-1186, PR5566, G008005054, and the Smith-Kettlewell Eye Research Foundation.

REFERENCES

1.   Bach-y-Rita, P., Collins, C. C., Saunders, F., White, B., &
      Scadden, L. A. (1969). Vision substitution by tactile image
      projection. Nature, 221, 963-964.

2.   Beauchamp, K. L., Matheson, D. W., & Scadden, L.A. (1971).
      Effect of stimulus-change method on tactile-image recogni-
      tion. Perceptual and Motor Skills, 33, 1067-1070.

3.   Boys, J. T., Strelow, E. R., & Clark, G. R. S. (1979). A
      prosthetic aid for a developing blind child. Ultrasonics,
      (January) 37-42.

4.   Brabyn, J. A., Collins, C. C. & Kay, L. (1981). A wide band-
      width CTFM scanning sonar with tactile and acoustic display
      for persons with impaired vision. Proceedings of the Ultra-
      sonic International 1981, Brighton, England.

5.   Collins, C. C. (1967). Tactile image projection. Proceedings
      of the National Symposium on Information Display, 8, 290.

6.   Collins, C. C. (1970). Tactile television: Mechanical and
      electrical image projection. IEEE Transactions on Man-
      Machine System, MMS-11, 65-71.

7.   Collins, C. C. (1971). Tactile vision synthesis. In T. D.
      Sterling, E. A. Bering, Jr., S. V. Pollack, & H. G. Vaughan,
      Jr. (Eds.), Visual Prosthesis: The Interdisciplinary Dia-
      logue. New York: Academic Press.

8.   Collins, C. C. (1973). Tactile image perception. Proceedings
      of the IEEE Intercon. Technical Papers, 37/3, 1-4.

9.   Collins, C. C. (1975). Fluid Mechanical Tactile Oscilloscope
      to Augment the Five Senses. U.S. Patent 3,914,800, October
      28.

10.   Collins, C. C. (1978). Study of fast feature recognition for
      blind mobility. N.S.F. Grant #PFR-7906299.

11.   Collins, C. C. & Bach-y-Rita, P. (1973). Transmission of
      pictorial information through the skin. Advances in Biolo-
      gical and Medical Physics, 14, 285-315.

12.   Collins, C. C. & Deering, M. F. (1984). A microcomputer
      based blind mobility aid. Proceedings of the Sixth Annual
      Conference IEEE Engineering in Medical & Biological Soc.,
      Los Angeles.

13. Collins, C. C. & Madey, J. M. (1974). Tactile sensory replacement. Proceedings of the San Diego Biomedical Symposium, 13, 15-26.

14. Collins, C. C. & Saunders, F. (1970). Tactile television: Electrocutaneous perception of pictorial images. In D. Reynolds & A. Sjoberg (Eds.), Neuroelectric Research. Kingsport, Tennessee: Kingsport Press.

15. Collins, C. C., Scadden, L. A., & Alden, A. B. (1977). Mobility studies with a tactile imaging device. Proceedings of the Conference on Systems and Devices for the Disabled, Seattle.

16. Deering, M. F. & Collins, C. C. (1981). Real-time natural scene analysis for a blind prosthesis. Proceedings of the 7th International Joint Conference on Artificial Intelligence.

17. Frost, B. J., & Nakayama, K. (1983). Single visual neurons code opposing motion independent of direction. Science, 220, 744-745.

18. Gibson, J. J. (1950). The Perception of the Visual World. Boston: Houghton Mifflin.

19. Hubel, D. H. & Wiesel, T. N. (1962). Receptive fields, binocular interaction, and functional architecture in the cat's visual cortex. Journal of Physiology, 160, 106-154.

20. Loomis, J. M. & Collins, C. C. (1978). Sensitivity to shifts in position of a tactile point stimulus: An instance of cutaneous hyperacuity. Perception & Psychophysics, 24, 487-492.

21. Nakayama, K. & Loomis, J. M. (1974). Optical velocity patterns, velocity-sensitive neurons, and space perception: A hypothesis. Perception, 3, 63-80.

22. Saunders, F. A. & Collins C. C. (1971). Electrical stimulation of the sense of touch. Journal of Biomedical Systems, 2, 27-37.

23. Strelow, E. R. & Boys, J. T. (1979). Canterbury child's aid: A binaural spatial sensor for research with blind children. Journal of Visual Impairment & Blindness, 73, 179-184.

24. Strelow, E. R. & Brabyn, J. A. (1980). Locomotion of the blind controlled by natural sound cues. Perception, 11, 635-640.

25.   Werblin, F. S. & Dowling, J. E.   (1969). Organization of the
       retina of the mudpuppy. Necturus maculosus, II.   Intracel-
       lular recordings. Journal of Neurophysiology, 32, 339.

26.   White, B. W., Saunders, F. A., Scadden, L. A., Bach-y-Rita,
       P., & Collins, C. C. (1970). Seeing with the skin. Percep-
       tion & Psychophysics, 7, 23-27.

COMPUTER VISION REQUIREMENTS IN BLIND MOBILITY AIDS

Michael F. Deering

Schlumberger Research, Palo Alto

There are many different approaches to blind mobility aids. All have in common the transformation of raw environmental data into a form suitable for non-visual perception by the blind user. However, when this transformation involves no direct "understanding" or complex interpretation of the data by the transforming device, the blind user is still faced with the formidable task of perceiving the data in some "analog" (iconic) form, and must extract the complex structure of the external world from low level cues. Examples of such systems in the past include tactile systems such as Collins (2) and Collins & Madey (3). While these systems have met with some success indoors (4), the outdoor environment has proven too complex for direct mapping of image data to the skin. Alternate imaging techniques such as ultrasonic systems (e.g. 1) reduce some of the information but have their own limitations. Others have gone in the direction of preprocessing the visual image before presentation to the blind (12), though the output still is a form of image.

For the past several years we have experimented with mobility aids that use the techniques of computer vision to provide the blind user with mobility data at as high a level of abstraction as possible. We are headed more in the direction of creating a mobility aid that acts like a sighted human assistant than in the direction of directly replacing sight with another sensory modality. This paper reviews this past work and describes issues that blind mobility aids based upon vision must address. It then considers the computational requirements of such vision systems, concluding that real time systems must use special VLSI vision chips. Finally a design for a next generation VLSI-based aid is described.

DESCRIPTION OF THE CURRENT BLIND GUIDANCE AID

Over the last decade a blind mobility aid based on computer vision has been under development at the Smith Kettlewell Institute of Visual Sciences. An overview appears in Deering and Collins (8), and a complete description in Deering (7). To focus our research, the environment of suburban sidewalks was chosen as a prime domain of application. The task was to guide a blind user in navigating down a typical sidewalk. Specifically the device must keep the user on the sidewalk away from the edges, and warn of any large objects or obstacles blocking or practically blocking the path ahead. We believe that this task is representative of the general needs for image processing for blind aids, and this task will remain the focus of the rest of this paper.

Motivation

Several goals motivated the construction of our system. The prime one was that we wished to explore how far computer vision techniques could be exploited for aiding the blind. Another goal was to study different blind user interface techniques in real time. Certainly from the computer vision end it would have been simpler to have run some non real-time programs on a large mainframe computer, but this would not have provided us with feed back from blind subjects. We also desired to know how far inexpensive technology could be pushed. Thus we chose to build a portable real-time device.

The System

Figure 1 displays our device in operation. It is configured as a wheeled cart of equipment trailing behind the user, connected by cables. The solid state camera can be seen over the subject's shoulder; the rack behind contains the computer processing hardware. The aid interacts with the user via computer generated synthetic speech and a 16 element linear tactile display. The tactile array is a skin-tapping device worn as a belt around the forehead or waist, each element corresponding to a particular angular direction, and the frequency of taps of an element corresponds inversely to the distance of the feature being pointed to. (For prototype it was convenient to wear the tactile display as a headband, rather than a more cosmetically acceptable inner belt arrangement.) Each of the 16 elements represents a roughly eight-degree directional indicator.

Operation

In the past blind subjects have complained that devices are too "chatty," and so we strove to minimize the amount of communi-

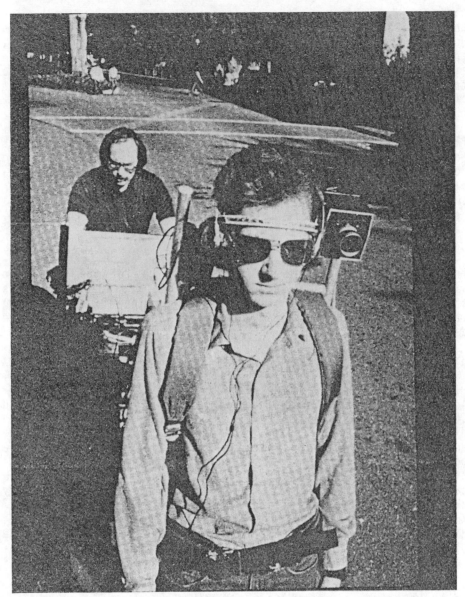

Figure 1. Front view of subject wearing device. The headband is
the 16 element tactile display, the headphones are for the speech
synthesizer output, and the solid-state camera cn be seen over the
subject's shoulder. The computer rack can be seen in the background.

cation. When the user is headed straight down the sidewalk, and there are no obstacles present, the system is mostly quiescent. However, should the user veer toward one edge of the sidewalk, the system "flashes" the edge of the sidewalk on the appropriate side of the display, and adds the single spoken word "edge." The frequency of the flashing indicates how close the edge is in travel time.

If a large obstacle is blocking the path ahead, the system flashes the appropriate directional display element, and presents the word "box" as a generic obstruction indicator. (The word "obstacle" has too many syllables.) If the obstacle is not com- pletely blocking the path ahead, and there is sufficient room for the user to pass by it, the object may be functionally called a "pole." Thus objects are semantically labeled by their mobility category, not necessarily their visual category.

The system has a number of configuration parameters, includ- ing such geometric constraints as the height of the user. To simplify the initialization of the device, the user is always started out in the middle of the sidewalk, pointed straight along it. This restriction is only due to the prototype nature of the device.

Hardware

The computational hardware consists of a 68000 32 bit micro- processor obtaining video input from a 64 x 64 element solid state camera. A secondary Z80 system handles most I/O: disk, TV display, speech output, and experimenter keyboard input. The entire system is battery powered and wheeled. Figure 2 shows the computational hardware. The system has a form of artificial ves- tibular system for providing information about the motion of the camera from frame to frame. This information is used to simplify the important computer vision "camera transformation problem." Knowing how much the camera has rotated since the last image was digitized makes it very easy to register the new frame with the old. This registration is needed to allow objects to be accurate- ly tracked from frame to frame.

Software

The task of the vision software is to analyze a sequence of input images, identifying and tracking visible three-dimensional objects. The vision processing algorithm that we developed can be classifed as a motion analysis system, as it is similar to other such systems. Lavin (16) worked with synthetic computer generated images. The images simulated an airplane flying over a range of mountains. Tsuji (21) analyzed dynamic line images from

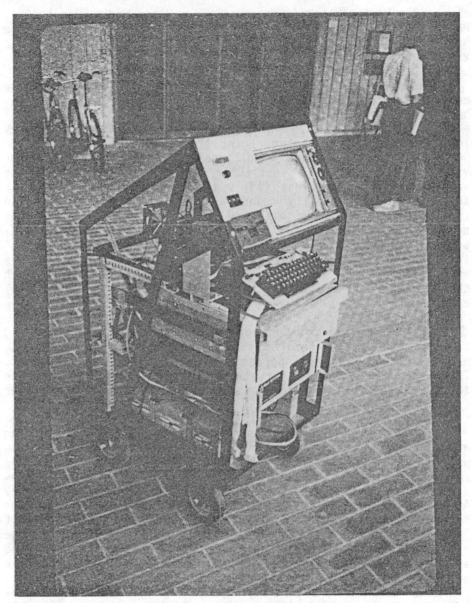

Figure 2. Side view of computer rack. From top to bottom the components are the CRT & floppy disk, keyboard, 68000 & Z80 box, camera controller box, and the battery system.

cartoons. Moving blocks were segmented and tracked by Roach (20). He assumed that the camera transformation was not known, while Nevatia (19) and Williams (22) did assume such knowledge in their vision programs.

The scene analysis algorithm uses semantic models of the environment to interpret edges in the multi-frame image data as borders of various objects, as well as to assign distance estimates to these objects. The input is a 64 x 64 x 6 bit gray image taken from the vantage point of the shoulder of the blind pedestrian twice a second. Additional input information was provided by an artificial vestibular system. Effectively, this vestibular system provides fairly exact information on how far the camera has physically moved from one frame to the next (in three dimensions), along with how much the camera has panned or tilted. In computer vision terms this is called "the three-dimensional transformation of the camera since the previous frame." It allows us to know exactly from what physical vantage points each frame of image data was taken, and also tells us what path the blind user is following. The processing of each frame proceeds as follows:

Initial processing. An edge detection operator is applied to each input image, resulting in an edge map image. This edge map is thinned, and edge points are grouped into line segments. Then arcs of circles are fit to the line segments. Other than its high speed, this process is functionally similar to other systems such as Perkins (11).

Segment to object matching. Up to this point the processing has proceeded bottom-up, extracting structure from the image without top down guidance. Now the direction of processing is reversed, and predictions of edges (generated by analysis of previous frames) are used to identify edges in the current frame. Any edges not identified by this top-down processing are subjected to more general world domain rules. As each edge in the current input image is accounted for, the distance to that edge can be estimated. For example, if an edge is identified as being the edge between the sidewalk and the bottom of an object, then via our knowledge of the three-dimensional equation of the ground plane we can quite accurately determine the three-dimensional location of the edge in space. The calculation to compute this location involves mathematically projecting the edge found on the camera plane back out into three-dimensional space until it intersects our estimate the ground plane. (This is called "back projection" in computer vision terms.) Thus when we finish identifying edges in the current scene, we have a sparse three-dimensional model of the universe in front of the user. This world model of objects can then be used to provide mobility information to the blind user. The model is also used to make predictions about where to expect edge segments in the next frame, thus both saving processing time _and_ making the segmentation more accurate.

Figures 3 and 4 display an example of a single frame of processing from Deering (6).

Limitations

While the device has successfully guided blind users along real world sidewalks, correctly performing the desired task, it is still severely limited. While conditions did not have to be ideal for the device to operate, it could not operate in the shade, and some sidewalks were so complex that the system would become quite confused. Because of the edge point-based initial segmentation algorithm, the system could not correctly function if too many or too few edges were present. This could readily occur if a grey sidewalk was bordered by a faded asphalt street: there simply was too little contrast present for the edge of the sidewalk to be visible. The same problem arises with some of the objects encountered on the sidewalk. Simple objects such as a paper bag might not show up, let alone somewhat camouflaged objects, like the Dalmatian that once got in front of the camera. In general, the resolution was too coarse: objects had to be fairly large to be seen at all. While the speed was close to the target rate of one frame a second, the blind users indicated that a faster rate would be better (at least two frames a second).

Other limitations of the device were due to its prototype nature. While curbs could be detected, there was not a mode for crossing streets. A real device would also include a self-initializing mode, and better ability to track moving objects. The hardware, while mobile, was certainly not portable by the operator. It is technologically feasible to overcome these limitations, but this was not done in our prototype as they would have added overhead not necessary for the main experiments.

WHAT VISION TASKS ARE NECESSARY FOR A USEFUL DEVICE

To be effective, a computer vision-based mobility aid must have a number of specific capabilities. Based upon experience with our first device, desirable capabilities and properties of vision based systems can be listed. Failings of our current device are indicated with respect to some items. (Most of these recommendations are aimed particularly at mobility aids, but many are applicable to any computer vision based blind aid.)

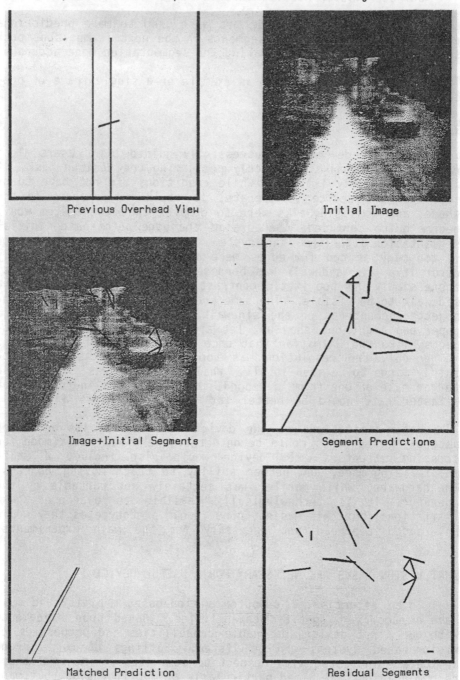

Figure 3.   Example of a single frame of processing.

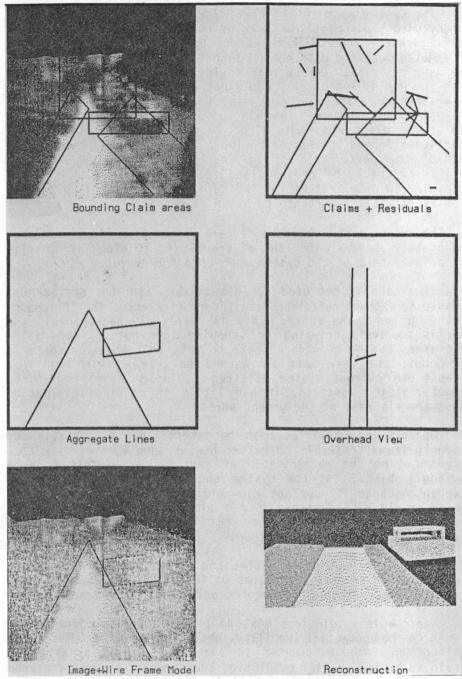

Figure 4.   Example of a single frame of processing.

The system must at all costs remain in frame to frame synchrony with the world; some part of the internal world model must be valid every frame. There cannot be any lengthy interruptions of updated mobility data coming into the system, if it is to keep the user on track. Our current device would sometimes lose touch with the world, and usually could not regain its grasp. Some form of vestibular system is very useful to keep user motions from confusing the program. The exact knowledge of the location of the ground plane must always be known. Many of our distance heuristics depend upon such knowledge, and it is fair to say that much of the performance of our current system is due to its ability to track the ground plane fairly accurately. It is interesting to note that Gibson indicated that ground plane perception is of vital importance to human flyers (9).

The system must be able to discern information about the space immediately ahead in the line of travel: is it blocked? This is the primary task of the system when used for travel.

If a cane is not used as an auxiliary aid, the system must be able to extract quite accurate information about the "flatness" of the ground plane ahead. This is absolutely necessary if the user is to avoid tripping or stepping into holes. Generally, flat areas can be considered safe to walk on. Whenever there is any doubt, the user must be warned to proceed with caution. Because our current system utilized a simple (fast) edge-based computer vision approach, it had little or no hard information about the flatness of the ground ahead.

Objects and obstacles must be internally representable and frame to frame trackable no matter how strange looking they are. A car need not be recognizable as anything other than a large (moving?) object, but the system should not refuse to see an elephant because it does not know what it is. In this sense the system should behave rather like a simple animal: a rat may not know enough to distinguish an automobile from an elephant, but it knows that both should be avoided.

The system must be real-time and it must completely examine and understand several new frames of image data each second. Any frame rate lower than this cannot track moving objects adequately.

Reasonable resolutions must be provided. All objects large enough to be potential mobility obstacles must be discovered (half of an inch or greater in size in critical areas). To obtain such high spatial resolution the camera can sweep the area ahead. This time multiplexing is the equivalent of a pointable fovea. The current device had a resolution of approximately a degree per pixel. This is much too low. At a distance of 20 feet, an object needed to be almost a foot wide to be seen at all.

Simple Computational Consequences of the Above Demands

Let us compute the pixel processing rate entailed by the above demands. If a 256 x 256 CCD camera is used at a frame rate of 4 frames a second, a quarter of a million pixels must be examined every second. This allows four microseconds of time per pixel, or stated in terms of present computer capabilities, time for eight computer instructions per pixel. Unfortunately powerful computer vision algorithms require hundreds to thousands of conventional computer instructions to process each pixel. The conclusion is straightforward: real-time computer vision requires special purpose custom VLSI vision chips.

Resolution Constraints

The resolution constraints depend upon a number of factors. Here the resolution constraints of stereo imaging are given in terms of the stereo baseline, the desired stereo resolution (depth resolution), the distance at which this resolution is desired, and the number of pixels (across) of the camera. The result is the maximum field of view that the camera can have and still have the same stereo acuity (without taking Vernier effects into account).

$$\text{Field of View} = \arctan \frac{\text{BaseLine} \times \text{Pixels} \times \text{StereoResolution}}{4 \times \text{Distance} \times (\text{Distance} + \text{StereoResolution})}$$

As an example, if with a 256 x 256 camera one wishes to spot a one inch high uneven sidewalk tile at a distance of five feet with a stereo baseline of six inches, then the field of view of the camera has to be less than 8 degrees, or about 0.03 degrees per pixel. (Due to perspective the required stereo resolution for this task is 1.5 inches, because that is the depth discontinuity caused by a one inch rise.) If the one inch feature is to be noticed at a greater distance, then an even smaller field of view is necessary. Note that cones in the human fovea have a resolution of about 0.01 degrees. (In this case human eye cones can be thought of as equivalent to computer camera pixel sensors.)

THE CURRENT STATE OF COMPUTER VISION

Computer vision algorithms and hardware have advanced a great deal since our original work was started in 1975, and the question arises how could we improve upon our device in the future. At this point it is very important to separate computer vision technology into three classes. The first and most advanced class contains high-level theories of how computer vision could work, but for which no working programs yet exist. This class is very necessary for pushing the limits of the field, but is yet too far off to be of practical value. The second class consists of working or mostly working computer vision systems, but which take minutes to hours of computer time per frame. This class provides existence proofs that a particular vision algorithm works, and quantitative evidence of how well it works. Unfortunately in their current form, these programs can be thousands of times too slow for real application. Finally we come to the third class of computer vision algorithms and systems, those for which hardware exists that allows them to run in real time (processing one or more frames of image data per second).

When designing our current device we took a chance and selected what were at the time advanced, non real-time algorithms from the second class, and hoped that we would eventually be able to speed them up as hardware technology improved. With a lot of tight machine code hacking, we won that bet, and in light of advances in VLSI technology are prepared to make it again. That is, we believe that many of the current crop of computer vision algorithms can eventually be put on a real-time basis with suffi-cient VLSI support. But there still is a question of the time-table. It is quite possible that the processing sophistication needed for a successful general purpose blind aid, even with the aid of VLSI, will be beyond a reasonable cost range for a decade to come. This was one of the motivations for building our current device, to find out the level of complexity of processing that is needed for a blind aid.

Some examples of current computer vision systems of interest are Gennery (13) and Moravec (18). These efforts are proceeding in a similar direction to the requirements of a blind aid system. The current U.S. Government program in strategic computing (5) has a strong program for autonomous vehicle research. This proposal makes very interesting reading, as many of the technolo-gical requirements for such a vehicle are identical to those of a next generation vision-based blind guidance device. Thus much of the technology development funded by this effort will be of use to blind aid researchers.

Most existing industrial computer vision systems are focused upon fixed camera industrial automation applications. The images analyzed are typically two-dimensional and do not form an image sequence. The main applications are in industrial inspection of machine parts, sub-assembles, semiconductor dies, etc. However, even these simple applications are forcing the development of sophisticated VLSI chips for image processing and computer vision (see 10). As these devices reach the market, they may also be useful for blind aid applications.

A NEXT GENERATION BLIND GUIDANCE AID

Taking all of the above into account, what would a next generation computer vision-based mobility aid look like? In this section some initial thoughts are laid out. This work is all very tentative, and it must be stressed that the new system described has not been built. It is hoped that a system similar to this may be constructed in a few years.

Image Input

One camera, of at least 256 x 256 resolution, would be set at a relatively wide angle (>70 degrees) for peripheral vision. Two other cameras of similar resolution would be used for a stereo system with a narrow field of view. The narrow field would be fixed somewhere in the range of 2 to 10 degrees, and would be "pointable" by the computer. Thus the vision algorithm could decide what portion of the wider 70-plus degree field of view it wanted to take a closer look at, independent of any motions by the blind user. Typically this artificial fovea would be sweeping across the path immediately ahead, verifying that it is suitable for walking upon. This does not necessarily require three separate cameras: one camera chip could be optically multiplexed. The frame rate of the images should be at least 4 frames a second.

Initial Processing

The raw images would be initially processed by a stage of low-level noise removal and simple feature detector steps, all in VLSI hardware. A number of simple feature operators are possible in VLSI. Convolution hardware can be programmed for selective enhancement of edges, points, corners, etc.

Stereo Matching

Image data from the narrow field of view cameras is to be processed as a stereo image. The feature outputs from the low level processing stages of the two cameras would be correlated, looking for stereo matches. There is a vast literature in the computer vision field for stereo processing, but presently no robust general solutions exist, let alone real-time implementations. For the purposes of a blind aid, the general stereo problem need not be solved. It is sufficient to verify flatness of a region of interest. If the region is not flat, additional information about its exact shape may be desirable but is not absolutely necessary. It is enough to know that the surface is not ideal for walking upon. Preliminary work on a simplified stereo matching algorithm for the restricted environment is underway. The algorithm is designed around known VLSI capabilities.

Object Recognition

The high level scene reconstruction and recognition loop of our current system, with a few modifications, can be used again in this next generation system. The high level algorithm was always limited by the inexact low level segmentation in our current system, and should perform even better with better input data. Rather than deal just with edge lines, much of the input would be in the form of surface patches, representing information about the surfaces of objects in the outside environment, not just the edges of those surfaces. The final result would be a much more detailed and accurate work model, with a corresponding increase in the accuracy and reliability of the mobility information to be presented to the blind user.

In the past the low levels of computer vision have been so slow that no one has worried much about how to speed up the higher levels, but now that VLSI has brought the low levels to real-time performance, it is worth considering what can be done to improve the symbolic computations that a computer vision system must do. The general issue of speeding symbolic computation is addressed in Deering (7), and it is likely that at some point in the future multi-microprocessors specialized for symbolic processing will be available to speed the higher levels of computer vision algorithms.

Blind User Interface

The current interface seems quite adequate, and in any case is easily modified in software. Certainly better-quality speech synthesis is available, and it should be possible to have a stereo speech circuit insert a relative delay between the speech going into each of the user's ears, so as to add a directional component. Thus the computer could "throw" its voice, and warnings of objects would seem to come from the objects themselves. (A simple CCD delay line circuit for this task has been designed but not completed.)

CONCLUSION

Computer vision techniques can be successfully applied to the domain of blind aids. Researchers from both fields should

find interesting synergies between their work. Advances in the
state of the art in machine vision will enable the construction
of even more capable aids. However, mobility aids for the blind
will require large amounts of computational power, and robust
usable aids will have to wait until VLSI-based vision systems are
available. There are still several difficult computer vision
problems to be solved before we can achieve our goal of extending
the reach of the blind beyond the end of the cane.

ACKNOWLEDGEMENTS

The 68000 based blind mobility system research was done in
conjunction with Carter C. Collins, who was Principle Investigator
on NSF Grant No. PFR-7906299 from the Science and Technology to
Aid the Handicapped Program. This prior work was performed at
Smith Kettlewell Institute of Visual Sciences, part of the
Institute of Medical Sciences in San Francisco, and at the University of California at Berkeley.

REFERENCES

1.   Brabyn, J., Collins, C. C., & Kay, L. (1981). A wide band-
     width CTFM scanning sonar with tactile and acoustic display
     for persons with impaired vision (blind, drivers, etc.).
     Proceedings of the Ultrasonic International 81, Brighton,
     U.K.

2.   Collins, C. C. (1970). Tactile television: Mechanical and
     electrical image projection.   IEEE Transactions on Man-
     Machine System, 11, 65-71.

3.   Collins, C. C. & Madey, J. (1974). Tactile sensory replace-
     ment. Proceedings of the San Diego Biomedical Symposium,
     13, 15-26.

4.   Collins, C. C., Scadden, L. A., & Alden, A. B. (1977). Mo-
     bility studies with a tactile imaging device. Proceedings
     of the Conference on Systems and Devices for the Disabled,
     Seattle, 170-174.

5.   DARPA (1983). STRATEGIC COMPUTING New-Generation Computing
     Technology: A Strategic Plan for its Development and Appli-
     cation to Critical Problems in Defense. Defense Advanced
     Research Projects Agency.

6.   Deering, M. (1982). Real-Time Natural Scene Analysis for a
     Blind Prosthesis. Ph.D. Thesis, University of California at
     Berkeley, November 1981. Available as Fairchild Technical
     Report No. 622, August.

7.   Deering, M. (1984). Hardware and software architectures for
     efficient AI. Proceedings of AAAI-84, Austin, Texas, August.

8.   Deering, M. & Collins, C. (1981). Real-Time natural scene
     analysis for a blind prosthesis. In Proceedings of IJCAI-
     81, Vancouver, B.C., Canada, 704-709.

9.   Gibson, J. (1950). The Perception of the Visual World.
     Boston: Houghton-Mifflin.

10. Kurokawa, H., Matsumoto, K., Iwashita, M., & Nukiyama, T.
     (1983). The architecture and performance of Image Pipeline
     Processor. In Proceedings of VLSI '83, Trondheim, Norway,
     August, 275-284.

11. Perkins, W. (1978) A model based vision system for indus-
     trial parts. IEEE Transactions in Computing, Vol. C-27,
     126-143.

12. Pun, T. & de Coulon, F. (1981). Image processing for visual
    prosthesis. Proceedings of the IEEE Conference on Pattern
    Recognition and Image Processing, 120-126, Dallas, Texas.

Computer Vision Papers with Application to Mobility Aids

13. Gennery, D. (1977). A stereo vision system for an autono-
    mous vehicle. Proceedings of IJCAI-77, Cambridge, Massachu-
    setts, August, 576-582.

14. Gennery, D. (1980). Modeling the Environment of an Exploring
    Vehicle by Means of Stereo Vision. Ph.D. Dissertation,
    Stanford Artificial Intelligence Laboratory Memo AIM-339,
    Stanford University, June.

15. Gennery, D (1982). Tracking known three-dimensional objects.
    Proceedings of AAAI-82, Pittsburgh, Pennsylvania, August,
    13-17.

16. Lavin, M. (1979). Analysis of scenes from a moving view-
    point. In P. Winston & R. Brown, (Eds.), Artificial Intel-
    ligence: An MIT Perspective. Cambridge, MA: MIT Press.

17. Moravec, H. (1977). Towards automatic visual obstacle avoid-
    ance. Proceedings of IJCAI-77, Cambridge, Massachusetts,
    August, 576-582.

18. Moravec, H. (1982). The CMU rover. Proceedings of AAAI-82,
    Pittsburgh, Pennsylvania, August, 377-380.

19. Nevatia, R. (1976). Depth measurement by motion stereo.
    Computer Graphics & Image Processing, 5, 203-214.

20. Roach, J. & Aggarwal, J. (1980). Determining the Three-
    Dimensional Motion and Model of Objects from a Sequence of
    Images. University of Texas at Austin Laboratory for Image
    and Signal Analysis research report TR-80-2, June.

21. Tsuji, S., Osada, M., & Yachida, M. (1980). Tracking and
    segmentation of moving objects in dynamic line images. IEEE
    Transactions in Pattern Analysis and Machine Intelligence,
    Vol. PAMI-2 6, 516-522.

22. Williams, T. (1980). Depth from camera motion in a real
    world scene. IEEE Transactions in Pattern Analysis and
    Machine Intelligence, Vol. PAMI-2, 6, 511-516.

23. Witkin, A. (1980). A statistical technique for recovering
     surface orientation from texture in natural imagery. The
     First Annual National Conference on Artificial Intelligence,
     1-3.

24. The November, 1980 issue of IEEE Transactions on Pattern
     Matching and Machine Intelligence, Vol. 2, No. 6, is a
     special issue on motion and time-varying imagery. These
     computer vision papers describe systems containing vision
     algorithms relevant to blind mobility aids.

     The following two books contain a good description of prac-
     tical vision algorithms:

25. Ballard, D. & Brown, C. (1982). Computer Vision. New Jer-
     sey: Prentice Hall.

26. Pavlidis, Theo (1982). Algorithms for Graphics and Image
     Processing. Computer Science Press.

COMPUTER VISION FOR THE BLIND

Julius T. Tou and Malek Adjouadi

University of Florida

During the past half century, considerable efforts have been devoted to the study of improving the hazardous and discouraging world of the blind. In this attempt, the needs of the blind both from the social point of view and from the scientific and techno- logical end of the spectrum were defined and explored. Advances have been made in the areas of social adjustment, rehabilitation, communication, and learning skills. However, relatively little progress has been made in the areas of research on guidance aids for the blind. Today, mobility needs of the blind are still met by the traditional cane and the dog-guide. In the words of Zahl (24), "a civilization with such skills as target detection, remote guided aircraft, etc. should be able to develop guidance aids for the blind more knowing than the cane, more dependable than the dog."

During the past two decades, a great deal of scientific research and development on guidance aids for the blind has been reported. The trend has been to the application of electromag- netic radiation or sonic energy, using predominantly infrared, laser, or ultrasonic waves (4,8,13,14,17,22). The result is a series of reasonably simply devices which, although useful in certain ways, offer limited capabilities for obstacle detection and range sensing and are hindered by subtle problems pertaining to the orientation and position of the signal-emitting source and the surface characteristics of the object which reflects the signal (21). Due to this limited environment-sensing capability, spatial judgments with the aforementioned devices are difficult to make. Furthermore, for some, but not all devices, guidance is reduced to going from one detected obstacle to another. The other approach to this problem is the design of tactile vision systems (3,6,19,15,19) which convert visual information before it is conveyed to the blind. Aside from the biophysical problem which results from relating the skin-impressed tactile patterns with the spatial resolution of the skin and from perceptual integration of these tactile patterns, this approach suffers two major drawbacks: (1) loss of the depth information and (2) indecipherability of vibrotactile patterns when the processed image is somewhat complex. A more recent research project has been the development of a real-time vision system for the blind (7, see also Deering, this volume). However, due to the model-based nature of this system, its application is limited to the real-world environment of city sidewalks only. To satisfy the model-based concept, special viewing conditions are imposed. Although these conditions and constraints seem to have limitations to meet practical requirements, this system has great merit for it has shown that such an undertaking is technologically feasible.

Visual Aids to the Blind

A human being is equipped with sensory organs for smell, taste, touch, hearing and vision. Via cognitive transformation, the sensory information is converted to certain languages which are natural to human sensory processors. These sensory organs possess a wide range of information processing capabilities. While the smell and taste sensors can process very limited information, the sense of vision possesses an enormous information processing capability (10). When our smell or taste sensors are impaired, we may be inconvenienced. However, the loss of vision is a disastrous blow to a human. That is why considerable efforts have been devoted to the study of visual aids for the blind.

The design of visual aids for the blind may be pursued along two major directions:

(1) Enhancing the information processing capability of other sensory organs of the blind;

(2) Providing the blind with limited artificial seeing capability.

The enhancement of the information processing capability of other sensory modalities may be accomplished by training the person to cope with problems created by the loss of vision, or by designing devices to convert primitive visual information into other sensory information such as auditory or tactile information. This effort represents the majority of research and development work on guidance aids for the blind which has been conducted in the past. The approach that we have taken in the design of computer vision for the blind is to provide the blind with limited artifical seeing capability through the design of machines to perform scene analysis and image interpretation and to provide verbal scene descriptions.

Computer Vision Approach

We have conceived a computer vision/audio system to serve as a guidance aid for the blind pedestrian. Our design of computer vision for the blind takes a broad approach which involves scene analysis, image interpretation, and voice conversion in order to provide the blind with limited artificial seeing capability. This system, which is modeled in two versions as shown in Figure 1, consists of a camera which serves as the necessary link between the real-world environment and the microcomputer of the system, a camera interface unit, a microcomputer, a knowledge base, and a voice converter. The camera interface unit digitizes the picture and transfers the digital data to the microcomputer system at video rates. The microprocessor of the microcomputer system is programmed to perform all the necessary image processing applications to interpret the viewed scene. The knowledge base is introduced to facilitate real-time processing and recognition of objects. In the design of version I, the microcontrol device serves as an access mechanism to select the appropriate read only memory (ROM) address which contains the proper digitized words. These digitized words are transformed into natural-voice sounding words by the voice converter represented by the synthesizer-filter pair. In the design of version II, the voice conversion is performed by a much simpler scheme which consists of a tape recorder equipped with automatic indexing accessed via the image data-to-tape index conversion interface. In both versions, the resulting auditory information is transmitted to the user via earphones or a speaker. The computer vision system interprets the scene in the immediate vicinity of the blind pedestrian. The description of the scene is converted to voice output. This system was conceived under the assumption that the user is not deaf. For the blind-deaf, we propose to use a tactile array instead of a voice converter. This array will display the trajectory of the safe path only, thus eliminating to a great extent the problems of tactile vision addressed earlier. The range information in this case can be supplied by taps (each tap will represent a step length of about 45 cm).

The major problem in the design of a computer vision system for the blind, given the complex nature of such an undertaking,

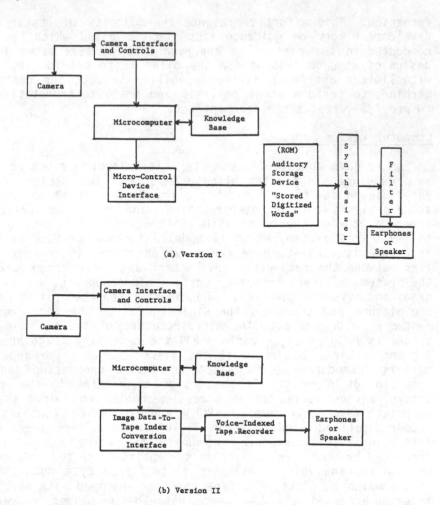

(a) Version I

(b) Version II

Figure 1. Architecture of the Blind Vision System

is real-time processing of scenes. Our approach to this problem
consists of two modes of operation. Mode 1 provides a general
feel of the viewed environment and plans a safe path for the
blind. Scene analysis is performed directly on the digitized
image. Mode 2 is designed for the purpose of identifying obstacles when the need arises and resolving ambiguities which may
arise from mode 1. Our goal is to provide a sense of direction
and to plan a safe path for the blind to follow in real time.
Computer programs are developed to identify staircases, crosswalks, curbs, depressions, doorway entrances, and other obstacles
which can either cause physical harm or can be of use to the

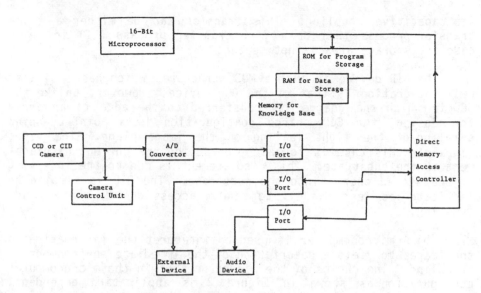

Figure 2. Microcomputer Hardware Configuration for the Blind
Vision System

blind. The concept of knowledge base is introduced as a means to
strengthen identification and interpretation of images and to
lead toward real-time processing. Experimental results will be
discussed in this paper.

System Architecture

The basic requirements for aiding the blind pedestrian are
(1) directional guidance, (2) obstacle avoidance, (3) orientation
information, (4) range information, and (5) object identification.
To meet these requirements, we propose the following system
architecture:

Hardware Configuration. The proposed hardware configuration
of the vision/audio system for the blind, as shown in Figure 2,
consists of three major components:

(a) A miniature camera is used to convert the scene in front of
a blind pedestrian into images. The camera can be either a
charge coupled device (CCD) camera or a CID camera (18).

The CCD device is a metal oxide semiconductor (MOS) structure. Incident photons on the silicon substrate generate charges
on the photosensitive array. These charges are carried via
conducting electrodes to the output gate where they are detected

via capacitive coupling. This transfer can be either a frame transfer process (FT) or a line transfer process (LT) in which case the storage area is not needed.

The CID device is also a MOS structure, which has a similar cell integration as that of the CCD device. However, unlike the CCD in which the charge is transferred to the edge of an array for sensing, the CID charge configuration is a point-by-point sampling of the light falling on the image plane. The video signal in this case is formed by detecting the current displacement in the substrate. This displacement is due to the injecting of the stored charge into the substrate. The CID is simpler to fabricate and lends itself to random access due to the x-y addressing.

(b) A microcomputer is used to interpret the information in the images to yield a description of the immediate environment of the blind. The choice of the microprocessor in the microcomputer configuration as shown in Figure 2 is application dependent. Since we are addressing the image processing issue, it is appropriate to select the more powerful 16-bit microprocessors. Unlike the 8-bit microprocessor, the 16-bit microprocessor allows more instructions, thus more powerful processing, and can address more memory space; in so doing it provides two features quite necessary in the image processing field. Examples of these 16-bit microprocessors are the Zilog Z-8000, the Motorola MC68000, and the Intel 8086.

The storage requirement necessitates the use of both read only memory (ROM) and random access memory (RAM). The ROM's obvious use is in program storage because of their nonvolatile characteristic. They are available in access speed varying from 100 ns to 1000 ns with a density of up to 65536 bits per chip. The RAMs are generally used for data storage and the data they hold is usually subject to continual change. This fact is due to the RAM's volatile characteristic, i.e., loss of data with loss of power.

To obtain an idea of the storage requirement in image data processing, we need to assess both the image data density and the density required by the various image processing software routines. For the image data, an image of size N x N with 2^m gray levels requires a storage area of N x N x m bits. For our experiments, images of size 200 x 200 with 2^6 gray levels are more than adequate in resolution for achieving good image interpretation. The required storage area is a function of the application and the results sought for this application.

The direct memory access (DMA) controller is an important part and plays a significant role in the microcomputer configuration in that it permits access to the memory without recourse to the microprocessor. This DMA is extremely useful for applications where the required data transfer is higher than the processor can support. This aspect of the DMA is particularly needed for our design since we would like to transfer image data as fast as possible and efficiently without any bus conflict.

The Input/Output ports constitute the communication link between the external devices and the processor. They are basically small external memories whose registers are linked to the outside world.

(c) A voice converter transforms the scene descriptions into auditory information. In version I, the idea of speech generation from a set of digitized words has been treated at great length in the field of speech synthesis. The design concept has actually been put to practical use in the case of talking calculators for the blind. The advantage of this design is the broad and varied range of sentences which can be reconstructed from the stored digitized words. In version II, many tape recorder manufacturers now offer recorders with automatic indexing. Figure 3 illustrates the use of such a device in the visual/audio transformation process. The automatic indexing is simply a sophisticated control process over the familiar tape counter found in all tape recording machines.

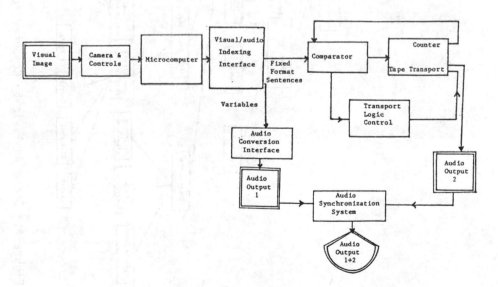

Figure 3.   Visual/Audio Conversion System

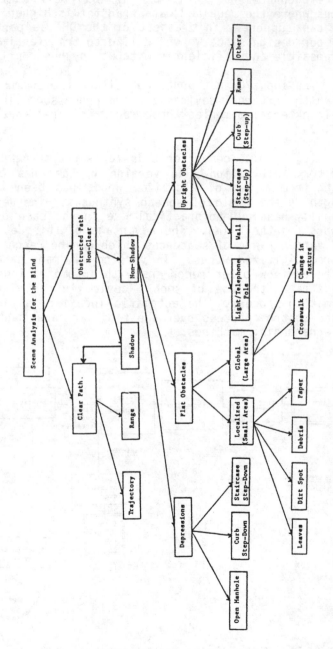

Figure 4.   Scene Analysis by Computer for the Blind

As shown in Figure 3, the computer results are first indexed via the indexing interface. This index is then compared via the comparator to the actual tape position. This comparison is fed to the transport logic control which initiates the necessary Reverse, Fast Forward, Stop, and Play Functions to retrieve the desired audio information. In our design, the audio information is divided into unchanging recorded sentences such as: "Your path is clear for X steps" and "You may turn left after X steps," and into variables (x) which will supplement the range information. Such a design necessitates an audio synchronizing process.

Software requirements. Before one can develop software modules for the interpretation of scenes, one first needs to establish a hierarchy of logically sequential events which take place in the overall image interpretation process. The conceptual hierarchy of our design is shown in Figure 4. Of course, once this hierarchy has been established, some of these events can be performed in parallel to enforce real-time processing. In our software implementation, the vision system will first determine whether the path in front of the blind is clear or not. If it is clear, the system will trace a safety trajectory for the blind to follow. In conjunction with the trajectory tracing, range of the obstacle-free path is generated. If the path if found not clear, the system will determine whether there is shadow or not. If a shadow is found on the path, the system declares that it is a safe path for the blind to walk through. If a non-shadow is found, it must be an object. The system then determines whether the object is flat or upright. If it is relatively flat, the object may be newspaper, debris, dirt, texture change of the pavement, etc. If it is an upright object, the system will then initiate the identification process which will classify such objects as staircase, crosswalk, curb, depression, wall, or other obstacles. A detailed description of the software modules which achieve the above stated tasks is given in the following sections.

Scene Interpretation

Software development for scene interpretation and understanding constitutes the central task in the design of the proposed vision/audio system for the blind. Figure 5 illustrates the functional organization for the system software. Scene analysis is automatically performed in the Mode 1 and Mode 2 types.

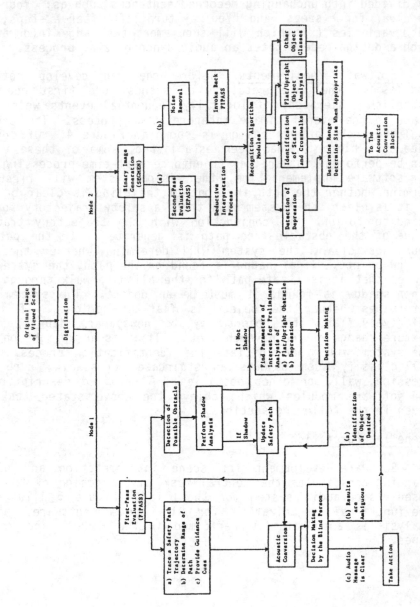

Figure 5.   Scene Interpretation Process

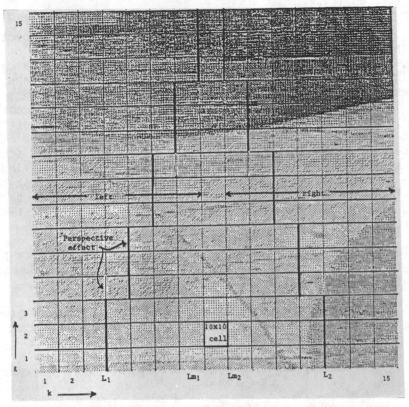

Figure 6. First-Pass Evaluation Partitioning Scheme

Before the blind pedestrian starts to walk, the vision/audio
system takes several pictures of the scene in his vicinity and
performs image analysis, interpretation and recognition. The
blind person stands still for a moment to wait for instructions
from the system. We may call this period the initialization
phase. During the walking phase, the system determines a safety
path for the blind pedestrian by performing the first-pass evaluation. When an obstacle is detected, the system issues a warning
signal to the user and asks him/her to walk slowly or take a
pause so that the system may have sufficient time to complete
image analysis and intepretation. We may call this period the
warning phase. Thus, the proposed vision/audio system processes
the image in real time during the walking phase, performs image
analysis and interpretation within 10 seconds during the warning
phase, and conducts image interpretation and recognition within a
fraction of a minute during the initialization phase.

First-Pass Evaluation

In the first-pass evaluation we make a basic assumption that the initial position and the immediate surrounding of the blind, an area which can be circumscribed by the reach of a cane, constitute a safe (obstacle-free) area. Furthermore, we take into consideration the perspective effect which we describe in Appendix 1. We do not have to process all the scene in front of the blind because we make use of the fact that above a certain height of the scene we are actually viewing the horizon. This fact becomes apparent when we discuss the range finding scheme which supplements this first-pass evaluation. This range finding scheme is treated in Appendix 2. To facilitate the first-pass evaluation, the image in front of the blind pedestrian is partitioned by a virtual grid as shown in Figure 6. The first-pass evaluation performs the following analysis:

(a) Walking Straight Ahead. This step is performed to plan a safety path for the blind pedestrian. The system makes the following computations:

(1) Compute the regional average gray level as a reference value. The regional average gray level is given by

$$G_r = [\sum_{k=L_1}^{L_2} \sum_{\ell=1}^{3} G(k,\ell)]/N_i$$

where $G(k,\ell)$ represents a 10 x 10 cell average gray-level value, and N_i is the number of cells in the safe area.

(2) Compute the step average gray level for each step along the path

$$G(\ell) = [\sum_{k=L_1}^{L_2} G(k,\ell)]/L_2-L_1)$$

(3) Check for safety conditions

(a) $G_r - T \leq G(\ell) \leq G_r + T$

(b) $G_r - T \leq G(k,\ell) \leq G_r + T$ $k=Lm_1,\ldots, Lm_2$

The range $(k=Lm_2,\ldots, Lm_1)$ may vary depending on the type of camera used, the safety factor specified and the perspective effect estimated. If the above conditions are satisfied, the path for the given step is declared obstacle-free. The audio output in this case is of the form "Your front path is clear for X steps."

(b) Making a Left or a Right Turn. This step is performed when an obstacle in the direction of travel is detected. For the convenience of computer analysis, three types of turns are considered:

(1) A turn to detour a small obstacle. This situation happens when the obstacle is small and the area beyond this obstacle is clear.

(2) A turn to avoid a large obstacle. This situation may lead to a new direction of travel.

(3) A turn to avoid a dead end.

In either case a or b or c, we simply determine the number of consecutive cells in the step preceding the obstacle satisfying

$$G_r - T \leq G(k,\ell) \leq G_r + T$$

where $k = Lm_1,..., 1$ for left turn and $k=Lm_2,..., 15$ for right turn. The mid-point of this range of cells is declared as the point of next destination. The audio output in this case is of the form "Turn to left/right after X steps."

(c) Permissible Left or Right Turns. This step is performed to determine whether a turn is permissible.

(1) Check for permissible left turn. A left turn is permissible, if

$$G_r - T \leq G(k,\ell) \leq G_r + T \qquad k=1,..., Lm_1$$

The audio output in this case is of the form "You may turn left after X1 steps."

(2) Check for permissible right turn. A right turn is permissible if

$$G_r - T \leq G(k,\ell) \leq G_r + T \qquad k=Lm2,..., 15$$

The audio output in this case is of the form "You may turn right after X steps."

(d) Determining the width of left and right clearances. It may be desired, for the cases of permissible left or right turns, to supply the width of the clearances to the left or to the right environment. The audio output can be of the form "Left clearance is X steps away and is Y steps wide" or "Right clearance is X steps away and is Y steps wide."

(e) Determining Additional Information About the Environment.

(1) Check for permissible veer to the left. This operation is performed to let the user know how the environment to his/her left is changing with respect to the initial position ($\ell=1$). This is achieved by checking the number of successive cells at the given step satisfying the condition

$$G_r - T \leq G(k,\ell) \leq G_r + T \qquad k=Lm_1,\ldots, 1$$

Compare this number with that of the initial step ($\ell=1$) and indicate a veer proportional to the difference of these two numbers. The audio output can be of the form "You may veer left X steps."

(2) Check for permissible veer to the right. The reasoning here is similar to that of left veer except that the condition is now

$$G_r - T \leq G(k,\ell) \leq G_r + T \qquad k=Lm_2,\ldots, 15$$

The audio output can be of the form "You may veer right X8 steps."

(3) Estimate the nature of the obstacle. The obstacle may be small or large, flat or upright, depression or hump, shadow or nonshadow. Some of these tasks take place in the second-pass evaluation. However, in order to speed up the process of shadow discrimination and depression detection, we make use of the scanning mechanism of the first-pass evaluation to store at least two intensity distributions of the pixels of the image records inclusive of the area declared obstacle-free. These stored records are then used as a basis for comparison with the pixel intensity distribution inclusive of the area where an obstacle is detected by the first-pass evaluation. The objective is then to extract occluded information from the new peaks that appear in the pixel intensity distribution for the task of depression detection, or to determine continuity in the pixel intensity distribution except for a shift in the magnitude, thus obtaining preliminary means with which we can identify shadows.

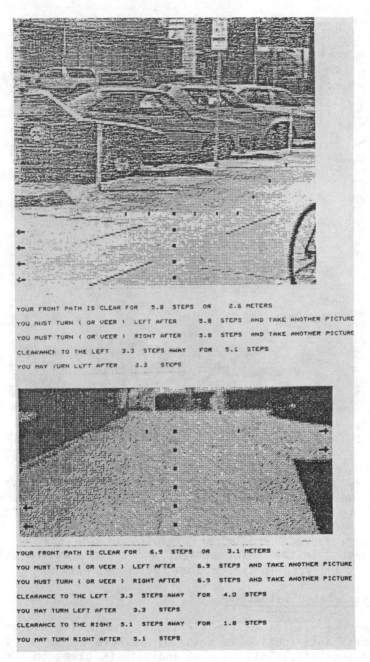

Figure 7. Continues overleaf

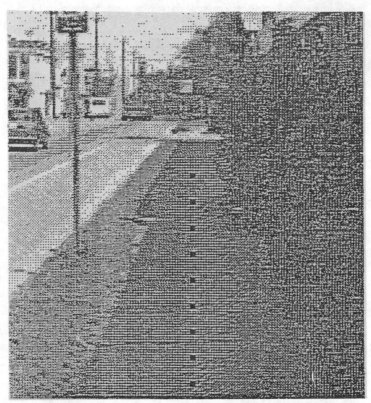

Figure 7.   Results of the First-Pass Evaluation

Computer results of the first-pass evaluation using several
scenes are shown in Figure 7. In these first-pass evaluation
results, we should indicate that the safety markers generated by
computer is a nonlinear function of distance, and the blind
person's position is 1.5 m or 3.3 steps away from the edge of
the picture frame. Preliminary results of the shadow analysis
are presented in the next section, and the depression detection
problem is analyzed in the section following that.

Second-Pass Evaluation

When the results of the first-pass evaluation are ambiguous
or object identification is desired, we have recourse to Mode 2
of scene analysis. This mode of analysis is based on the binary
image which is generated via an adaptive segmentation technique

(SEGMEN). The threshold value T fed to this segmentation module is computed as $(T_c-T_0)/2$ where, T_c is the mean gray-level value of a small area within the clear-path surface, and T_0 is the mean gray-level of a small area within the assumed object surface or,

$$T_c = [\sum_{x=j_1}^{j_2} \sum_{y=k_1}^{k_2} G(x,y)] /Q_{W_1}$$

$$T_0 = [\sum_{x=j_3}^{j_4} \sum_{y=k_3}^{k_4} G(x,y)] /Q_{W_2}$$

where

$G(x,y)$ is the gray level at picture point (x,y),

Q_{W_1} denotes the total number of pixels within the considered window W_1 in the clear path area, and

Q_{W_2} denotes the total number of pixels within the considered window W_2 in the area of the assumed object.

The second-pass evaluation, which takes place following binary image generation, constitutes the central task of Mode 2. This evaluation is designed primarily for the identification of obstacles, but it also resolves false alarms of the first-pass evaluation which can be caused by the presence of debris, leaves, dirt spots, etc. It is based on two modes of analysis: one is fast but rough, providing only the category to which the object may belong, and the other is slower but more thorough, providing identification of the object. The fast-mode of analysis is based on the determination of the aspect ratio describing an object. The slow-mode analysis is based on a deductive interpretation technique containing various interpretation schemes which lead to the selection of the desired recognition algorithm. This deductive interpretation program is under development (1). The procedures of fast-mode analysis are summarized as follows:

(a) A virtual grid is superimposed on the generated binary image containing the obstacle detected by the first-pass evaluation. Figure 8 illustrates a grid example. The unit of the grid is called a cell. The kth cell is denoted by C_k, k=1,2,3,...

(b) Find the object cells which covers the object. The cells not covering the object are called background cells. This step determines the extent of the obstacle in the grid. Since each cell is defined by a square of 10 x 10 pixels, the intensity of each cell $G(C_k)$ may have a value in the range [0, 100].

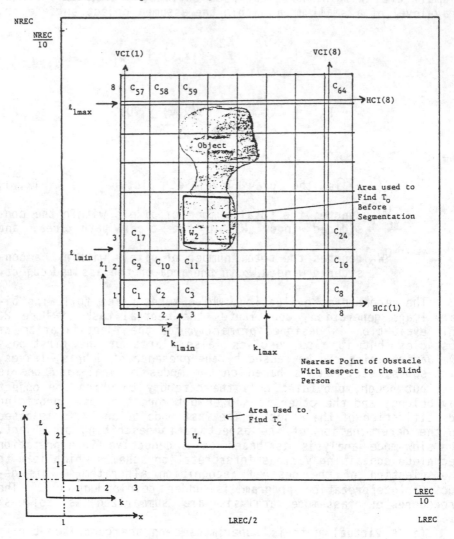

Figure 8. A Simple Illustration of the Superposition of a Grid Over an Obstacle Detected by the First-Pass Evaluation

(c) Quantize the intensity values of $G(C_k)$ in order to (a) distinguish between object and debris or dirt spots or leaves, and (b) facilitate image interpretation. A quantization example is given below:

$$G(C_k) \leq 10 \qquad\qquad C_k = 0: \text{debris, dirt spots,}$$
$$\qquad\qquad\qquad\qquad\qquad\qquad \text{leaves}$$
$$10 < G(C_k) \leq 35 \qquad\quad C_k = 0.25$$
$$35 < G(C_k) \leq 55 \qquad\quad C_k = 0.5$$
$$35 < G(C_k) \leq 75 \qquad\quad C_k = 0.75$$
$$G(C_k) > 75 \qquad\qquad\quad C_k = 1$$

(d) Compute the horizontal cumulative intensity HCI and the vertical cumulative intensity VCI of all rows and columns of the grid:

$$HCI(\ell_1) = \sum_{i=1}^{n_1} C_{i+n_1(\ell_1-1)}$$

$$VCI(k_1) = \sum_{j=1}^{n_2} C_{k_1+n_2(j-1)}$$

where n_1 and n_2 represent the number of horizontal and vertical cells respectively. We use notation (k_1,ℓ_1) to avoid confusion with notation (k,ℓ) used in the first-pass evaluation. In Figure 8, $n_1=n_2=8$.

The computed values of HCIs and VCIs provide the means with which we can assess the obstacle as described below.

(e) If either all HCIs=0 or all VCIs=0, a false alarm is issued by the first-pass evaluation; i.e., it is only debris, dirt spots, or leaves, otherwise an obstacle exists.

(f) Determine the size and location of the object.

(1) Overall size is given by the area

$$A = (\ell_{1\,max} - \ell_{1\,min})(k_{1\,max} - k_{1\,min})$$

where $\ell_{1\ min}$ and $\ell_{1\ max}$ are the minimum and maximum values of ℓ_1 for HCI>0 and $k_{1\ min}$ and $k_{1\ max}$ are the minimum and maximum values of k_1 for VCI>0.

(2) The location of the object is determined by the value of ℓ_1 for HCI>0 closest to $\ell=1$ and the value of k_1 for VCI>0 closest to the midpoint of the record length (LREC) of the original image, i.e., LREC/(2*10).

(g) Compute the aspect ratio λ given by

$$\lambda = \frac{VCI(k_1)_{max}}{HCI(\ell_1)_{max}}$$

The object is categorized according to the value of λ:

$\lambda > 1$ [tree-trunk, light pole, mail box, fire hydrant,...]

$\lambda \simeq 1$ [square or circular shaped objects]

$\lambda < 1$ [car, curb, bench, step,...]

For certain objects, λ is orientation-dependent. In such cases, the object may be misclassified. We are currently developing interpretation algorithms which are orientation-invariant. Size invariance may be achieved in this case by making use of the range information derived in Appendix 2. Experimental results are shown in Figure 9. Figure 10 illustrates application of first-pass and second-pass evaluation techniques to initialization, walking, and warning phases mentioned earlier in this section.

Shadow discrimination. One of the most difficult problems in scene interpretation is the correct discrimination of shadows from a pile of debris, some elevated obstacle, a depression, or a covered manhole. We have conducted some preliminary analyses of the shadow problem.

The generalized process for shadow analysis is shown in Figure 11. The decision making is based on the integration of the histogram analyses, the power spectrum analysis, the cross

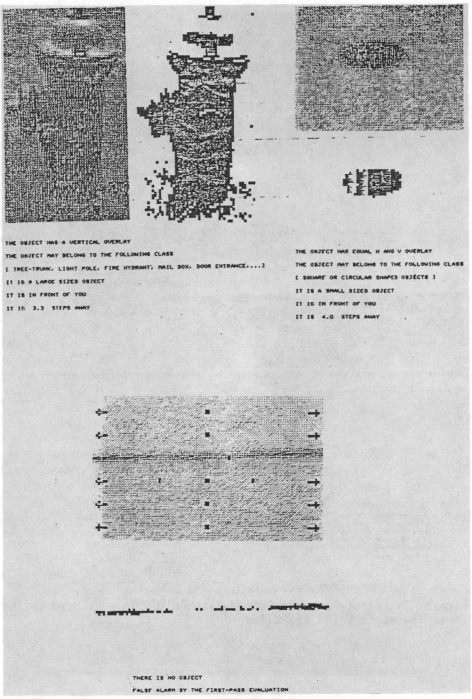

Figure 9.   Results of the Second-Pass Evaluation

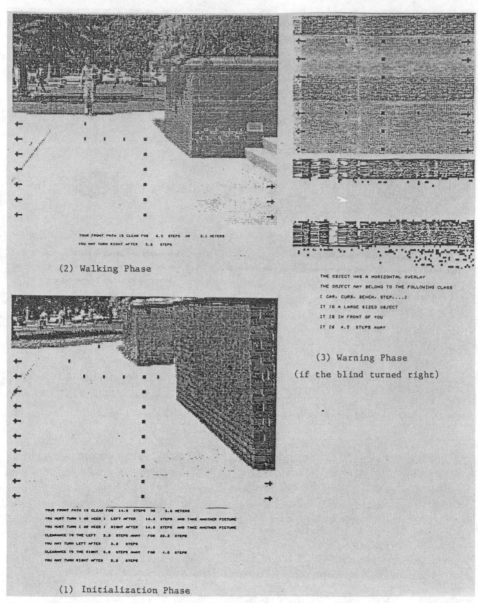

(2) Walking Phase

(3) Warning Phase
(if the blind turned right)

(1) Initialization Phase

Figure 10.   First-Pass and Second-Pass Evaluations as Used in the
Three Phases to Guide the Blind

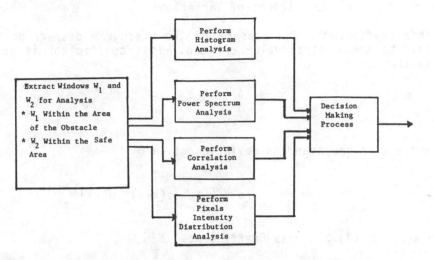

Figure 11. Generalized Process of the Shadow Analysis

correlation function, and the pixel intensity distribution. In
each of these analysis, the objective is to characterize the
effect inherent to shadows. The decision-making process can be
enhanced further by supplementing it with such knowledge as (a)
shadows are normally not free-standing, (b) shadows normally have
fuzzy edges, and (c) whether we are moving toward a shadowed area
or coming out of one.

   (a) Histogram Analysis. The parameters of interest in this
analysis are

   (1) Mean Value

$$\mu + \sum_{x=0}^{k} x\, p(x)$$

in which k represents the quantized gray level and $p(x) = N(x)/Q$,
where Q represents the total number of pixels in the image and
$N(x)$ denotes the number of pixels with gray level x.

   This parameter is important in the obvious sense of detecting a shift in the mean value going from a shaded area to a
lighted area or vice versa. Without the knowledge pointed out in
the case mentioned above or without the use of, say, a photodiode
to measure the ambient light intensity change, the direction of
this shift is meaningless to the decision-making process.

(2) Coefficient of Variation

This coefficient is a measure of the histogram dispersion relative to the central value or mean. This coefficient is defined as the ratio

$$\delta = \frac{\sigma}{\mu}$$

where σ is the standard deviation given by

$$\sigma = [\sum_{x=0}^{k} (x-\mu)^2 p(x)]^{1/2}$$

(3) Skewness Coefficient

This parameter, which is the third central moment, is the measure of the degree and direction of histogram asymmetry. It is given by

$$0 = \frac{s}{\sigma^3}$$

where s is the skewness given by

$$s = \sum_{x=0}^{k} (x - \mu)^3 p(x)$$

In this histogram analysis, experimental results as illustrated in Figure 12 have shown that besides the obvious shift in the mean, the coefficient of variation and the skewness coefficient vary only slightly when going from a shaded area to a lighted area of the same texture, but they experience larger variations when going from one area to another with different texture.

(b) Power Spectrum Analysis. We have presented thus far the parameters used in measuring the shadow effect on the gray level intensities. The results of histogram analysis which support the assumption that textural properties are preserved under the shadow effect can also be verified by power spectrum.

In terms of Fourier Transforms, by mapping the spatial domain of an image to its frequency domain we learn that the spectral energy concentrated at low frequencies represents those spatial areas of the image which vary slowly and smoothly in gray

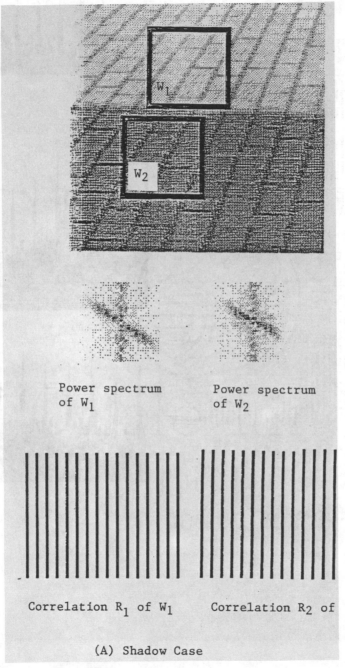

Power spectrum
of W_1

Power spectrum
of W_2

Correlation R_1 of W_1 Correlation R_2 of

(A) Shadow Case

Figure 12.   Continues overleaf

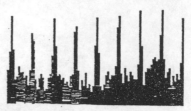

PID within W_1

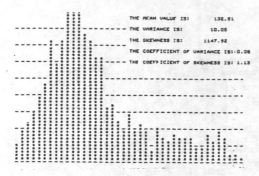

THE MEAN VALUE IS: 132.51
THE VARIANCE IS: 10.05
THE SKEWNESS IS: 1147.92
THE COEFFICIENT OF VARIANCE IS: 0.08
THE COEFFICIENT OF SKEWNESS IS: 1.13

Histogram analysis of W_1

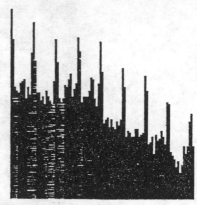

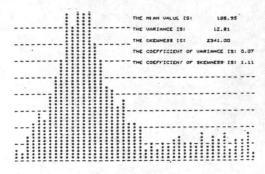

THE MEAN VALUE IS: 186.95
THE VARIANCE IS: 12.81
THE SKEWNESS IS: 2341.00
THE COEFFICIENT OF VARIANCE IS: 0.07
THE COEFFICIENT OF SKEWNESS IS: 1.11

PID between W_1 & W_2

Histogram analysis of W_2

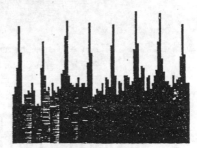

PID within W_2

Figure 12.   Continued

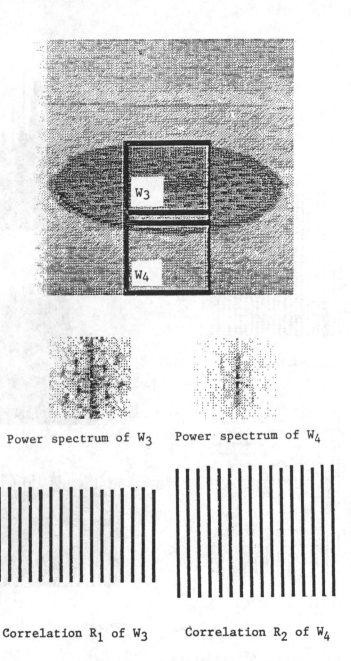

Power spectrum of W_3 Power spectrum of W_4

Correlation R_1 of W_3 Correlation R_2 of W_4

(B) Non-Shadow Case

Figure 12. Continues overleaf

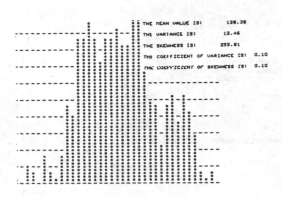

THE MEAN VALUE IS: 138.38
THE VARIANCE IS: 13.46
THE SKEWNESS IS: 253.81
THE COEFFICIENT OF VARIANCE IS: 0.10
THE COEFFICIENT OF SKEWNESS IS: 0.10

Histogram analysis of W_3

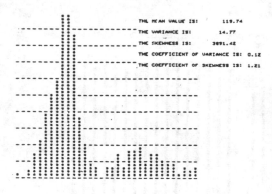

THE MEAN VALUE IS: 119.74
THE VARIANCE IS: 14.77
THE SKEWNESS IS: 3691.42
THE COEFFICIENT OF VARIANCE IS: 0.12
THE COEFFICIENT OF SKEWNESS IS: 1.21

Histogram analysis of W_4

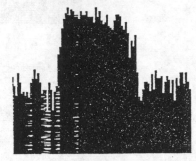

PID within W_3

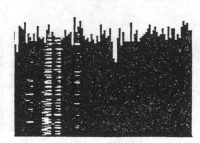

PID between W_3 & W_4

PID within W_4

Figure 12.   Shadow Discrimination

level intensities, while the spectral energy concentrated at high
frequencies represents the spatial areas which exhibit edges or
display abrupt changes in the gray level intensities. This knowledge allows us to distinguish a surface of fine texture from a
surface of coarse texture. Indeed, since shadow formation does
not change the texture of a surface but only darkens its intensity, the edges on the surface and the smoothness or coarseness of
the surface remain unchanged. This translates into obtaining
similar power spectra if we are to compare a lighted area with a
shadowed area. Experimental results have proved this conjecture
as shown in Figure 12. The slight changes are due to the blurring effect of shadow and to the darkening effect which translates
into a weight factor in the magnitude of the power spectrum. To
visualize the procedure we make use of power spectrum to discriminate shadow from other objects. Consider a pavement upon
which a shadow of a tree or a light pole is cast. The first-
pass evaluation will indicate an obstacle at the location of the
shadow. The step we take from here on is to determine the power
spectra of two windows, one in the lighted and the other in the
shaded area. The results are then analyzed in the decision-
making process shown in Figure 11. Detailed work on Fourier
Transforms and their use in texture discrimination is given in
Brzakovic & Tou (5). For a comprehensive study on Fourier Transforms and their application see Gonzalez and Wintz (9).

(c) Cross-Correlation Function.

We have made use of two correlation functions in shadow analysis.

(1) Correlation Measure 1

$$R_1(d_1,d_2) = \frac{\sum_j \sum_k F_1(j,k)\, F_2(j-d_1, k-d_2)}{[\sum_j \sum_k F_1^2(j,k)]^{1/2} [\sum_j \sum_k F_2^2(j-d_1,k-d_2)]^{1/2}}$$

where F_1 and F_2 denote the two images and d_1 and d_2 stand for the
shifts.

(2) Correlation Measure 2

$$R_1(d_1,d_2) = \frac{\sum_j \sum_k F_1(j,k)\, F_2(k-d_1, k-d_2)}{\sum_j \sum_k [F_1(j,k)]^2}$$

Experimental results illustrated in Figure 12 have shown that both R_1 and R_2 have a uniform distribution over the considered shifts d_1 and d_2, and certain statistical parameters are repeatable when any shaded area is compared to a nonshaded area of the same texture. The same outcome is not experienced in the case where two areas of different textures are analyzed. For results of the pixel intensity distribution analysis mentioned earlier, the reader is referred to Figure 12. Some limitations of the overall shadow analysis exist, however. These limitations are due to (a) the effect of distance, i.e., the recognition of shadow is limited to the case where the shadow is viewed at a short range, and (b) the darkness of the shadow. A shadow that is too dark conceals any texture information.

An approach to detecting depressions. Depressions or dropoffs constitute a serious obstacle for the blind pedestrian. Unfortunately, they also represent a complex image interpretaton problem. In the human visual system, many visual cues such as stereopsis, occlusion, context in the viewed scene, and textural properties are used for the detection of depressions. These tasks are performed by the human visual system with relative ease. In image processing, analysis of any of these tasks is by no means a simple information processing problem (11,16,20).

Our approach to this problem makes use of an image correspondence technique to extract occluded information in a simple yet efficient manner. The image correspondence technique is generally used to recover the third dimension in the two-dimensional picture by matching a given object in two or more frames. In our approach, we are neither interested in a perfect match nor in the recovery of the third dimension, but simply in extracting occluded information with a subsequent frame. The procedure of our approach is as follows:

(a) When the first-pass evaluation discovers that an obstacle is not a shadow, the system selects a window W_1 covering the obstacle.

(b) The user moves a short distance d towards the obstacle and the camera takes another picture.

(c) In this new picture, the system determines a window W_2 which still views the obstacle. This is done by assessing the effect of displacement d on both the width between any arbitrary two points (a,b) and the depth covered (see Figures 13 a-b). Since W_1 and W_2 are windows of digitized images, let us first define the conversion factor which relates a film image whose dimensions are in millimeter (mm) to the digitized image whose

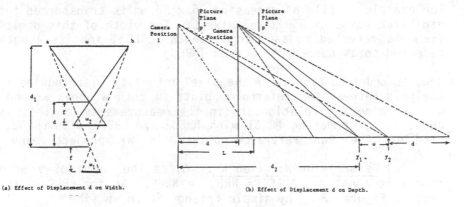

(a) Effect of Displacement d on Width.

(b) Effect of Displacement d on Depth.

Mapping of the Reference Points

Example Illustrating Moving Towards
A Curb (Step-Down)

(c) Effect of Displacement d on the Picture Frames.

Figure 13. An Approach to Extract Occluded information for the
Detection of Depressions

size is measured by pixels (p). Conversion factor is defined
as

$$\beta = \frac{1}{resolution}$$

In our digitizing device, a resolution of 100 μm is used.   That
is, for each 100 μm (10^{-6} meters), the intensity of light passing
through a point of the film is read and stored as a pixel. β is
thus given by

$$\beta = \frac{1p}{100 \times 10^{-6} \ mm} = 10p/mm$$

For example, a film of dimension 35 x 25 mm is transformed into a digitized image of 350 x 250 pixels. The width of this digitized image is referred to as record length (LREC), and its length is referred to as number of records (NREC).

Now, in order to facilitate the pixel intensity distribution (pid) analysis between two reference points in both windows W_1 and W_2, we determine the relationship in the measurements of these windows, i.e., comparing NREC1 with NREC2 and LREC1 with LREC2, and find how the two reference points in W_1 project onto W_2.

(a) <u>Determining W_2 given W_1</u>: Since the depth of view of a camera is constant, NREC2 = NREC1 = NREC. As for LREC's, referring to Figure 13-a, by simple triangulation we find

$$\omega_2 = \omega_1 \cdot \frac{d_1}{d_1 - d} \quad \text{or} \quad LREC2 = LREC1 \cdot \frac{d_1}{d_1 - d}$$

d is equal to 1 step or 0.45m, and d_1 is determined in the first picture by the range finding scheme of the first pass evaluation.

(b) <u>Projecting the reference points</u>: points y_{11} and y_{12} of W_1 as shown in Figure 13-c are chosen so that y_{12} coincides with the last record number, and y_{11} to be near the detected obstacle. Referring back to Figure 13-b, we find that

$$y_{22} = NREC - P_\ell^2 (d) \cdot \beta$$

$$y_{21} = P_\ell^2 (d_2 - d - L)$$

where P^2 denotes picture plane projection in frame 2. The equation for $P_\ell (*)$ is derived in Appendix 1.

Experimental results are shown in Figure 14. Similar analysis can be peformed using binary images. In this case, although the occluded information is easier to extract, additional time is needed for binary image generation. This analysis depends upon the discovery of occluded information. A depression is detected if occluded information is found in the second picture. However, this result is not conclusive. Further investigation of this problem is underway.

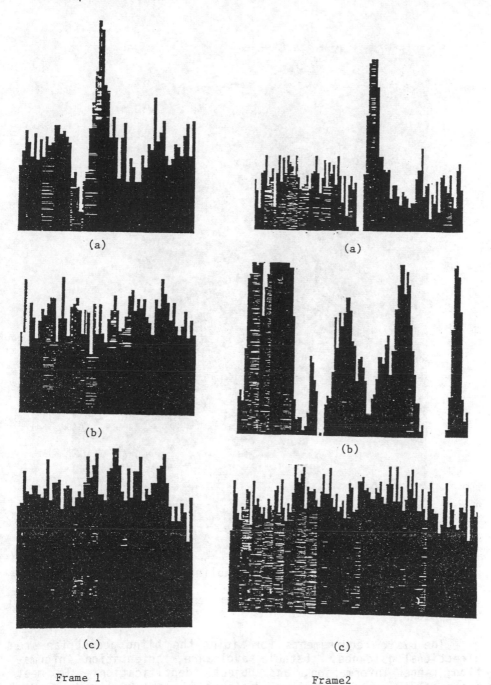

(a)   (a)

(b)

(b)

(c)   (c)

Frame 1   Frame 2

Figure 14. Pixel Intensity Distribution for the Detection of
Occluded Information.

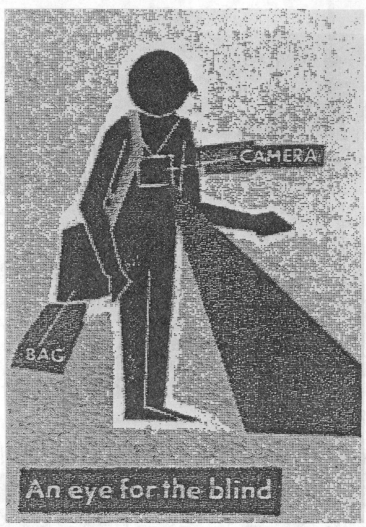

Figure 15.   Artist Rendition of the Blind Vision System

CONCLUSIONS

The basic requirements for aiding the blind pedestrian are directional guidance, obstacle avoidance, orientation information, range information, and object identification. To meet these requirements, we have designed a computer vision/audio system to serve as a guidance aid for the blind pedestrian. The design of visual aids to the blind may be pursued along two major directions: (1) enhancing the information processing capability of other sensory organs of the blind and (2) providing the blind with limited artificial seeing capability. To accomplish the latter we have designed machines to perform scene analysis and image interpretation and to convert scene descriptions into voice.

Scene interpretation and image understanding are performed in two modes of operation. Mode 1 is to provide a general description of the environment viewed by the camera and to plan a safety path for the blind. This mode is accomplished by the first-pass evaluation. Mode 2, which makes use of the second-pass evaluation, is designed for the purpose of (a) identifying objects when necessary and (b) resolving ambiguities caused by the first-pass evaluation. Case (b) also requires further analysis of the first-pass evaluation following resolution of ambiguity by the second-pass evaluation.

Before the blind person starts to walk, the vision/audio system takes several pictures of the scene in his/her vicinity and performs image analysis, interpretation, and recognition. During this initialization phase, the blind person stands still for a moment to wait for instructions from the system. During the walking phase, the system determines in real-time a safety path for the blind pedestrian to follow. When an obstacle is detected, the system enters into the warning phase and asks the blind to walk slowly or to take a pause so that the system is allowed sufficient time to complete image analysis and interpretation. This paper concludes with discussions of shadow discrimination and depression detection. The proposed computer vision/audio system has been implemented on a PDP11/40 minicomputer. Research is planned to make full use of the knowledge base, to generate a wide-angle view of the vicinity of the blind pedestrian by integrating left, front, and right views for the purpose of optimizing safety paths determination, and to design a portable vision/audio system for the blind on the basis of the techniques presented in this paper. The ultimate design is illustrated in Figure 15.

APPENDIX 1: Perspective Effect

The perspective effect used in the first-pass evaluation is based on a simple mapping scheme of the real-world environment onto the picture plane. Given the camera parameters, we simply determine the geometrical relationships of the measurements of depth and width in the real world with their projections onto the picture plane. The advantages of taking this effect into account are (a) that our analysis conforms to our view of the real world; (b) this effect helps speed up processing since only the vicinity of the blind is considered at any given level of the virtual partitioning, but it also helps produce better results by not covering too big an area; and (c) if an obstacle is detected in the global view of our analysis, we can easily estimate its actual width and length.

To establish the aforementioned geometrical relationships, we make use of the properties of similar triangles. Referring to Figure 1-A, we have derived that the picture plane projection of any segment of depth (d) at a given level (ℓ) of the partitioning ($\ell=1,2,...,$ n; n is the number of partitions considered) is given by

$$P_\ell(d) = \frac{dhf}{[\, f+L_1+(\ell-1)d \,](f+L_1\ell d)}$$

where f denotes the focal length of the camera, and h represents the camera height from the ground plane. L_1 represents the distance from the camera's picture plane to the nearest point viewed by the camera. Referring to Figure 1-B, on the basis of similar reasoning, we find that the picture plane projection of a given width (w) at a given level (ℓ) of the partitioning is given by the relationship

$$P_\ell(w) = \frac{fw}{f+L_1+(\ell-1)d}$$

With these two projections, given the camera parameters and camera viewing position, we can easily determine the perspective effect. However, at this stage of our work, we have implemented this perspective effect to conform with the partitioning scheme used in the first-pass evaluation. Thus, offset error up to 10 pixels or the size of each cell of the partition can occur. This error, however, has no effect on the practical usefulness for which this perspective effect is intended. This error may affect the estimate of the width of the obstacle detected by the global view analysis, but in no way does it affect the safety of the blind.

Attention can be drawn at this point to the fact that if one desires a more thorough analysis by the first-pass evaluation, one can implement this perspective effect even at levels of the partitions themselves by making them smaller in width and depth with increasing level.

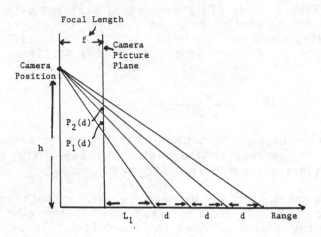

Figure 1-A. Picture Plane Mapping of Range

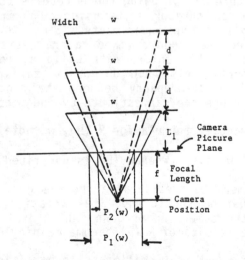

Figure 1-B. Picture Plane Mapping of Width

APPENDIX 2: A Range Finding Scheme

The specialized range finding scheme described here is devised to conform to the virtual partitioning scheme used in the first-pass evaluation. The objective is to map at each level (ℓ) of this partitioning the real-world measurement of range as illustrated in Figure II-A. This mapping is achieved using geometrical properties of similar triangles. Given the camera parameters and viewing position, the range R from the initial position of the blind to a given level (ℓ) of the partitioning is given by:

$$R_\ell(D) = \frac{hf}{h-g-\ell D}$$

D denotes the size of each partition, h and f are as defined in Appendix 1, and L represents the distance between the camera position and the nearest point viewed by the camera.

To estimate parameter L, we need to set both the camera height h from the ground, and the view angle of the camera (θ) with respect to the ground as shown in Figure II-B. To determine the variation of L with respect to θ, we have conducted an experimental study using a COHU Camera equipped with a 28-135 mm lens coupled to a display system via the camera control unit and an 8-bit digitizer. We set the camera lens to 28 mm and the camera height at 1.25 m. The result of the variation of L with respect to θ is shown in Figure II-C. Using these results together with the results obtained on outdoor shots using a 35 mm camera, we decided to let L=1.5 m for our experiments. Since we have not at this stage of research designed a fixed camera system which can be carried by the blind to conform with L=1.5 m condition, the picture examples shown in this paper do not all satisfy this condition. There exists a discrepancy between the range evaluated by computer and the range one can estimate by judgment.

Now, from the above formula for $R_\ell(D)$, we note that (a) at step ℓ where $\ell=(h-g)/D$, i.e. when $R_\ell(D)$ is undefined, the incident ray of the camera becomes parallel to the ground plane and the first-pass evaluation should end; (b) variation of L translates into tilting the camera up or down, which explains why for some values of L the results of $R_\ell(D)$ become meaningless; (c) experimental results suggest that smaller scale partitioning translates into more depth (range) covered in the first passs evaluation. This fact can be proved by simply using two different values D_1 and D_2 for D where, $D_1 < D_2$; (d) uphill or downhill type

environments can cause either an underestimation or an overesti-
mation of the range respectively. This fact is easily demonstrated by simply tilting up or down the groundplane of Figure
II-A.

    In estimating the range or in making any type of image
analysis concerning guidance of the blind for that matter, we
should be aware of the deviation errors which can be generated
due to the camera unstable viewing conditions and the occasional
shift of the blind from the right path. In such cases, we must
estimate these errors and either compensate for them or include
them in the decision-making process, and we should also make sure
that the image-based guidance scheme for the blind can tolerate or
compensate for these errors (2).

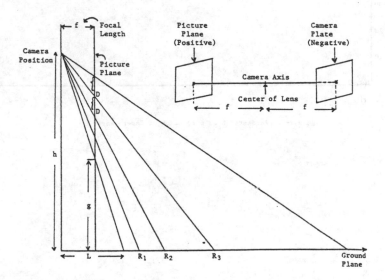

Figure 2-A. Estimating Range from Equal Partitioning of the Picture Plane.

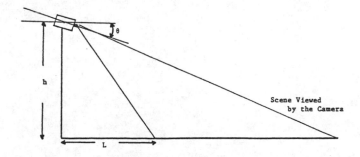

Figure 2-B. Estimating L from the Camera Viewing Position.

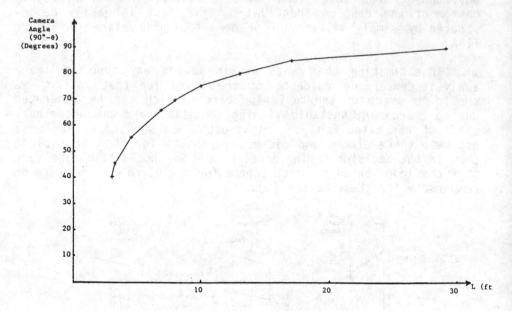

Figure 2-C.   Parameter L as a Function of Camera Angle θ.

REFERENCES

1. Adjouadi, M. & Tou, J. T. (1982). Automatic staircase and crosswalk identification for a vision system to aid the blind, CIR Technical Report.

2. Adjouadi, M. & Tou, J. T. (1984). A new approach to guiding the blind via computer vision techniques, 7th International Conference on Pattern Recognition, Montreal, Canada.

3. Bach-y-Rita, P. (1972). Brain Mechanisms in Sensory Substitution. New York: Academic Press.

4. Brabyn, J. A., Collins, C. C., & Kay, L. (1981). A wide band with CTFM scanning sonar with tactile and acoustic display for persons with impaired vision. Proceedings of Ultrasonics International Conference, 81, Brighton, England.

5. Brzakovic, D. & Tou, J. T. (1984). Boundary determination of object surfaces via textural information. 7th International Conference on Pattern Recognition, Montreal, Canada.

6. Collins, C. C. (1978). Visual substitution in blind mobility. Proceedings of the 7th International Conference of Ergophthalmology, Nagoya, Japan.

7. Deering, M. F. (1982). Real time natural scene analysis for a blind prosthesis. Fairchild Technical Report, No. 622.

8. Dodds, A. G., Carter, D. D. C., & Howarth, C. I. (1981). The Nottingham obstacle detector: Development and evaluation, Journal of Visual Impairment & Blindness, 75, 203-207.

9. Gonzalez, R. C. & Wintz, P. (1977). Digital Image Processing. Addison-Wesley.

10. Gregory, R. L. (1978). Eye and Brain. New York: McGraw-Hill.

11. Grimson, W. E. L. (1981). A computer theory of human stero vision. Philosophical Transactions of the Royal Society of London. Vol. B292, 217-253.

12. Guarniero, G. (1974). Experience of tactile vision. Perception, 3, 101-104.

13. Heyes, A. D. (1982). A 'Polaroid' ultrasonic travel aid for the blind? Journal of Vision Impairment & Blindness, 76, 199-201.

14. Kay, L. (1984). Acoustic coupling to the ears in binaural sensory aids. Journal of Visual Impairment & Blindness, 78, 12-16.

15. Loomis, J. M. (1981). Tactile pattern perception. Perception, 10, 5-27.

16. Marr, D. & Poggio, T. (1979). A computational theory of human stereo vision. Proceedings of the Royal Society of London, Vol. B204, 301-328.

17. Maure, D. R., Mellor, C. M., & Uslan, M. (1979). AFB's computerized travel aid: experimenters wanted. Journal of Visual Impairment & Blindness, 73, 380-381.

18. Melen, R. & Buss, D. (Eds.) (1977). Charge Coupled Devices: Technology and Applications. IEEE Press.

19. Moricca, L. S. & Slocum, R. V. (1977). Pattern recognition on the forehead: an electronic scan system. Journal of Visual Impairment & Blindness, 71, 164-167.

20. Poggio, T. (1984). Vision by man and machine. Scientific American, 250, 106-116.

21. Ray, R., Birk, J., & Kelley, R. B. (1983). Error analysis of surface normals determined by radiometry. IEE Transactions on Pattern Analysis and Machine Intelligence, 631, 645.

22. Strelow, E. R., Kay, N., & Kay, L. (1978). Binaural sensory aid: case studies of its use by two children. Journal of Visual Impairment & Blindness, 72, 1-9.

23. Tou, J. T. (1979). Zoom thresholding technique for boundary determination. International Journal of Computer and Information Science, 8.

24. Zahl, Paul A. (Ed.) (1950). Blindness: Modern Approaches to the Unseen Environment. Princeton University Press.

SENSORY AIDS TO SPATIAL PERCEPTION FOR BLIND PERSONS: THEIR DESIGN AND EVALUATION

L. Kay, FRSNZ

University of Canterbury

A recent review of electronic aids for the blind (7) showed how little progress toward a widely usable electronic aid for mobility had been made over a period of 25 years. The range of devices of widely varying technology, information gathering capacity, and market price shows that engineers have not been idle, but somehow have failed to reach their goal--that of providing the blind traveler with a highly acceptable electronic aid to spatial perception. That is, an aid which can be obtained readily by individuals generally with limited income, an aid which they would freely choose to use in order to get about in their daily lives or relate more effectively to their immediate environment.

By what measures can such a statement be justified? The non-electronic long cane is provided throughout the world by welfare organizations to all blind persons who need an aid to travel, and extensive training in its use is given by qualified instructors. Very few of those trained in long cane travel receive additional training in the use of an electronic travel aid. The percentage is not known, but from the very low level of sales of devices the proportion can be said to be negligible -- an adequate measure by any standard.

The reasons for this are many: Price, device effectiveness, ease of use, reliability, flexibility in application, time to learn, and relative merit of aid versus the Long Cane are but a few factors which finally determine the reality that electronic aids to travel have failed to satisfy a perceived market. Unfortunately, this failure has not provided the data from which engineers can design new aids that might meet a blind person's

needs better. The philosophy of the engineering innovator therefore remains unchanged: think of a better solution. This process
is generally one of studying the limitations of existing devices
in the light of numerous reports and thinking of an alternative
approach. Simplicity and low cost are criteria which are most
commonly used because these are criteria most commonly discussed
by the market. They are not necessarily the most important
criteria. What are our options?

THE BASELINE

In the 25-year period during which electronic aids have been
under development, the Long Cane method of travel has advanced
from an atmosphere of strong resistance among blind persons and
instructors (1) to one of almost universal acceptance by the
blind and the mobility teaching professional, a person who is
able to determine that the Long Cane will be the primary aid to
travel by a blind client. There are good reasons for this acceptance. Travel with and without the cane is observed to be so
different that no one can seriously question the validity of the
decision to teach all blind persons to use the Long Cane to the
best of their ability in the time allotted to training. The cane
is cheap, about $30; the training is expensive, 150 hours at $30
per hour including all overheads (an estimate by the writer),
making a total of $4530 per person to be provided by some social
system.

Whatever the travel performance of a blind Long Cane user
might be, that performance would be significantly reduced without
the cane. However, there are no data on the use of the Long Cane
after training which can be used to assess the change in lifestyle
brought about by such training, and so the long-term value of Long
Cane travel training is virtually unknown. Since this is the
baseline to which sensory aid engineers have to work, some special
attention to this area is long overdue. There are of course research groups that have studied Long Cane travel and made comparisons with travel using electronic sensory aids in combination with
the Long Cane, but the information obtained from this research
gives little insight to the real problem of sightless travel.
Too many variables are involved which limit the usefulness of the
findings in an engineering sense.

Design Criteria

The designer of a sensory aid to spatial perception, basing
his work on the literature and interviews with users of existing
aids, must find the field confusing, and he is mentally forced to
adopt criteria which fit his perception of the problem.

Much will depend upon his engineering background and special interests -- communications, sonar or radar, computers, etc. This paper is an attempt to analyze the field as it is today and to draw attention to pathways which might lead more effectively to the goals we have sought for over one quarter of a century.

Whatever the discipline involved in the search for these goals, be it special education, psychology, physics, or engineering, an end product has to be designed by the engineer. He has to make it work reliably; it must be a profitable product to the manufacturer. Both of these criteria define success in reaching the goal; all other evaluative procedures are secondary to these two primary criteria. The scientific approach of first finding what will meet the needs and then attempting to make a commercial product requires that society meet whatever cost arises out of this process.

Unless the reliability factor and the profitability factor are dealt with, failure to meet the blind man's need is inevitable. Not only must the engineer look carefully at user factors if he is not to fall foul of the "rejection factor," but the educator, psychologist, and sociologist, or others who are involved in the application of aids, must address themselves to the profitability factor in their search for sensory solutions.

Experience over the past 25 years has shown just how wrong most workers in this field have been. Devices have reached the marketplace but show little if any profitability. Their workability is questioned. We don't have a satisfactory predictor of usability, workability, or profitability and hence seem unable to escape from the stranglehold of prejudice surrounding sensory aids supply and use.

Only the engineering designer can break out, and to do so he has to pay great attention to those interest areas which are ever ready to caution his approach.

SOME BASICS

Other than through physical contact or touch, spatial information can be gathered only through electromagnetic or stress waves: both forms of wave energy are well understood and used in a variety of applications as well as employed by animals as a sensing means. Visual and infrared light, radar (particularly millimetre wavelength), sonar (also millimetre wavelength), and audible sound are in common use in technology and are applicable to the sensing needs of the blind. With the exception of audible sound, all are capable of providing images of space.

Image Forms

Recent advances in technology have broadened the concept of an image. When restricted to optical systems an image was conceived as a two-dimensional scene representation of three-dimensional space. The TV screen is a common example of a 2D image of 3D space, but our ability to perceive a 3D space from it through scene familiarity and monocular visual cues often masks this simple fact. Machine vision is now commonly used in various forms of remote sensing, from satellite sensing of Earth's features to robot sensing of its work space. The images are processed by a computer to extract features of interest.

Echo location systems such as radar and sonar are now included as ways of imaging space. These systems also produce 2D images, but in contrast with optical-type systems they are inherently 2D, gathering spatial information in terms of distance and direction of objects.

It is easy to understand why optical type systems have in the past attracted attention as a sensing means for the blind. Great familiarity exists through our experience with vision. Unfortunately two factors have worked against successful exploitation of the potential of optical systems. 2D images are very difficult for machine systems to interpret, and even though powerful computers are used, picture processing time to recognize simple features in a scene can involve many seconds. High speed processing is restricted to images from environments which have been artificially reduced to two dimensional planes, as in robot vision systems.

Today, and for the foreseeable future, optical machine vision is well beyond the economic structure of the blindness system to support as a means to spatial perception in the blind. Existing robot vision systems cost between $10,000 and $50,000.

In contrast to 2D vision systems, which lack distance information, echo-location systems inherently provide both distance and direction information but exhibit greatly reduced object detail in their images. Since the optical and echolocation images are orthogonal they can be complementary; this may be seen to have powerful potential for speeding up robot perception of a work space.

3D information can be obtained rapidly from a combination of the two imaging methods, as illustrated in Figure 1.

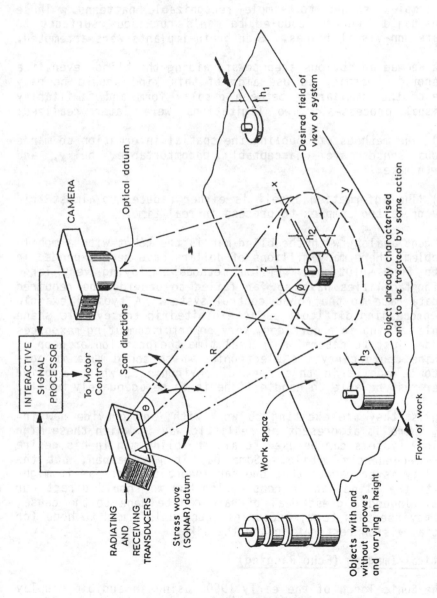

Figure 1. The interactive use of a camera and a scanning sonar can speed up the picture processing of object images in an industrial application of robots.

Optical Imaging

Various workers during the late 1960's and the 1970's saw the possibility of optical information, in a heavily processed form, as the basis for a visual prosthesis. Early work on optical image processing created the belief that the microcomputer of the future (late 1970's, early 1980's) could provide the means to reduce complex scenes to simple recognizable patterns. These patterns could then be coupled to man's cutaneous surfaces to stimulate non-visual images. Even brain implants were attempted.

It seemed an obvious step toward aiding the blind, even if a "long shot." Learning to use aids of this kind should be easy because of the similarity between display form and familiarity with visual processes. Two limitations were later realized:

1) The methods of coupling the spatial information to man's cutaneous senses are unacceptably uncomfortable, bulky, and costly to make;

2) The information itself is either reduced to almost tri-viality or is too complex to process in real time.

A good analogy with the blind man is the robot with a mobil-ity problem. Here many millions of dollars have been expended in order to find solutions. Vision methods employing very large computing facilities have so far failed to provide the required input data rate to the robot control system. A typical example of the processing difficulties is exhibited in the dynamic scene of people walking in a corridor. Very powerful computing resources are needed just to determine in real time the position of people. No machine could carry the electronics which could make it pos-sible to be mobile in this sort of environment, which a blind traveler must be able to handle if he is to be adequately mobile.

Whilst they are exciting to work with, and provide new in-sights, there is at present no realistic way in which these high technology systems can be used to aid the blind man in his desire to be independently mobile. Some day it may happen, but the possibility is so remote that one can ignore the work as it might relate to the blind man in considering how we should direct our efforts. Indeed a great deal of harm can be done to the cause, if one may use this term, encouraging the uninformed to hope for artificial vision restoration and the like.

Non-Optical Imaging (Echo Ranging)

The Sonic Torch of the early 1960s using an audible display and its spinoff, the Sonar Camera (Polaroid) of the late 1970s in

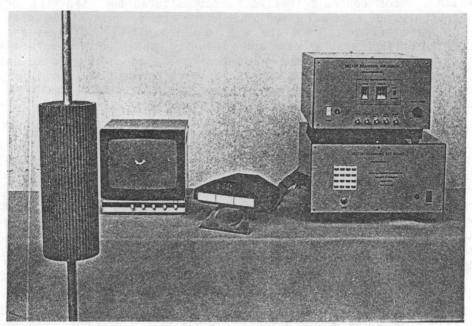

Figure 2a. Sector scanning air sonar with focussed beam used to image the frontal view of a 20 cm. diameter cylinder covered with corrugataed paper).

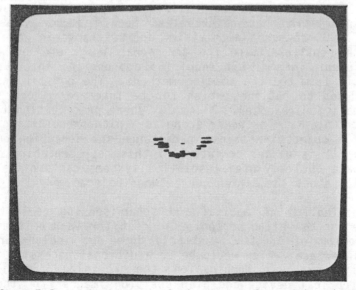

Figure 2b. Enlarged picture of the image formed by the scanning sonar. Note only the surface "seen" by the sonar beam can be imaged in cross-section when a semicircle is obtained.

which a motor controls the focus, demonstrated the usability of ultrasonics as a sensing medium. There are now many industrial uses for ultrasonics, but the way in which ultrasonic waves are used to collect spatial data and allow its subsequent interpretation is not obvious. Some engineers have used ultrasonic waves in water, body tissue, and metals for a very long time, but it is only recently through ultrasonic medical diagnostics that the public has become aware of its great potential.

Recently Kay (7) demonstrated the first "in air" real time 2D imaging system using ultrasonic waves as an alternative means for sensing a robot work space. This work arose in part because blind children had exhibited an ability to use the Trisensor in reaching exercises and discriminating between objects which exceed the adaptive ability of robots in these actions. A high resolution focused imaging sensor was constructed to show that the high picture detail obtained in medical ultrasonic imaging could now be obtained in air up to a distance of about 1 m. The system as demonstrated operated up to a range of 0.6m with a radial resolution of 1.7mm and an azimuth resolution of 7mm over an arc of 60 degrees. Figure 2 shows an image of a 20 cm diameter pole covered with corrugated paper. To present this same image detail to a blind person a matrix of vitrotactile stimulators is required having 60 elements covering the azimuth arc and 200 to represent radial distance, a total of 12,000 elements, each with a grey scale of at least 20 dB dynamic range.

Such an interface is not possible in any practial sense. The spatial information has nevertheless been reduced by a linear factor of 7000 compared with vision due to change in wavelength. Because the optical image and the sonar image are orthogonal, very different information requiring appropriate interpretation is possible from the two imaging methods. The optical scene has to be reduced to outlines which can be interpreted only when a single shape is presented. A complex scene presentation is not a realistic concept. The sonar scene is a plan presentation of the location of objects in terms of distance and direction from the observer. It is easier to interpret this representation of geometric space but only high resolution systems can provide usable information about the difference between objects.

A combination of optical and sonar sensing could be very effective for the blind person. The cost for each unit might be in the region of $30,000, and this does not include any man-machine interface, which would be an additional necessity for use with a blind man. In combination, the provision of both scenes from the optical device and plan position images from the sonar has powerful features for a machine in terms of providing faster processing rates. However, there is no way that this type of device could be provided for the blind person at present. The total cost, quite apart from size and interface complexity, determines impracticability.

REALISTIC SOLUTIONS

Simple Sensors

These can be considered because the Long Cane method of travel has shown how well people can travel using little distal information about their environment.

Twenty-five years of thinking has left us with a few low-cost sensors either in the marketplace or seeking to find a place. These generally provide binary echo information about the environment. Some designers have incorporated microprocessors into the signal processing so as to simplify the information coupled to man. The primary goal seems to be to improve Long Cane travel by incorporating secondary aids into the travel scheme. The potential of such devices to aid a blind person is nevertheless limited to the obstacle detector concept. Little progress towards the provision of an effective general purpose spatial sensor is likely along this pathway.

Sophisticated Sensors

These can be defined as sensors which provide image information about more than one object at a time. The concept of resolution must be invoked whereby it is possible to perceive two or more objects simultaneously and know their positions relative to the sensing system.

The Sonicguide (6) is the most simple form of sophisticated sensor under this definition. Spatial information in terms of radial distance is converted to a linear relationship in the audible frequency domain (see Figure 3). The only processing carried out on the echo information is multiplication, which converts the ultrasound to audible signals. The user further processes the new audible information through the cochlear filtering action to complete the process. When a machine is used, as in the scanning air sonar, a bank of filters is employed which must then be followed by a machine perception system. The radial resolution available to a machine system (i.e., the ability to resolve two objects in different azimuth directions) using the Sonicguide principle, is two wavelengths (8mm). That is, a machine can determine that there are two echo sources separated radially by 8mm. Man, using the Sonicguide, is able to achieve the same resolution although not as two separate targets. Two

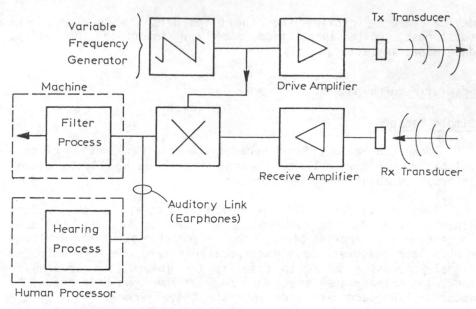

Figure 3.   CWFM sonar for blind and machines.

echo sources spaced radially by 8mm can be perceived as two
sources by the tone complex that is set up. This type of tonal
complexity, using sound-timbre signatures, also forms the basis
of object recognition.

    Direction information is obtained by the loudness difference
in the left and right channels. For two objects at the same
distance, interaction between the two produces false indications
in the form of a phantom object perceived between the two (5).
When the objects are spaced radially the radial resolution also
varies with the radial motion of one object relative to the
other (3).

    The Sonicguide display is sensitive to many variables of de-
sign, and in the process of commercialization from the research
designs, certain critical features were changed which have significantly detracted from the original performance criteria. Two
threshold levels of performance are very important.

    1) Azimuth Motion Perception. In the process of commercial-
ly producing this device the direction cue was reduced (i.e., the
ability to detect left-right differences was reduced) to satisfy
a number of technical and cosmetic criteria, thus raising the
threshold of azimuth motion perception. This has caused confusion
to the blind traveler by reducing his ability to detect azimuth
motion.

2) Object detection and recognition require a high signal to noise ratio. There should be no noticeable background noise. Instead the commercialization increased the vertical field of view which introduced backscatter from the ground, producing a constant masking noise of little value to the user. Even so, a few blind persons have found the Sonicguide usable over long periods of time (3-4 hours per day over 10 years or more).

I believed that these changes--not well understood by the field--have resulted in conclusions about the display which are particular to a commercial product, the Sonicguide, and not the general principle of this form of display.

A recent example of this is seen in the work of Shingledecker (9). An attempt was made to measure the difference in performance of a Long Cane traveler aided by a) an electronic aid with a simplified display of spatial information, and b) an electronic aid with a "rich" display of spatial information (the Sonicguide). The hypothesis was: whilst traveling with the Long Cane the simple display should have less effect on the execution of a secondary task than that of a rich display of spatial information, but performance using the Long Cane alone would be poorest. The results confirmed the hypothesis. The question of mental overload was a prime factor under consideration. However, a contaminating factor in this study was that the aid with a rich display of spatial information suffered from having a background of noiselike signals because of excessive signal from the ground. This noise carried virtually no information which deserved attention, yet it masked important signals which were required for spatial awareness. This overlay of noise is not inherent in this type of device and was not a feature of the early prototypes (6). The results of this type of experiment are thus valueless unless the effect of the masking signals can be assessed.

Background noise from ground returns can also explain some of the adverse comments about the use of an auditory display. If the display can be characterized by continuous background noise, as described by Shingledecker (9), then two serious criticisms are valid. Natural echo location and the use of ambient noise for orientation can be seriously impaired. This was not the situation when the experimental aids were used during evaluation (6). Indeed, so much attention was given to background noise that 40% of aids supplied were rejected by O & M instructors for having too much self noise--a noise level well below the backscatter noise often experienced from the ground when the head was pointing down to "look" along the ground.

Some reappraisal of the Sonicguide design is required to overcome its present shortcomings.

The Trisensor

One of the limitations of the binaural system as used in the
Sonicguide which restricts its general use arises from poor spatial resolution, an important factor in spatial image formation.
Children using the Sonicguide (4) and even the later Canterbury
Children's Aid (10,11) must have experienced difficulty in discriminating between objects forming their environment. A simple
test of spatial resolution (8) shows that both devices lack adequate resolution for use in a home environment. Out of doors in
pedestrian areas, stationary objects are generally sufficiently
well spaced for them to be resolved by a traveler using a binaural
display. Also, moving pedestrians produce flow patterns which
have been shown to provide significantly increased resolution
(3).

To overcome these resolution problems, the Trisensor was designed (8) to have an independent narrow central beam as well as
two wide peripheral beams for sensing the environment. This
design allows two user tasks to occur simultaneously. For example,
it is possible to:

1) Demonstrate a high resolution capability by counting rods
closely spaced in azimuth angle at the same radial distance; and

2) Track an object moving through the field of view.

As might be anticipated, the unexpected appearance of a
moving object in the field of view immediately attracts attention,
detracting from the counting process, but the ability to immediately continue counting exists. This may be likened to the
visual process of attention being caught by peripheral moving
stimuli under similar circumstances.

The addition of two overlapping peripheral beams to the central narrow beam at the acoustic output of the sensor in order to
provide a binaural characteristic has only a small effect on the
resolution capability of the central beam. In the present design,
subjectively tested deterioration is about 10%.

A particular feature of the Trisensor is that object recognition in the central field is enhanced relative to the peripheral
fields by system design.

A wide variety of choices of sensory parameters is available
in the Trisensor so that experimenters and teachers alike can be
given the opportunity to explore these variables with children
who either seek better performance in their spatial awareness
training programs or require reduced information input in the

early stages of learning. These factors will be discussed in
separate papers. (See Hornby, Kay, & Satherley; Easton; Muir,
Humphreys, Dodwell, & Humphreys; and Strelow & Warren, this
volume).

GENERAL DISCUSSION

Both optical and ultrasonic two-dimensional images of a blind
person's environment can be formed by present day technology. The
images are largely orthogonal, providing different information,
and the different wavelengths of the two forms of propagation
provide, in the optical case, high resolution shape, discrimination, and, in the ultrasonic case, discrimination between objects. When the interface between man and machine is considered,
a very significant reduction in information results, to the point
where only simple patterns can be sensed. Under these circumstances the ultrasonic image in the form of a plan of objects
ahead is easier to use than the optical image of a scene processed
down to a few lines (2).

Both imaging systems are expensive, well beyond the level
affordable by agencies for the blind or by blind individuals. It
is most unlikely that a viable mobility system will be developed
using imaging methods which resemble the visual image of sighted
persons or the images which can be presented on a visual screen.

The alternative is the use of audible information coded to
carry spatial information which, when matched to the human auditory processing system, enables a blind person to respond quickly
to the acoustic spatial image formed. This approach leads to
much less costly devices which are easily carried, with minimal
inconvenience. They do, however, invoke new imaging concepts
which are little understood either by the engineering creators or
the psychophysical specialists who study them. They have therefore been received with caution and considerable reserve.

Two areas of controversy exist which act as deterrents to
use of these devices:

1) They require sensory attention to a channel (hearing)
already used for communication with the world;

2) A wide range of signal complexity can be provided which
may either be under-using the auditory channel capacity, or
overloading the perceptual system to the detriment of other
information-processing requirements.

Some experimenters suggest that the auditory system should not be used. Others find that significantly reducing the auditory neural processing by some form of pre-processing leads to a better arrangement for the blind user. There remains a group who feel that given the correct auditory coding, man is capable of processing rich spatial information from a sensor integrating it with spatial information from other sensory inputs as well as receiving and understanding communication from other persons. All have evidence in support of their viewpoints.

The writer clearly belongs to the last group. The Trisensor has been shown to provide a means to give children a rich experience in spatial awareness, even those with low I.Q. in the region of 60 (Hornby et al., this volume). This experience could not be provided by any other means, today or into the foreseeable future.

It follows that any other method is depriving blind persons of spatial experience. The argument for using other aids or no aids must be very convincing to be acceptable.

REFERENCES

1. Bledsoe, C. W. (1980). Originators of orientation and mo-
    bility training.   In R. L. Welsh & B. B. Blasch (Eds.),
    Foundations of Orientation and Mobility. New York: American
    Foundation for the Blind.

2. Brabyn, J. A., Collins, C. C., & Kay, L. (1981). A wide
    bandwidth CTFM sonar with tactile and acoustic display for
    persons with impaired vision. Proceedings of the Ultrasonic
    International. Brighton, England.

3. Do, M. A. & Kay, L. (1976/77). Resolution in an artificially
    generated multiple object space using auditory sensations.
    Acoustica, 36, 9-15.

4. Ferrell, K. A. (1980). Can infants use the Sonicguide? Two
    years experience of Project VIEW. Journal of Visual Impair-
    ment & Blindness, 74, 209-220.

5. Kay, L. (1966). Ultrasonic spectacles for the blind. Pro-
    ceedings of the Conference on Sensory Devices for the Blind.
    St Dunstan's, England, 275-290.

6. Kay, L. (1974). A sonar aid to enhance spatial perception
    of the blind: Engineering design and evaluation. Radio and
    Electronic Engineer, 44, 40-62.

7. Kay, L. (1984).   IEE Review - Electronic aids for blind
    persons: an interdisciplinary subject. IEE Proceedings, 131,
    pt. A., no. 7, 559-76.

8. Kay, L. & Kay, N. (1983). An ultrasonic spatial sensor's
    role as a developmental aid for Blind Children. Transactions
    of the Opthalmological Society of New Zealand, 35, 38-42.

9. Shingledecker, C. A. (1983).   Measuring the mental effort
    of blind mobility. Journal of Visual Impairment & Blindness,
    77, 334-339.

10. Strelow, E. R. (1980). The use of the binaural sensory aid
    by pre-school and school age blind children. Department of
    Electrical Engineering, University of Canterbury, and De-
    partment of Psychology, University of Auckland, New Zealand.

11. Strelow, E. R. (1983). Use of the binaural sensory aid by
    young children. Journal of Visual Impairment & Blindness,
    77, 429-38.

PHYSICAL PRINCIPLES UNDERLYING BLIND GUIDANCE PROSTHESES WITH AN
EMPHASIS ON THE ULTRASONIC EXPLORATION OF A REGION OF SPACE

R. Stuart Mackay

Boston University
California State University, San Francisco

This chapter constitutes a summary of a few physical principles which can have relevance to the production of guidance
prostheses for the blind. Mention will be made of several which
perhaps warrant further consideration for special circumstances.

Accelerometers can now be built that are small, light, and
inexpensive, and if the moving weight is properly suspended upon
a suitable diaphragm or spiral flexure, then movements in transverse directions will not be coupled as signals into the main
axis. It is usually assumed that the use of such devices in
inertial navigation systems requires complex stabilized platforms,
but it can be shown that if the signals from two of these mounted
upon a pendulum are suitably combined, then the output gives a
unique indication of how far one has moved (2), and this can be
converted to a spoken indication by presently readily available
circuits. Similarly, the measurement of turning actions does not
require torsion pendulums or complicated gyros, but can be
indicated by the change in cooling of a heated wire upon which
impinges a jet of air. An indication of the new position of a
person could be a helpful result in some cases.

The evaluation of other prostheses might also be helped by
accelerometers placed upon the subject, the signals from them
being readily telemetered to some central data-gathering location.
Thus the root-mean-square ac signal from an accelerometer seems
to be a measure of the smoothness or hesitancy and uncertainty in
the progress of a person (6). Telemetering pressure foot-plates
in the soles of shoes might provide similar information, and we
have studied drunkenness this way. We have also studied aspects

of stress by monitoring both acid secretion and peristaltic patterns with a comfortable conveniently swallowable radio transmitter (6), and these might be used in prosthesis comparisons to supplement heart rate information. Further discussion of these general matters is found in an accompanying paper (see Mackay, this volume).

However, obviously one of the most critical problems of mobility in both familiar and unfamiliar surroundings is the sensing of obstacles and voids or drop-offs. Various electromagnetic modalities, including visible light, infrared, and radio have been considered for this purpose, as has the use of ultrasonic energy. A number of the considerations are the same in all cases, and the remainder of the discussion will be devoted to examples involving high frequency sound waves. The problem of exploring a region in space using the mechanical disturbances of sound has received considerable attention in the literature on medical imaging, and most of the remaining examples are taken from a book on that subject (7).

ULTRASONICS

Choice of Frequency

Frequencies above about 20,000 cycles per second (20 kHz) are usually considered to be inaudible to humans, and that is the range of frequencies which will interest us here. The attenuation of sound is about three orders of magnitude higher in air than in water. Thus, according to classical considerations, a drop in amplitude of about 12% (1 dB), which can be perceived by the ear, would occur under the following conditions:

ATTENUATION OF SOUND

Frequency (kHz)	Transmission Distance	
	In Air	In Water (km)
1	5 km	10,000
10	50 m	100
100	50 cm	1

In practice these ranges generally are not realized because of inhomogeneities in the sound-conducting medium: winds, ground effects, etc.   Attenuation depends upon temperature and upon relative humidity in air. The attenuation constant in decibels per foot in air increases as a straight-line function of frequency on a log-log scale, with the value being up to a hundred times as much if the air is not dry (11). Thus, to achieve useful signals in air with minimum power might seem to call for the lowest possible frequency, keeping in mind that low frequencies are neither well generated nor well-received by small transducers. We would expect adequate signals under a variety of conditions up to 50 kHz, even in a strong wind.

However, another consideration requires the use of the highest possible frequency. The interaction of a wave with a structure depends upon the relative size of the structure compared with a wavelength. Remembering that wavelength is velocity divided by frequency, it is immediately obvious that to detect small objects requires a short wavelength or a high frequency. (This is, of course, true for electromagnetic radiation as well as for sound waves.) Objects can be good reflectors if they are larger in size than a wavelength, and they will generally reflect back little energy if they are much smaller than a wavelength. A mirror must be at least several wavelengths across and smooth to less than a wavelength. Such an object can reflect incident energy off in a particular direction, which may not be in the direction of the sender, and thus such specular reflections can lead to large objects' being invisible. A small object cannot send out a beam of sound in a particular direction, and if acting as a reflector, will return it weakly in all directions. Similarly, a sound source must be several wavelengths across if it is to generate a directed beam, and a receiver, if several wavelengths across, can "look" in a particular direction, while a small source will transmit in all directions or, if acting as a receiver, will receive about equally well from all directions. These simple ideas will have applicability in a number of the systems to be mentioned presently.

A vibrating plunger will radiate sound in a pattern confined largely to the region indicated in Figure 1. It is seen that there are two regions, a near field and a far field, with properties and transitions depending upon the relative size of the transducer compared to a wavelength. If the sound is being propagated in air, then the wavelength is calculated by dividing the velocity of sound in air by the frequency, the former being approximately 344 m/sec, largely independent of frequency, and the velocity increases, minimally, about 0.61 m/sec for each degree C increase. In Figure 1, if the vibrator is instead acting as a receiver of sound, then the geometrical pattern of sensitivity has about the same form. Curved materials can act as a lens to focus the pattern. The same sorts of considerations apply also to radio, laser light, infrared radiation, etc., beams of which can be used in other guidance prostheses for the blind.

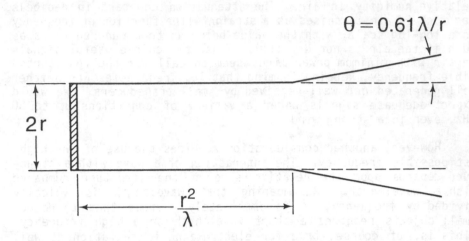

Figure 1.   Approximate extent of pattern of radiation from a
vibrator moving left and right along the axis, showing a near and
far field region.   Though shown as a disc of radius r, the pattern
is similar for other shaped vibrators, and a square avoids some
nulls along the axis.

For an object to be a good reflector of sound, its acoustic
properties must be different from the surroundings.   Specifically,
the acoustic impedance, which is the product of density and sound
velocity in the material, must be different for the reflector
from the material in which the reflector is immersed.   Thus it is
as difficult to detect a thin balloon in air as it is a bag of
water immersed in water, using only reflected sound waves.   However, a balloon filled with gas under water or a water-filled bag
in air are both as noticeable as a piece of steel in either place
since in all cases there are good reflecting conditions.

Ultrasonic Transducers

In medical and oceanographic applications of high frequency
sound, the source and receiver are often pieces of piezoelectric
material that will give out sound upon application of an electrical signal or will convert returning sound into an electrical
signal.   However, sound does not go well between air and these
relatively stiff, heavy materials because of the very different
acoustic impedances.   Thus, for airborne sounds a different sort
of source or receiver is used in order to work with reasonably
low intensities.   There was a time when detectors of high frequency sounds in air, for example those emitted by bats, were
sensed with a microphone in which a thin metal diaphragm was

tightly stretched and its motion sensed in response to the passing sound. To obtain maximum sensitivity and frequency response,
the diaphragm had to be as thin as possible and stretched as
tightly as possible. Obviously at some point the diaphragm would
tear, and it was stated that the absolute limit of sensitivity
had been reached as determined by the strength of materials available. However, this was a technical, not actually an absolute,
limit, as an alternative principle was developed. In this alternative method of construction (4), a block of metal with a grooved
or roughened surface has placed against it a thin sheet of plastic
whose outer surface has a thin film of metal deposited upon it,
allowing sound to vibrate the two conducting surfaces with respect
to each other with much more sensitivity than if the intervening
space were fully filled with even a highly compressible solid.
Such microphones were first mentioned in a 1929 patent and are
used in devices ranging from Kay's blind guidance "sonicles" (3)
to the Polaroid automatic focusing camera, and both groups have
made contributions to the construction of such transducers.
Again, as in many cases, such a good detector of sound can also
be used as a good producer of sound in the same range of frequencies, and these are employed as the sound source in the various
ranging systems.

Pulse Sonars

Application of a short electrical impulse to a transducer
releases a click of high frequency sound which can explore the
surroundings by reflecting back from them as a series of echoes
returning in succession from increasingly distant objects or
interfaces. Scanning the beam along to different directions or
positions allows building up an impression or image as in Figure
2 (7). Here is seen an outgoing click of sound returning in
succession four echoes from four interfaces or transitions between
different materials. When the click is emitted, a dim electron
beam is started upward across a television-like display tube, as
at the upper right in the figure; each returning echo is converted
into an electrical impulse that momentarily brightens the beam to
produce a spot of light. Successive emitted clicks while scanning
to the right produce a cross-sectional image. A medical example
is given in Figure 3 (from 8) which shows an ultrasonic image of
the author's eye and beyond, formed at an ultrasound frequency of
15 MHz. This medical example shows that not all regions are fully
detected, since some echoes are reflected to the side and go unnoticed. The iris of the eye is acoustically rough and seen in
its entirety since echoes return from it in all directions from
every point. In the lower part of Figure 2 is indicated what
actually would be displayed unless a compound scan allowed observation of every point from all angles, thus filling in the entire
outline. (This effect would be called "glint" in a visible light

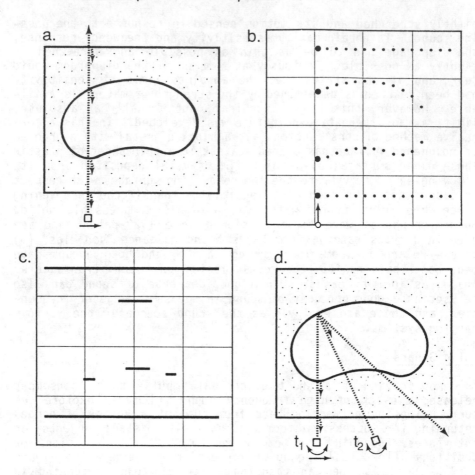

Figure 2. Pulsing a transducer and collecting the returning echoes allows formation of a cross section image. Due to specular reflections the image will actually have parts missing if a more complex pattern of viewing is not used as at the bottom.

image.) The same problem is found in exploring a street scene with sound waves as in exploring the body. A blind guidance device aimed at a smooth glass store window set at an angle to the beam will receive back little or no warning since the echo will bounce to one side in a specular fashion dictated by the usual optics rule that the angle of reflection equals the angle of incidence. This applies when the reflector is smooth to less than a wavelength, which for sound waves includes many surfaces that are considered rough when viewed by the shorter wavelengths of visible light. The sense in which this limitation is absolute should be clear.

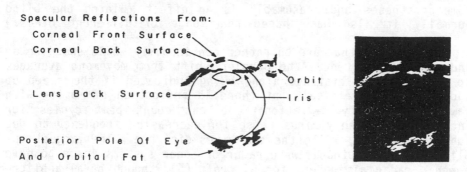

Figure 3.   Image of a human eye showing some parts completely and others only partially due to use of a simple sector scan.

The finest detail detected in a scene is about a wavelength of the exploring beam at best and may be limited to worse than this by the instrument design.   This is an absolute limit.   In some cases exploring with the longer wavelength of ultrasound rather than light automatically removes the clutter or fine detail, and may be an advantage.

Continuous Wave Sonars

The use of sharp impulses allows discrimination of one instant from another in the returning sound sequence or pattern. If instead the sound is on steadily and the frequency is continuously being changed, then a different frequency corresponds to each instant rather than each instant having a different amplitude of "on" or "off" depending upon momentary presence or absence of the impulse.   In such frequency modulated (FM) systems it is possible to provide a greater average signal amplitude with a continuous emission rather than having periodic moments of high intensity, and zero the rest of the time.   Also, background noise can be less troublesome with the narrower bandwidth receivers of FM systems which need not have as many frequencies present at once as with a sharp pulse.   In some cases, the FM equipment is simpler or allows more convenient displays of the result.   One type of data processing is to beat the momentary outgoing frequency with the momentary returning frequency to yield an audible difference frequency that changes with the distance to the reflector.   This is done in Kay's devices, and the returning signal is also altered somewhat in a noticeable fashion by the character of the reflector, being different, for example, for a concrete wall and for the many irregular points constituting foliage.   (It is known that sound passing through or over vegetation is attenuated and that the variation of attenuation with frequency indicates something about the nature of the materials. This can be used in some prostheses and presumably is an effect guiding the blind normally; it also has shaped the songs of different birds.)

In systems that are on rather continuously while sweeping up and down in frequency, the Doppler shift from movement averages to zero, leaving distance alone being indicated if the sweep up and down is symmetrical, but there is indication of motion with sawtooth frequency deviation; one can count beat cycles for increasing frequency minus those for decreasing frequency to get subject velocity, while the sum gives distance. The largest application of continuous wave radar or sonar systems seems to have been in radar altimeters for aircraft (5), though naval applications also have been made (10).

Scanning Sonars

Mechanical scanning of a radio or sound transducer to build up an image of a region of space can be quite rapid, but for some purposes it may be considered slow or cumbersome. In that case, it is possible to activate in succession a series of differently oriented or positioned transducers to give the same effect as mechanical motion. It is also possible to subdivide a single large transducer having a desirable pattern of directivity in such a way that it can "shift attention" to various directions without actually moving.

This concept of a "phased array" was introduced to medical engineering groups by Figure 4 (from 8). A row of transducers are all simultaneously recording their received signals, and each receives everything coming from all directions since each is smaller than a wavelength (as in Figure 1, a small object can neither direct a beam outward nor concentrate attention in a particular direction). The recording of all signals on a moving film or magnetic tape, which is then viewed through a tilted slit, is simply a way of combining the signals from successive transducers with a small time delay between each so that only echoes coming from one sideward direction will all add together, while sounds from any other direction will combine their signals at random to yield noise (see 7). One can provide electronic time delays to sweep the direction of attention from side to side rapidly, or one can have attention directed to all directions at once along separate channels so that even a single click can yield an entire image. (Probably the first such suggestion for looking in all directions at once was in a patent for radar systems for detecting cannon shells by Mercer & Richmond, 9, that had been applied for in 1955.)

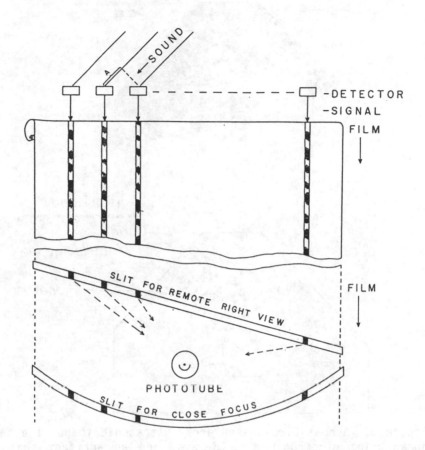

Figure 4. A phased array method in which recording steadily
from several spaced detectors allows concentration in any direction, or indeed from any range, by adjustment of time delays.

Such systems can have directions of sensitivity other than
the expected one for the same reasons that a diffraction grating
produces several orders of a spectrum. These can result in arti-
facts such as are seen in Figure 5, which is an ultrasonic real-
time image of the kidney of an intact healthy human (from 7).
The proper image is to the right but there is some sensitivity by
the probe in that direction when the unit "thinks it is looking
straight ahead," and so a false pattern is displayed weakly in
the forward direction. Such effects are minimized by spacing
the transducer subdivisions by a half wavelength of sound. In
the medical applications this spacing would be a half wavelength

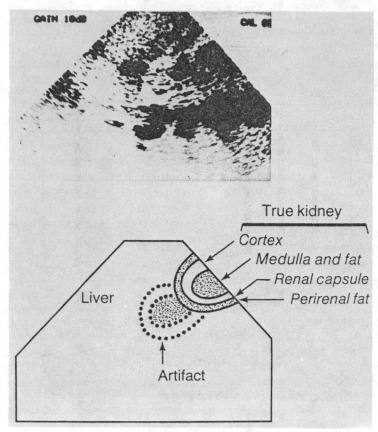

Figure 5.   A real-time phased array ultrasonic image of a healthy human using electronic time delays, and an artifact that seems to add extra structure.   This could be misleading in adding extra obstacles if used as the scanner in a blind guidance prosthesis, though head movement could help sort out reality from artifact.

in tissue, where the velocity is about that in water, while in a scanning prosthesis for the blind, it would be a half wavelength of sound moving at a velocity corresponding to air.   This also minimizes distracting meaningless returns that constitute one form of noise in such images.   A phased array air sonar that could serve as a prosthesis has been mentioned (1).

No matter how the scanning is done to determine spatial distribution, the other factors remain relevant.   Steady streaming of the air due to wind does not change the apparent frequency though it can change flight time. At an opening a sound compression can return as a rarifaction; that is, there can be a phase change. Wind-generated motion of leaves might be expected to produce noticeable modulation. A reflector moving in a constant frequency sound beam will return a slightly different frequency which one can beat against the original; one gets one cycle of the beat frequency (or Doppler frequency) each time the reflector approaches or recedes from the transducer by a half wavelength of the sound frequency. But swinging the transducer from side to side across a receding landscape can cause noise, and yet it generally will not introduce a large Doppler signal.

If the display of the signal from the probing beam goes to the ears then binaural hearing can invoke some of the same sorts of advantages enjoyed by the sighted having two eyes. A source of sound moving across a pair of detectors separately feeding the two ears will be perceived as if moving, and the same applies to a supersonic source (or its echoes) if they are made audible by beating the signal with a local oscillator (10). A large change in actual location results in a smaller change in apparent position. Similar ideas have been most fully developed by Leslie Kay, who has had a major program in studying the adjustment of parameters so that the output of such a system is adapted to an individual's perceptual parameters for maximum spatial accuracy even when several distinct targets are being detected at once (3).

The examples shown here are medical ultrasonic images of regions of the body, but the same considerations apply to the exploration of a street scene or building interior. In a visible display of such information to a sighted person, it sometimes aids the transfer of information to emphasize edges by either computer processing the image or other processing. (For more details, see 7.) An example of such a process is seen in Figure 6, where some of the negative second derivative of the brightness pattern is added to the original pattern to emphasize structure. In a television system with scanning this is done with simple differentiating circuits, while a similar effect normally takes place in the eye to a limited extent by mutual lateral inhibition between receptors. Perhaps this is true of most sensory modalities. An extreme example is pushing a finger down into a cup of mercury, where only the horizontal boundary will be felt. In any case, such image processing also seems warranted before creating tactile or other displays for the blind.

Edge modification appears useful in many images both to emphasize structure and to de-blur a degraded image, with the extreme being the conversion to a line drawing displaying only boundaries. Nonlinear response in the circuits also can change contrast, and either emphasize or de-emphasize small differences

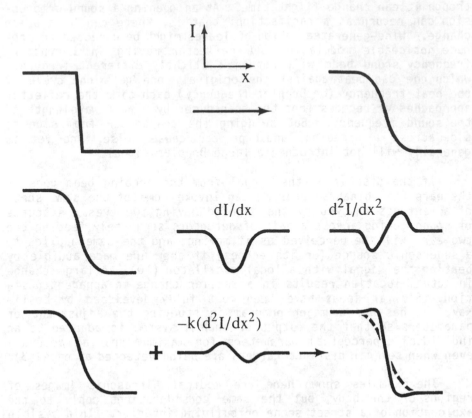

Figure 6. Mixing with an image some of its own negative second derivative is one form of processing that can sharpen edges after blurring or can emphasize structure in a sharp image. Here is shown intensity as a function of position, with a sharp edge becoming degraded in the image collecting system; processing can be by computer, by television circuits, or by optical means.

before display to either the sighted or the blind (see 7). Particular periodicities in images can also be extracted, emphasized, or rejected before display by either electronic methods or extremely fast optical processing (7), and these techniques should allow emphasis in a scene of elements of importance to the blind walker.

REFERENCES

1. Brabyn, J., Collins, C. C., & Kay, L. (1981). A wide band-
    width CT FM scanning sonar with tactile and acoustic display
    for persons with impaired vision. Proceedings of the Ultra-
    sonic International 1981. Brighton, England.

2. Bradner, H. (1969). Internal navigation without gyros.
    American Journal of Physics, 37, 169-170.

3. Kay, L. (1980). Air sonars with acoustical display of spa-
    tial information. In R. G. Busnel & J. Fish (Eds.), Animal
    Sonar Systems. New York: Plenum Press.

4. Kuhl, W., Schodder, G., & Schroder, F. (1954). Condenser
    transmitters and microphones with solid dielectric for air-
    borne ultrasonics. Acoustica, 4, 519-532.

5. Luck, D. (1949). Frequency Modulated Radar. New York:
    McGraw-Hill.

6. Mackay, R. S. (1970). Bio-Medical Telemetry. New York:
    Wiley.

7. Mackay, R. S. (1984). Medical Images and Displays. New
    York: Wiley.

8. Mackay, R. S., Eilers, G., Horowitz, J., & Marg, E. (1962).
    Ultrasonic echo imaging in eye research. In Proceedings of
    15th Annual Conference on Engineering in Medicine and Bio-
    logy. Paper VII-9. IEEE New York.

9. Mercer, W. R. & Richmond, M. (1965). Non scanning panoramic
    radar system. U.S. Patent 3,218,639. Applied for May 3,
    1955.

10. National Defense Research Committee (1946). Principles and
    applications of underwater sound. Summary of Technical Re-
    port of Division 6, NDRC Vol. 7, Washington, D.C.; reprinted
    by Dept.of Navy, Headquarters Naval Material Command (1968),
    pp. 259-260.

11. Sivian, L. J. (1947). High frequency absorption in air
    and in other gases. Journal of the Acoustical Society of
    America, 19, 914-916.

THREE NEW BLIND GUIDANCE PROSTHESES AND WHAT THEY TEACH US

R. Stuart Mackay

Boston University
California State University, San Francisco

Over the years a number of devices for the guidance of the blind have been developed. However, there are still possibilities for fresh thought to suggest new approaches. Partially tested proposals are made here for a traversed distance indicator, a straight path guidance device, and a moving hazard indicator. The approaches can result in potentially practical devices, and they can also provide instructive new concepts in their analysis.

A conceivable alternative can be studied while watering a lawn. The hose nozzle can be held with one hand fixed against the upper body and maintained aimed at the center of the palm of the other hand with arm extended. As one twists from side to side the stream of water will be felt to move across the hand. Thus this could provide a way of monitoring or guiding travel straight down a street. It might be thought inconvenient for the blind to tow a hundred feet of hose or a fire truck after them, but it should be noted that a small jet of recirculated water has been scanned over the abdomen (covered with a rubber sheet) to attempt a pattern display (1).

Several ideas derive from the above thought, the general theme of the first two examples being inertial guidance as a possible aid to blind mobility. It is well known that the electrical signal from an accelerometer can be passed through an integrating circuit to give a voltage proportional to velocity, which signal can be integrated to give distance traversed or position. Such a method has certain inaccuracies, but preliminary experiments with reasonably rapid motion indicate that a simplified form can yield an uncertainty of a few feet in a hundred feet, where a blind walker could "pick up" the next landmark. The output indication of distance traversed could be readily displayed as a spoken word by simple modern electronic circuit chips.

An accelerometer usually consists of a weight on a spring, the deflection in response to motion being measured.   Such units can be made small enough with all their circuits to surgically implant in small animals to monitor their activity (3).   If the support of the weight is a flexure or spider (web) support then motion across the direction of interest has little effect.   Indeed, the r.m.s. or a.c. signal from such a unit may be helpful in evaluating the relative effectiveness of different blind guidance prostheses, the accelerometer being carried by a walking person and serving to measure the steadiness or halting aspect of progression (3).

The water hose concept suggests an alternative accelerometer (Figure 1) in which a jet of fluid (liquid or gas) cools a warm thermistor to a different degree depending on the location within the stream.   Changes in resistance indicate motion.   Angular velocity, as in the case of the hose, causes an effective shift of fluid impact in the reverse direction for the same reason that

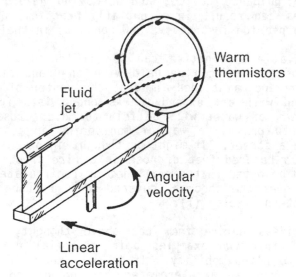

Figure 1.   Apparent path of fluid relative to support if the latter is moved in certain ways.   The fluid blows on four warmed thermistors whose spread relative to the stream size is here shown exaggerated, all four being in the stream at once to a varying degree.   The top and bottom thermistors can be omitted if only horizontal motions are to be monitored.

shooting a gun at a moving target causes the bullet to pass behind the target (necessitating leading the target). Transverse
velocity across the stream does not shift the impact since each
"droplet" has the same sideward velocity as the target, but
transverse acceleration causes a signal because the target moves
after the jet has left the orifice. If opposite thermistors are
connected in a Wheatstone bridge configuration, they will be
heated and a shift in stream will affect both in such a way that
their signals add, but a change in ambient temperature will cause
signals that tend to cancel in the output imbalance. The unit,
of course, would be enclosed so that ambient winds would not
shift the jet. This device could control a unit to tap the side
of a person deviating from a straight course, or it could have
more general application as an accelerometer.

Inertial methods are routinely used to guide submarines and
airplanes. In these cases of high precision it is common to
place the accelerometer on a horizontal platform whose orientation
is maintained by gyroscopes and a fancy servo system. If the
platform drifts from horizontal then the accelerometer will
"feel" a little of the acceleration of gravity and "decide" that
the vessel is speeding up (or slowing down). After integration
there can thus be an indication of increasingly high velocity by
a vessel that has not moved at all. Integration of the velocity
signal can then show the passage of great distance though there
has been no motion.

It is interesting to consider the signal from an accelerometer mounted across a pendulum hanging down along the direction
of gravity rather than placed on a horizontal platform. As the
vehicle supporting the pivot of the pendulum starts or stops
moving, the pendulum deflects forward or backward. A second
accelerometer might help monitor pendulum motion. The signal
from two accelerometers on one pendulum can be compared after
multiple integration. This relatively simple arrangement has
been analyzed (2) with the interesting result that if the signal
is monitored from before motion starts until it all stops, the
signal indicates the distance traversed independent of the nature
of the motion or of tilts, and independent of the period and
damping of the pendulum.

The use of digital integrators (a counter plus oscillator)
for stability would seem to supply a simple and cheap arrangement
for guidance of blind walkers, who might periodically halt and
have the device tell them how far they had come. In some designs
vertical bouncing of the pendulum can cause problems. Position
error in inertial guidance systems tends to increase with the
cube of the time due to multiple integration, and this is slow at
the start. There is also an 84 minute oscillation involving

gravity and earth curvature with stable platforms. Such problems should be minimal here because the time to walk a city block is not long. Present commercial units probably have a minimum cost of about $10,000 but their specifications are much more demanding. After hours of uncorrected inertial guidance an error of 0.1 mile is expected, or a fraction of a foot in 50 km; units for surveying are expected to involve tolerance of 0.2×10^6. Periodically reducing velocity to zero places a bound on part of the error so that final error in position does not grow impossibly.

Another problem in blind mobility is determining the presence of moving hazards such as automobiles. One might thus consider sending out a wave which would reflect from the surroundings. The returning reflection would have the same frequency as the outgoing wave if there was no reflector motion, but comparison with the original signal would show a difference in frequency or a beat frequency due to the Doppler shift if there was any movement either toward or away from the detector. The wave could be on continuously, though if pulsed, the reflections would also contain information about the distance to various surrounding objects (5). The wave could be a mechanical disturbance (e.g., ultrasonic) or it could be electromagnetic, that is, radio, laser light, or infrared.

The concept raises an instructive question. If the sensing device jiggles somewhat as it is held, or if its aim is swept from side to side across a scene at different distances, will there be a big signal of motion since the point of reflection will be approaching or receding? This could be ruinously distracting whether the output were electronically processed to give an indication or whether one merely listened to the beat frequency between outgoing and returning signals (which should be zero if there was no target movement along the direction of aim).

An equivalent situation is shown in Figure 2 (from 4). Here is shown the effect of moving a tilted target across a beam, rather than sweeping the beam across a receding landscape. The target seems to rapidly approach the source, and the path length is shortened many wavelengths. However, there may be excess noise during the motion, but there is not a Doppler signal of motion. If the surface is not rough, no signal will return in the direction shown. If a signal does return as shown, then a series of small reflector points effectively, enters the beam and moves straight across it rather than having a coherent pattern moving down; only the latter generates a beat note or difference frequency by returning a steady frequency without random jumps in phase (see also 5).

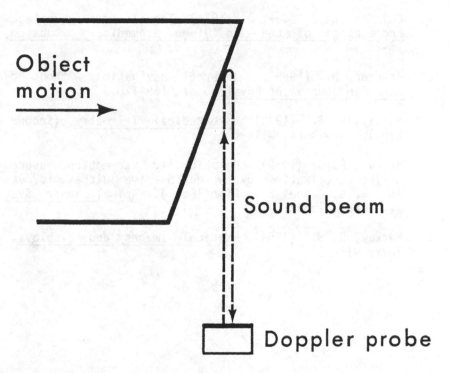

Figure 2. A continuous wave Doppler device (radar or sonar) will not give a large Doppler signal when scanned over a receding landscape in which there is nothing moving toward or away from the detector, just as motion of a tilted reflector across the beam will not give a Doppler signal (From 5).

This somewhat surprising conjecture was verified with a continuous wave radar set that could detect automobiles. It did not produce large troublesome signals when swept across a receding landscape or when aimed up along a street. Translation of the detector along its beam did give an indication of velocity of the holder.

Each of the systems mentioned may or may not prove of benefit to the blind, but at least they seem to provide useful concepts for consideration.

REFERENCES

1. Collins, C. & Madey, J. (1974). Tactile sensory replacement. Proceedings of the San Diego Biomedical Symposium, 13, 15-26.

2. Bradner, H. (1969).   Internal   navigation   without   gyros. American Journal of Physics, 37, 169-170.

3. Mackay, R. S. (1970). Bio-Medical Telemetry. (Second Edition). New York: Wiley.

4. Mackay, R. S. (1980). Dolphin air sac motion measurements during vocalization by two noninvasive ultrasonic methods. In: R. G. Busnel & J. Fish (Eds.). Animal Sonar Systems. New York: Plenum.

5. Mackay, R. S. (1984). Medical Images and Displays. New York: Wiley.

MICROPROCESSOR TECHNIQUES APPLIED TO ULTRASONIC PULSE/ECHO TRAVEL
AIDS FOR THE BLIND

Anthony D. Heyes

University of Nottingham

The design of electronic mobility aids at Nottingham is a
fairly modest enterprise; no attempt is made to provide a surrogate for vision. Instead we follow the philosophical approach
pioneered by the late J. Alfred Leonard simply to provide the
blind pedestrian with information useful for mobility. The
process is one which involves alternate periods of prototype
development and evaluation, the evaluation serving to test the
hypothetical conjectures embodied in the new prototype. The
construction of prototypes used to be a huge problem, and by far
the most time-consuming part of the research program. This is no
longer the case; the availability of microprocessors suitable for
use in light-weight portable devices has transformed the whole
process. It is now possible, using the same hardware, to produce
a succession of different aids simply by changing the software
stored in the onboard memory. Conjectures relating to, for
example, alternative displays, or new information processing
algorithms, may now be transformed into working prototypes at a
rate guaranteed to saturate the evaluation capacity of the most
diligent team of evaluators.

Our work at Nottingham has led to the development of an extremely versatile aid/research tool capable of being programmed to
collect, analyze and display information to the blind pedestrian.

The Sonic Pathfinder

Our starting point was the desire to build a microprocessor
implementation of the Sonic Pathfinder (3). The Sonic Pathfinder
is a spectacle-frame-mounted ultrasonic pulse-echo device with an

auditory display. The prime function of the aid is to detect and indicate the distance of any obstacle which lies directly in the blind pedestrian's path. In the absence of any obstruction ahead, it reverts to its secondary function of indicating the presence and range of obstacles to the left and right of the travel path. Like the simpler hand-held Nottingham Obstacle Detector (2), the aid represents the distance of the nearest object in terms of the notes of the musical scale, one note being assigned to each of the one-foot range zones. Again, like its predecessor, the aid is a digital device; no attempt is made to provide an analog signal giving textural information. This is done to avoid information overload. Moreover, if a blind user really wants to distinguish between a tree and a lamppost he can reach out and discover this by touch.

The user listens to the display through two small earpieces, one mounted on each side of the spectacle frame in close proximity to, though not actually in contact with, the ear. Time division multiplexing is employed between the three receivers and the two earpieces so that the distance of any object which lies, within range, to the left of the main travel path is signalled only in the left earpiece whilst an object to the right is signalled only in the right earpiece. An object which lies directly ahead produces a signal at both earpieces and, in this way, creates a central sound image. In the absence of any obstacle within the area viewed by the aid the display is totally silent.

With the aid, the pedestrian is able to walk parallel to the inner shore line -- the hedge or wall -- by keeping the repeating note at the 'inner' ear at a constant pitch. He is at the same time able to tell when he passes a tree or lamppost on the outer shore line by the interposition of the occasional note in the other ear; such objects are vital landmarks for the blind. If he encounters an object lying directly ahead, the side information is no longer provided and information relating to the central hazard is presented to both ears. As an additional 'attention grabber', the central display is arranged to have a repetition rate four times that for the side information -- some 16 times a second. Only when the hazard is no longer in the path does the aid revert to giving side information.

Early prototypes of the aid were made using Complementary Metal Oxide Substrate (CMOS) integrated circuits. A number of these prototypes have been evaluated using blind volunteers (1). The results were encouraging although some shortcomings were identified. For example, although users were advised to switch the aid from long range to short range -- i.e., from eight feet down to four feet -- when trying to negotiate narrow openings, they tended not to do so. The main reason for changing to a

microprocessor based system was the hope that software information processing algorithms might be developed which would enable
an automatic adjustment of the range.

The Hardware

Of prime importance was the need to design a system having a
low power consumption and capable of being programmed to produce
output frequencies as high as 40 KHz. After two false starts,
using the RCA804 and the Z80 microcomputers, the decision was
made to use the Intel 80C35. The Intel 80C35 is a member of the
Intel MCS-48 family of single chip microcomputers. The 8048 has
factory masked onboard Read Only Memory (ROM) and is suitable for
a finalized product. The 8748 has onboard Erasable, Programable
Read Only Memory (EPROM) and would have been ideal for my work if
only I had had the necessary EPROM programmer. The 8035 has no
onboard ROM for program storage and must be used in conjunction
with an external memory, e.g. the 2716, and an associated latch,
the 74HC373. All family members are available in low power consumption CMOS versions. In addition to the 80C35 and its associated components the device uses a Darlington driver, to buffer the
outputs; an LS404 as a four stage 40 KHz receiver amplifier; a
4052 as a two pole analog switch, one pole being used to select
the current receiver transducer and the other to short out one of
the earpieces when the side receiver transducers are in use, or
neither earpiece when the center receiver transducer is in use;
and a hex switch, to select various software options. Reference
should be made to Heyes (3) for a detailed circuit description.

The spectacle frame supports a row of five ultrasonic transducers and two earpiece outputs. Use has been made of cheap,
readily available 40 KHz ultrasonic transducers. Three receivers
are used, one centrally mounted, one on the left splayed outwards
by 20 degrees, and one on the right similarly splayed. In order
to cover a wide enough arc, two transmitters are used. These are
mounted either side of the central receiver but splayed conver-
gently, rather than divergently, to avoid the 'hole in the middle', by 10 degrees.

The Software for the Sonic Pathfinder

In order to produce a 40 KHz output from the 80C35, one bit
of one of the output ports must change state every 12.5 microseconds. In order to achieve this critical timing from the
software it is necessary to have a clock period which is a 'whole
number fraction' of this interval, a 'whole number fraction'
being the reciprocal of an integer. Using a 6 MHz crystal to
control the internal oscillator of the microprocessor, a clock
interval of 2.5 microseconds is obtained, giving five clock

periods during this critical time. Since each of the program
instructions has an execution time of either one or two clock
cycles, this gives enough time -- with a little in hand. Driving
the two transmitters from the single output is not a good idea.
Using two such transmitters at the same frequency produces a
diffraction pattern resulting in the aid having 'corridors of
insensitivity'. This was overcome by using two separate bits for
the transmitter outputs and reversing the phase of one of them,
with respect to the other, halfway through the transmitter pulse.
The transmitters are active for 0.6 msecs, they begin in phase
and end out of phase.

During the transmitter pulse and for a short time afterward
the receiver must remain off. This, the 'dead time', is necessary
to prevent the receiver from triggering due to cross-talk. For
short range pulse-echo systems it is necessary to set this time
to a minimum value. However, this minimum is critically dependent
upon component and wiring layout and is therefore difficult to
pre-set. Using the microprocessor it has been possible to write
a software routine which uses the first 24 transmission pulses
after switch-on to 'dynamically' determine and set the minimum
usable 'dead time'.

The elapsed time between the transmitter pulse and the re-
ceipt of the first echo determines the musical note displayed to
the user. The notes are obtained from a software timing loop,
the parameters of which are obtained from a 'look-up' table.

Interference from other ultrasonic sources has been largely
eliminated by the inclusion of a software controlled digital
filter: Recalling that the processor has a cycle time of 2.5
microseconds, the output of the analog receiver amplifier is
sampled every 4 cycles until a change is detected. Confirmatory
samples are then taken every 5 cycles, provided each one is the
inverse of its predecessor; if not, after a 3-cycle delay the 4-
cycle sample is resumed. This mixture of 3, 4, and 5-cycle
sampling ensures that any 40 KHz wave form is detected no matter
what its phase relationship to the internal clock of the processor. By requiring nine successful samples before an echo signal
is regarded as genuine, the digital filter has an effective bandwidth of 6 KHz cycles. This is more than adequate to compensate
for the Doppler shift introduced in the frequency when the user
is approaching the object from which the echo is received. For
example, at a walking speed of 5 mph the received frequency is
40.5 KHz.

Priority is given to objects in the center of the user's path
-- Center Echo Priority -- by failing to increment the register
used to control the 4502 multiplexer whenever a central echo is
detected.

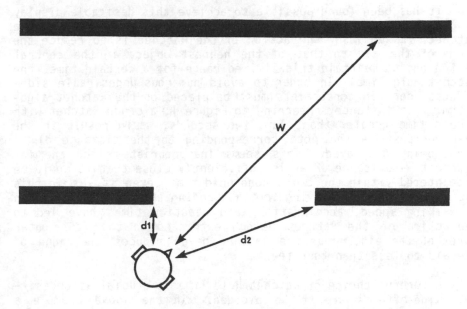

Figure 1.   Plan view of user approaching an open doorway.

More Speculative Information Processing Algorithms

The difficulties encountered during the evaluation by users trying to negotiate narrow gaps may be illustrated with reference to Figure 1. The figure depicts a plan view of a subject standing still and facing an open doorway leading into a corridor. Very small rotations of the head produce three different musical notes: A note of low pitch corresponding to the distance to the nearest doorpost $d1$, a note of higher pitch corresponding to the distance to the corridor wall w, and a note of intermediate pitch corresponding to the distance to the far doorpost $d2$. The Center Echo Priority algorithm ensures that these notes are presented to both ears, giving no obvious impression of the existence of a gap. Thus, very small head movements produce a jangling sound which is very difficult to interpret. (The user will only realize he is facing a gap when he notices that one of the notes has a higher pitch than the other two!) How much better the information display would be if the aid had a maximum range greater than $d2$ but less than w. If this were the case, small head rotations would produce a note of low pitch corresponding to distance $d1$, a note of higher pitch corresponding to distance $d2$, and a middle position in which these two notes are presented alternately to the left and right ears, giving an unambiguous indication of an opening in the centre.

It has been found possible to achieve this desirable display by the introduction of an algorithm which I have named the Ratchet. Essentially the action of the Ratchet is to reduce the range of the aid to that of the nearest object in the central region and to maintain this limited range for a certain time, the Ratchet Hold Time. In order to avoid numerous undesirable side-effects, certain constraints must be placed on the Ratchet algorithm. For instance, referring to Figure 1, a crude Ratchet with a hold time greater than, say, two seconds, would result in the near doorpost -- the note corresponding to the distance $\underline{d1}$ -- alone being displayed. This seems inappropriate since the far doorpost -- distance $\underline{d2}$ -- is sufficiently close that it could be encountered within the two second hold time, even if, as in this case, the subject is moving from a standing start. Consideration of walking speed, acceleration, and reaction times have led to the action of the Ratchet being restricted to the four outer zones of the aid. Thus the Ratchet never reduces the range of the aid to less than four feet.

A careful choice of Ratchet Hold Time is crucial if undesirable side-effects are to be avoided. In the above example a Ratchet Hold Time of two seconds was chosen, a duration long compared with the time taken for the user to make head rotations but short compared with the time required to negotiate the doorway and move into the comparative open space of the corridor. Although in these circumstances the choice of two seconds for the Ratchet Hold Time is appropriate, it does produce one unfortunate consequence. If a pedestrian is using the side signal of the aid in order to maintain a travel line parallel to the shore line at a distance of say three feet, and if he were momentarily to rotate his head toward the shore line, the Ratchet would immediately be invoked and the range of the aid set to four feet. (Four feet, not three feet, because of the restriction described above.) Thus from that moment, for the duration of the Ratchet Hold Time, the user has only the protection of an aid with a range of four feet. In these circumstances this is serious because he is not moving from a standing start, he may be traveling at four mph! The solution is to use a Ratchet Hold Time proportional to the time the invoking object remained in 'view'. Thus a quick 'glance' toward a near object would produce a hold time considerably shorter than would a prolonged 'stare'. It does, however, remain necessary to limit the Ratchet Hold Time to some maximum value -- two seconds seems to be approximately correct and has been chosen pending a more detailed evaluation.

Having made the Ratchet Hold Time dynamically determined, one has, in effect, produced an aid whose range is governed by the walking speed of the user. That is to say, instead of an aid with a range of eight feet, we have an aid with a range of

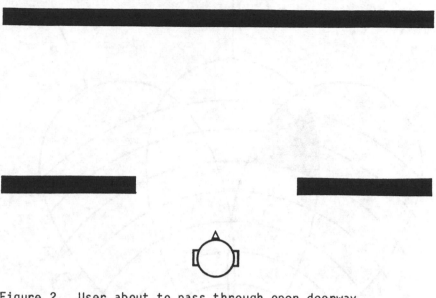

Figure 2.   User about to pass through open doorway.

two seconds! Rather an odd concept. However, given the information processing demands inherent in independent blind travel (4)
and the moment to moment problem solving nature of blind travel
it would seem highly desirable to have an aid which is limited
to providing information solely about those objects which would
be encountered during the next two seconds of travel.

Figure 2 illustrates what may happen when our blind subject
takes a pace forward. Large head rotations are now required to
bring the door posts into the central region of the aid, and
there is a high probability that the Ratchet will be released
before the doorway is negotiated. When this happens the aid
returns to having an eight foot range and the Center Echo Priority algorithm ensures that the musical note corresponding to the
corridor wall is displayed rather than the side information about
the door posts. The undesirable effect may be eliminated by yet
another information processing algorithm -- the Clamp.

The Ratchet can only be invoked and sustained by signals received in the central, forward facing receiver. The Clamp, on
the other hand, may be invoked and sustained by any signal, right,
left, or center. The Clamp operates for a fixed duration (1.2
seconds, pending a more detailed study) and has the effect of
reducing the aid to a single zone device. By increasing the
length of near zone to two feet and reducing the ranges of the

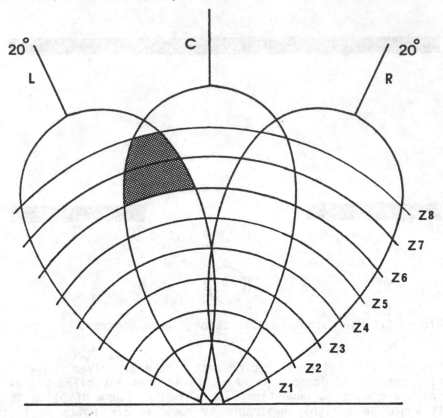

Figure 3.   Sonic Pathfinder input matrix.   Shaded area defined by: $C \wedge L \wedge (Z6 \cup Z7)$.

other zones so that the overall range of the aid remains equal to eight feet, the Clamp provides an effective solution to the problem described with reference to Figure 2.   The presence of one or the other door post in the side regions of the near zone prevents the far corridor wall from being perceived no matter how slowly the subject moves.   Only when he steps through the doorway is the user informed of the existence of the corridor wall. Indeed, it is only then that this information becomes relevant.

Because the Ratchet and the Clamp are additive, after introducing this second algorithm it became necessary to reduce the maximum Ratchet Hold Time to 1.5 seconds.

The existence of the Ratchet and the Clamp will not be perceived by the pedestrian during normal use of the aid.   The various durations used in the algorithms are tentative choices based on simple assumptions about human movement.   The user does not, contrary to what might appear to be the case from the above description, experience objects leaping in and out of his perception. There is only one unusual side-effect: Central objects in the range four to eight feet disappear if the user walks backwards!

Possible Future Trends

Finally, in order to emphasize the potential of the microprocessor in the context of aid design, I would ask you to consider the following: Figure 3 shows the polar diagram of the three receiver transducers. These overlapping areas may be treated as Venn diagrams. For instance, the shaded area is defined by the Boolean expression given at the bottom of the figure. This is the AND of the centre beam, the left beam and zones 7 and 8. Using the existing 8 range zones and 3 receiver transducers enables us to identify 40 unique areas -- the Boolean input matrix. I anticipate that the next step forward will be the development of algorithms which analyze the changing contents of the input matrix and select the important features for display to the user.

REFERENCES

1. Dodds A. G., Carter D. C., & Howarth C. I. (1984). The Sonic Pathfinder -- An evaluation. Journal of Visual Impairment & Blindness, 78, 203-206.

2. Heyes A. D. (1981). The Nottingham Obstacle Detector -- A technical description. Journal of Visual Impairment & Blindness, 75, 203-209.

3. Heyes A. D. (1984). The Sonic Pathfinder. Electronics and Wireless World, 90, 26-29, 62.

4. Shingledecker C. A. (1978). The effects of anticipation on performance and processing load on blind mobility. Ergonomics, 21, 335-371.

ACKNOWLEDGEMENTS
The work described in this paper was funded by the Department of Health and Social Security and carried out under the general supervision of Professor C. I. Howarth. Special thanks are due to the Unit technician, Carl Espin, who has helped in the manufacture of numerous prototypes.

TACTILE VISION SUBSTITUTION: SOME INSTRUMENTATION
AND PERCEPTUAL CONSIDERATIONS

Paul Bach-y-Rita and Barry Hughes

University of Wisconsin-Madison

The development of various sensory substitution devices and
aids for the blind has been based on the notion that the human
perceptual systems are remarkably flexible in their functional
capacities and that such devices, to be practically useful, need
make use of the functional similarities of other perceptual
systems to provide the effective information. Since their inception, optical-to-tactile conversion systems have capitalized
on the qualitatively similar functional characteristics of the
skin and the retina. The Optacon (Telesensory Systems, Inc.), a
device which permits the blind to read printed material, is an
example of a system which can be thought of as allowing a dynamic
form of 'tactile vision' for two-dimensional displays (lines of
print). The Tactile Vision Substitution System (TVSS) is an even
more appealing example since it was designed to transduce more
complex optical images into tactile stimulation and to be capable
of providing a far greater variety of environmental information.

We will briefly discuss several aspects of our ongoing research, including recent instrumentation development, a modification of the standard Optacon, and a 'time division multiplexing'
system which permits the sequential presentation of parts of
larger and more complex images and which has possible educational
and research applications. We will also consider certain theoretical aspects of sensory substitution and present some preliminary
data relevant to the issues of vibrotactile perception and mental
representation of two- and three-dimensional patterns in the
blind. In the process, we will suggest some of the more promising avenues for research that have been opened up through these
instrumentation developments.

INSTRUMENTATION DEVELOPMENT

The TVSS was developed to deliver visual information to the brain via arrays of stimulators in contact with one of several parts of the body (e.g., abdomen, back, thigh). Optical images were picked up by a TV camera and transduced into vibratory or direct electrical stimulation that could be mediated by the skin receptors. The visual information reached the information processing levels of the brain for analysis and interpretation via somato-sensory pathways and structures. After sufficient training with the TVSS, both perceptual and motor, subjects reported experiencing images in space instead of on the skin, an accomplishment that Epstein (this volume) refers to as distal attribution. They quickly learned to make perceptual judgments using visual means of analysis, such as perspective, parallax, looming and zooming, and depth judgments (1,2,3,4,5,27).

These findings were often replicated and led to a heightened optimism about the possibilities for flexible, general purpose tactile-visual substitution devices. However, the findings were often reported anecodotally; more feasible long-term developments clearly need to be based on rigorous experimental data. If we are to insist, for example, that we are producing a viable, if partial, substitute for the visual perceptual system, more needs to be learned about the extent to which vibrotactile information is perceived, represented, and acted upon like visual information, and where it is not, what qualitative or quantitative modifications to the information are required in order for behavioral equivalence to arise.

The Modified Optacon

Discussions with subjects who had been trained with the TVSS eight to 12 years ago (as adults) revealed that the most useful long-term result has been an understanding of certain visual concepts learned with this system (e.g., perspective changes with movement). In order to develop a practical system that could be widely used, development has concentrated on adapting commercially available equipment rather than developing new prototypes. We have modified an Optacon camera by adding a clip-on lens that permits spatial information to be delivered to the fingertip of the user. The camera and lens attachment are mounted on a lightweight helmet, thus permitting scanning and image stabilization to be controlled by the head and neck muscles rather than by the hand; this also frees one hand to manipulate objects (see Figure 1).

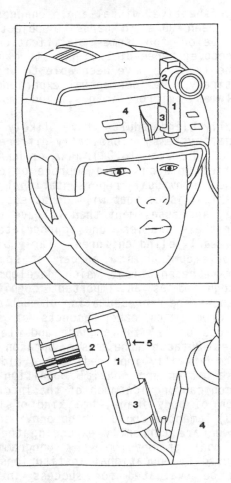

Figure 1. The standard Optacon (1), modified by a lens attachment, including an adjustable focus and a 21 mm diameter/33 mm
focal length lens (2), and attached to a lightweight headpiece
(4) by means of an angle-adjustable clasp (3). The Optacon is
modified by deactivating the internal light source. Zoom is
located at (5).

Preliminary work with four congenitally blind subjects (ranging in age from 13 to 26 years) has demonstrated that much of the
information provided by the original TVSS can also be accessed
and used via the modified Optacon. For example, as with the
TVSS, subjects have been able to recognize (often with little or
no instruction or feedback) vibrotactile patterns corresponding
to haptically familiar objects such as balls, cups, and various
geometric patterns. They have been taught to use monocular depth

cues such as perspective, visual angle changes, and motion parallax, and have been able to perceive object rotation in depth
(however, see below for some qualifications regarding their
abilities to recover three-dimensional structure from 2-D motion).
And as with the TVSS, we have been able to provide these subjects
with other entirely novel perceptual experiences such as flicker-
ing candle flames, mirror images, and moving human shapes.

Congenitally blind adults have likely developed (through
other perceptual systems) a basically different mental representation system of 3D space (18,24). How, or how quickly, experience
with the modified Optacon would improve or otherwise alter that
slowly developed nonvisual representational system remains an
important empirical issue that will doubtless require more experience, teaching, and assessment than we have been able to provide
thus far. For these studies, one appropriate subject population
might be young early blind children. Early blind children suffer
from delayed development in a number of spatio-cognitive areas
including self-representation, which developmental psychologists
have long recognized as an important cognitive acquisition in
that it influences the representation of much else in the environment, and is crucial to other aspects of self-identification,
including the use of 'I' in language and play (8,9). Early use
of the modified Optacon (the basic Optacon is widely used in
schools for the visually impaired) could aid in the development
of self-representation and spatial cognition in the blind. The
modified Optacon can provide much of the information necessary in
the replication of body image, the kind of information Fraiberg
and Adelson (8) lamented could not be provided by any sense other
than vision. We are currently extending these studies with the
more specific goal of developing a programmed training course
which can be used by educational institutions serving the blind,
and which can be evaluated for success in aiding longer term
visuospatial aspects of development.

Time-Division Multiplexing

The design of a high-resolution tactile-vision substitution
system must take into account the physiological differences
between visual and somatosensory systems. Although the latter is
far more capable of mediating sequentially presented information,
it is less capable of mediating parallel input (it cannot capture
an entire scene at an instant, such as is often done in tachisto-
scopic visual presentations). In an optimal sensory substitution
system, the information must be presented in a form most compat-
ible with the sensory system's processing characteristics.

Recent studies by Craig (6) have shown that the somatosensory
system is more capable of processing tactile patterns presented
in a static mode than had been suspected. While his work confirmed

our previous findings that a scanning mode was superior for presentations of 200 msec or longer, performance on a letter recognition task (using a computer-driven Optacon) was significantly better in the static mode for presentations of less than 200 msec duration. Letter recognition from static presentations was even possible (with approximately 40% accuracy) at durations as short as 4 msec, an effect we have been able to replicate in pilot work for upright as well as rotated letters.

We have developed a time-division multiplexing system (TDM) to take advantage of the sequential processing capabilities of the somatosensory system (14). With the TDM, a large or complex image is broken down into discrete 6 by 24 (144 point) segments, each of which is delivered to a fingertip stimulation matrix of the same dimensions. The TDM system utilizes a digital camera (MicronEye by Micron Technology, Inc.) to capture a 128 row by 256 column image. The image is stored on an IBM personal computer, and is accessed by a program allowing the user to select any 24 by 6 segment from the image for output to the Optacon. Artifically created images can also be stored and accessed. Individual frames can be selected manually by moving up/down or left/right) or can be automatically 'scanned' (row by row horizontally) by parameterizing the output from the computer (with independent specifications for frame overlap, presentation time and interstimulus interval).

There are limits to the perception of sequentially presented vibrotactile patterns. The earlier TVSS work suggested that subjects obtained most of the useful information during active scanning from the leading edge. Thus they attended only to parts of the stimulation at a time, with the total image having to be mentally synthesized over time. With the TDM system, the scanning 'unit' could now consist of all six columns, which in principle can increase the useful information available in any particular time period by making it available more rapidly. Of course, whether this increase in information can be handled by the somatosensory processing system in an efficient manner remains one of the major issues of our research.

With earlier versions of the TVSS, manual camera control was slow. Later versions of the TVSS and the modified Optacon significantly reduce this problem by using lightweight cameras mounted on the head, and the TDM effectively frees the perceiver from having to stabilize an image and from scanning in nonlinear paths. With the TDM, however, there is a different approach to the scanning aspect of perception: with the manual mode, scanning involves no head movements at all, but is completed by manual finger pressing of the control keys; and in the automatic mode scanning is not involved at all, the rate and direction are set

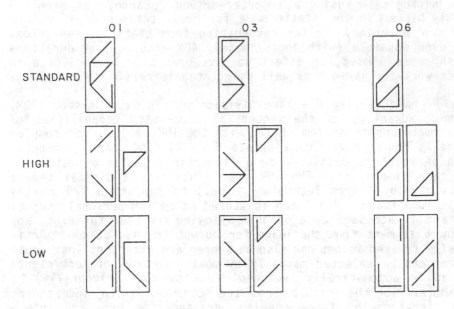

Figure 2.   Sample stimulus patterns used in mental synthesis.
Standard pattern broken into two 3-segment halves, with (High) or
without (Low) retention of triangle from Standard.

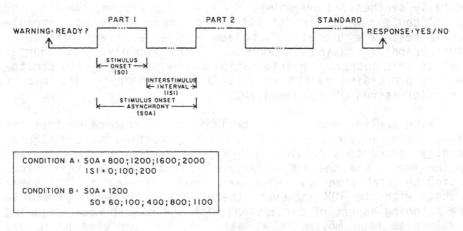

Figure 3.   Schematic of trial procedure for mental pattern synthesis, with independent variables used in different conditions.

by the parameterized computer output. Of course, this removal of an active component of perception, and the constraint of being able to scan only in horizontal or vertical directions and at a rate dictated either by the experimenter or by manual speed limitations, bring with them their own theoretical and empirical considerations, such as whether we are altering the most important aspects of tactile perception. The costs and benefits associated with the increase in potential information and the change in motor control remain to be assessed.

TDM Representation of Unfamiliar Patterns

An experiment using the TDM system examined certain aspects of mental synthesis and the structural representation of unfamiliar patterns. This experiment attempted to determine whether vibrotactile patterns are represented in any particularly obvious manner. This kind of research is relevant to work with the Optacon because, as noted above, the receptive field of the device is very small and relatively poorly resolved, and perception therefore involves scanning, remembering, and mental reconstruction of patterns. To briefly illustrate, consider how a vibrotactile image of a face might be mentally synthesized from the successive presentation of parts of the face. To maximize the efficiency of mental synthesis, would it be worthwhile, indeed necessary, to decompose the face into its structural components (eyes, nose, ears, etc.), or would any random breakdown of the image be sufficient? We examined this question using unfamiliar static vibrotactile patterns comprised of 6-line segments as the large image. Each of these standard patterns contained a triangle and three other lines. As illustrated in Figure 2, we broke these standards up into two three-line parts in one of two ways, by retaining the intact closed triangle, or by presenting maximally separated segments. These different methods of breakdown resulted in what we termed High and Low Goodness parts, following the approach taken by Reed (17) and Palmer (16) in a similar paradigm with visual patterns.

These parts were presented sequentially for equal but variable periods of time, and following an interval during which mental synthesis of the parts could occur, a standard pattern was presented for the same period of time (see Figure 3). The three subjects' task was to say whether or not the parts spatially combined to produce the standard. Three sighted subjects, viewing the Optacon's visual monitor, participated in a control condition. On 50% of the trials, which were randomly ordered, the correct response was Yes.

As is shown on Figure 4, there is a clear effect for pattern goodness on error rates: those patterns which are separated to

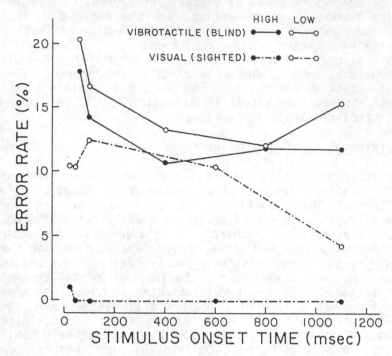

Figure 4. Mean error rate for mental synthesis task for blind subjects receiving vibrotactile patterns and sighted subjects receiving visual patterns.

minimize line connectedness and closedness are apparently more difficult to synthesize mentally than those which are separated so as to maximize structural goodness. While the error rates for both vibrotactile conditions are greater than those for the visual control condition, the basic influence of structural organization is apparent. This finding, if it holds up in more detailed experiments, suggests first that one of the most important design features of the TDM will need to be a means by which the scanning procedure can exploit the inherent structural representation of images. Second, it would suggest that mental representation of shape from vibrotactile stimulation is not unlike that from visual information.

THEORETICAL CONSIDERATIONS OF VISUAL AND VIBROTACTILE PERCEPTION

Since their inception, tactile vision substitution studies have given rise to a host of philosophical, theoretical, and empirical issues, of which the perceptual and mental representa-

tion of 3D space via vibrotactile stimulation is of primary
interest to us. An understanding of the <u>functional equivalence</u>
between visual and vibrotactual processing would have both basic
scientific and practical implications, the former because it would
bear on whether information for the various perceptual systems
ought to be considered modality specific or amodal, and the
latter because the data would suggest the possibilities and
constraints for vision substitution and other prosthetic developments. Additionally, basic research in tactile shape perception
has tended to focus on a small part of the overall problem, e.g.
the psychophysics of static letter recognition (see 6,7,21),
and has not, for reasons of technical and equipment limitations,
considered the issues of depth perception or dynamic pattern representation (either vibrotactually or in the blind). In the
remainder of this paper we will suggest how research with the
modified Optacon and the TDM system might bear on these issues.

Can We "See" With the Skin?

The TVSS and now the modified Optacon studies suggest that
it may be possible for the blind to see with their skin (27).
Although the early system was termed a tactile visual substitution
system, we have been reluctant to suggest that blind users of the
device are actually seeing. Others (e.g. 12,15) have not been so
reluctant, claiming that since blind subjects are being given
similar information to that which causes the sighted to see and
are capable of giving similar responses, one is left with little
alternative but to admit that they are seeing (and not merely
"seeing"). In <u>Molyneux's Question</u>, Morgan (15) offers two basic
arguments for this position. One, the structural nature of the
perceptual system does not offer any criteria for distinguishing
seeing from not seeing (e.g., the horseshoe crab is offered as
an example of a biological system with fewer receptors than most
mammals but which can nonetheless see). A decision as to whether
perception is seeing via a nonvisual perceptual system involves
considerations other than solely those of physiological hardware
and quantitative capabilities. It ought to be noted, nonetheless,
that there are a number of structural similarities between visual
and vibrotactile perception: (a) static and continuously transformed images are formed by a lens on a 2D surface; (b) the
receptor surface contains discrete elements; (c) the surface can
be voluntarily moved to scan the environment; and (d) the source
of stimulation is not in direct physical contact with the receptor
surface, so that perception can be subject to similar interruptions such as by object occlusion.

Morgan's second argument concerns behavioral equivalence: if
blind subjects receive (vibrotactile conversions of) optical
information that would satisfy criteria for seeing in the sighted

and respond in an indistinguishable manner, one might concede that the blind are seeing: "There is not the slightest reason to think that if two sensory messages give the animal <u>exactly</u> the same information, and lead to exactly the same behavior, they will be perceived differently--even if they come over completely different pathways" (15, p. 207). Using the modified Optacon is more like visual perception than typical tactile perception since under normal ecologically valid conditions the tactile perceptual system is neither pure (it usually involves concurrent kinesthetic information, which leads to its common designation as the haptic system) nor localized in one reception area (10). It would seem that the question of seeing with the skin centers on whether the modified Optacon provides "<u>exactly</u> the same information" as is provided to the visual system. If the decision is to be made on strict quantitative grounds, clearly it does not (e.g., color perception is not yet possible), but one might also ask if the ways in which it does not match are crucial? For example, can a colorblind person recognize patterns or faces? Do not sighted persons still see even under impoverished environmental conditions (e.g., fog or rain) where shapes and patterns are difficult to distinguish? Would we not say that a person with blurred tunnel vision (an analogy often drawn between TVSS perception and traditional visual perception) can see?

A KINETIC DEPTH EFFECT IN TACTILE PERCEPTION

While the above discussion concerns a philosophical issue it is, nonetheless, an issue with some important theoretical implications, including the extent to which perception is not merely a receptive accomplishment, but a cognitive one, based on such diverse factors as knowledge, beliefs, and inference as well. Consider, for example, the detection of rotation and the recovery of object structure from the tranformation of 2D projections (see also Epstein, this volume). The original demonstration of subjects' proclivity to perceive veridically the rotation of an object in depth from its flat and logically ambiguous 2D projection was made by Wallach and O'Connell (25, see also 26), who termed it the kinetic depth effect (KDE). What would a demonstration of the KDE from 2D stimulation of the skin (rather than one eye) mean for its candidate explanations? And what if it could be demonstrated in the congenitally blind? While past TVSS research demonstrated the ability of blind subjects to perceive rotation, it should be emphasized that from a theoretical stance, subject naivety and total inexperience is necessary (see below). We have considered these and corollary questions primarily in terms of the two major metatheories of perception, the direct realist account advocated by J. J. Gibson (e.g. 10,11,13,23) and the constructivist theories which have been popular since the time of Helmholtz and whose principles have been advocated most clearly by Rock (e.g. 19,20, see also 22).

For direct realists, the reason that a 2D stimulus pattern, which if static would be ambiguous with respect to 3D structure, produces under rotation the perception of a unique object rotating in 3D-space is that the combined change in the pattern's length and orientation constitutes the information necessary and sufficient for the perception of movement in depth. This information pickup of depth is 'direct' in that it involves no cognitive reasoning on the part of the observer about the possible causes of that particular changing pattern, no consideration of alternative solutions, no inference, and no guesswork.

For Rock, on the other hand, problem-solving is not only part of the perception of depth, it is a crucial and quite decisive part. In fact, his theory is explicitly grounded in the Helmholtzian notion of inference, that the stimulus underdetermines the distal object and that what is needed is some active problem-solving to arrive at a best guess about what is causing that effect. "The transforming stimulus poses the problem for the perceptual system as to what event in the world might be producing it. Hypotheses are generated that could do justice to the stimulus; that is, if such and such an event were occurring, it would produce just that stimulus" (19,20).

A demonstration of a kinetic depth-like effect in blind persons might not be accounted for by a theory resting on the subject's 'solving the problem' if by this is meant that subjects are held to (a) utilize consciously appreciated rules or hypotheses in arriving at the percept (i.e., to be able to verbally report having had a particular strategy, to have considered a possible alternatives, etc.), or (b) have learned through one or more previous encounters with rotating objects what 2D projections look like, and have arrived at the typical KDE effect via such memory. The KDE might not be predicted in blind persons because they have not presumably had any similarly passive and detached experience with transforming 2D projections of 3D distal objects; that is, they lack the knowledge necessary for any such problem-solving or remembering.

In an experimental investigation of the recovery of structure from motion the following questions suggest themselves: (1) Most basically, is an effect such as the kinetic depth effect possible when the proximal stimulus is on the skin rather than the retina? (2) Will subjects be capable of arriving at a percept of pattern motion in the 2D frontal plane as well as in 3-dimensional depth (i.e., will any stimulus ambiguity be perceived)? (3) Can there be a change in perception with such factors as practice, task familiarity, experimental instructions, and subject expectations, and would it be difficult to perceive 2D motion after having already perceived 3D rotation? (4) What are the minimal stimuli effective for 3D perception? (5) If rotation in depth is perceived, will subjects be capable of recovering the 3D shape of the distal stimulus from its 2D projection? (6) To what extent is the recovery of shape from motion possible in different special subject populations, especially the congenitally blind, the adventiously blind, and the sighted? And (7) if early blind subjects, those with no visually based memorial or perceptual systems, are nonetheless capable of perceiving in-depth rotations in ambiguous 2D transformations, what would be the theoretical implications for similar effects in the sighted?

The Study

Our initial investigation into the ability of three early and totally blind subjects to perceive rotation in depth from the 2D transformations provided by the modified Optacon have suggested that this indeed may be possible. During the initial phase, each subject was fitted with the helmet and camera and told that at head-height directly in front of him he would be able to detect a certain static pattern. These well-lit patterns, white pipe-cleaners bent into various 3D configurations and suspended like mobiles against a black background, were all that was detectable in an otherwise darkened room. Following adjustments to the Optacon's threshold and zoom settings which made the pattern as clearly perceivable to them as possible, the subject was asked to describe the shape. The experimenter then told the subject that he was to attend very carefully to the pattern, because it was about to begin moving, and to describe what he felt. Otherwise the subject was given no information at all regarding the true nature of the distal pattern. From their verbal descriptions, we attempted to determine if the subjects perceived any rotation in depth.

The first subject, after perceiving the various patterns changing at a variety of different rates, indeed made reference to "something spinning" with certain patterns. Asked to demonstrate what he meant by "spinning", the subject raised his hand and supinated and pronated his wrist. The patterns for which this reference to rotation occurred were of a distinctive sort: they were either short straight lines lying almost but not quite vertically, or asymmetrical configurations. No reference was made to spinning with any flat symmetrical patterns (e.g., a W, an inverted V, and an equilateral triangle). Still without any information regarding the true distal pattern, the subject was asked to state why he referred to spinning. His response was that the <u>sound</u> of the changing vibrotactile stimulation pattern gave the impression of rotation. Still without any information regarding the true distal arrangement, the subject was released for the day and asked to ponder the possible causes of the changing patterns.

In order to control for the possible confounding effects of the auditory information from the Optacon, the two subsequent subjects wore headphones into which was played a tape recording of the constant Optacon buzz at a volume where any actual change in the Optacon's noise was effectively masked. Nonetheless each subject still made reference to motion in depth. Again, this perception was distinct with obliquely oriented lines and irregular patterns, and especially at rotation rates above approximately 720 degrees per second. Interestingly, reference to rotation was also made on several symmetrical patterns. This perceived rotation differed in that subjects sometimes referred to a "flip-flopping" of the pattern, as if it were rotating 180 degrees and then reversing direction.

It is also worth noting that subjects were often perplexed when pressed for one particular answer; they often claimed to be able to perceive these changes equally easily as 2D transformations or as rotations in depth. After the first day, the subjects were told that the patterns were actually 3D objects rotating in space. On the second and third days they were required to reproduce physically various distal objects' shapes using a pipe-cleaner. While the verbal reference to the perception of rotation was common, the reproduction of the actual 3D shape was extremely difficult. Flat alphanumeric characters were easily made, but less familiar patterns were poorly reconstructed (with only one exception on one trial). An illustration of the difficulty of interpreting this performance occurred with a spiral-shaped distal object. After being presented with the rotating spiral, their attempts to construct a physical copy of that object invariably resulted in the production of a flat snake-shaped pattern. The pattern's third (depth) dimension was not represented in their constructions, although the correct number of curves was. However, when shown their reproductions rotating alongside the distal spiral, two of the three readily determined which was theirs: they recognized that their patterns presented a vertical line when rotated 90 degrees. Still, none could recreate the spiral. This is an interesting example of subjects' ability to perceive rotation in depth without being able to recover the structure of the distal object, a distinction which our research continues to explore.

CONCLUDING REMARKS

In this paper we have outlined some recent modifications to a commercially available optical-to-tactile transduction system. The addition of an inexpensive lens to the standard Optacon camera has resulted in the Optacon's becoming a more general-purpose device with many of the same capabilities as the TVSS but with several advantages, among them size, availability to blind users, reliability, and flexibility. However, there are some disadvantages associated with the modified Optacon relative to the TVSS systems: it requires the use of one hand as a receptor surface, the tactile array is quite small and of relatively low resolution, and it is less a mobility aid than an educational aid. Nonetheless, we have been able to replicate many of the successes of the TVSS, and have begun to develop an educational program that can be used with younger blind students who are at an age when the kinds of experiences available through the Optacon may be particularly important in a variety of development contexts.

In recognition of several basic psychophysical differences between visual and tactile systems, we have also begun to explore the ability of blind subjects to perceive static presentations at rapid presentation rates, to mentally synthesize sequentially presented pattern parts into wholes, and to interpret vibrotactile events. We have created a microcomputer based system that can store large images and represent them to subjects in constituent parts. Our current research examines some of the variables which crucially determine subjects' abilities to synthesize pattern shapes mentally from the presentation of parts. If we are to make any claims about the ability of such systems to substitute for vision, even if only partially, finding functional similarities in the processing of visual and tactual information will be necessary, and where differences exist, alternative means of getting visual information vibrotactually to blind subjects will be required.

ACKNOWLEDGEMENTS

We gratefully acknowledge the support of this research by The Foundation For Glaucoma Research, San Francisco. We have also profited from discussions with and the contributions of William Epstein, Sandy Schneider, Todd DeVries, Matthew Olaiya, Patrick Kwanashie, and Kevin Kirby.

REFERENCES

1. Bach-y-Rita, P. (1972). Brain Mechanisms in Sensory Sub-
    stitution. New York: Academic Press.

2. Bach-y-Rita, P. (1983). Tactile-vision substitution: Past
    and future. International Journal of Neuroscience, 19,
    29-36.

3. Bach-y-Rita, P. (1984). The relationship between motor
    processes and cognition in tactile vision substitution. In
    W. Prinz & A. F. Sanders (Eds.), Cognition and Motor Proces-
    ses. Berlin: Springer-Verlag.

4. Bach-y-Rita, P., Collins, C., Saunders, F., White, B., &
    Scadden, L. (1969). Vision substitution by tactile image
    projection. Nature, 221, 963-964.

5. Collins, C. C. & Bach-y-Rita, P. (1973). Transmission of
    pictorial information through the skin. Advances in Biologi-
    cal and Medical Physics, 14, 285-315.

6. Craig, J. C. (1980). Some factors affecting tactile pattern
    recognition. International Journal of Neuroscience, 19, 47-
    58.

7. Craig, J. C. & Sherrick, C. E. (1982). Dynamic tactile dis-
    plays. In W. Schiff & E. Foulke (Eds.), Tactual Perception
    --A Sourcebook. Cambridge: Cambridge University Press.

8. Fraiberg, S. & Adelson, E. (1978). Self-representation in
    young blind children. In Z. S. Jastrzembska (Ed.), The
    Effects of Blindness and Other Impairments on Early Develop-
    ment. New York: American Foundation for the Blind.

9. Friedlander, B. Z. (1978). [Untitled] In Z. S. Jastrzembska
    (Ed.), The Effects of Blindness and Other Impairments on
    Early Development. New York: American Foundation for the
    Blind.

10. Gibson, J. J. (1966). The Senses Considered as Perceptual
    Systems. Boston: Houghton Mifflin.

11. Gibson, J. J. (1979). The Ecological Approach to Visual
    Perception. Boston: Houghton Mifflin.

12. Heil, J. (1983). Perception and Cognition. Berkeley, CA:
    University of California Press.

13. Johansson, G. (1977). Spatial constancy and motion in visual perception. In W. Epstein (Ed.), Stability and Constancy in Visual Perception. New York: Wiley.

14. Kaczmarek, K., Bach-y-Rita, P., Tompkins, W. J., & Webster, J. G. Multiplexed tactile-vision substitution system. Manuscript in preparation.

15. Morgan, M. J. (1977). Molyneux's Question. Cambridge: Cambridge University Press.

16. Palmer, S. E. (1977). Hierarchical structure in perceptual representation. Cognitive Psychology, 9, 441-474.

17. Reed, S. K. (1974). Structural descriptions and limitations of visual images. Memory and Cognition, 2, 329-336.

18. Revesz, G. (1950). Psychology and the Art of the Blind. London: Longmans Green.

19. Rock, I. (1975). An Introduction to Perception. New York: Macmillan.

20. Rock, I. (1983). The Logic of Perception. Cambridge, MA: MIT Press.

21. Sherrick, C. E. & Craig, J. C. (1982). The psychophysics of touch. In W. Schiff & E. Foulke (Eds.), Tactual Perception--A Sourcebook. Cambridge: Cambridge University Press.

22. Ullman, S. (1979). The Interpretation of Visual Motion. Cambridge MA: MIT Press.

23. von Fieandt, K. & Gibson, J. J. (1959). The sensitivity of the eye to two kinds of continuous transformation of a shadow-pattern. Journal of Experimental Psychology, 57, 344-347.

24. von Senden, M. (1960). Space and Sight. London: Methuen.

25. Wallach, H. & O'Connell, D. N. (1953). The kinetic depth effect. Journal of Experimental Psychology, 45, 205-217.

26. Wallach, H., O'Connell, D. N., & Neisser, U. (1953). The memory effect of visual perception of 3-d form. Journal of Experimental Psychology, 45, 360-368.

27. White, B., Saunders, F., Scadden, L., Bach-y-Rita P., & Collins, C.C. (1973). Seeing with the skin. Perception & Psychophysics, 7, 23-27.

STUDIES OF THE USE OF SPATIAL SENSORS

INTRODUCTION

Examples of studies designed to evaluate the effectiveness of spatial sensors, to examine the training issues of aid use, or to use spatial sensors as research tools for the examination of other questions appear in this section.

One issue that has attracted major interest because of its practical considerations is the question of how the effectiveness of a spatial sensor designed for use in mobility should be assessed. The Blind Mobility Research Unit, at the University of Nottingham, has, under the leadership of J. Alfred Leonard and then John Armstrong, conducted a number of evaluation programs in which a particular device was assessed as an aid to street travel. In his paper, Dodds discusses these issues, describes his approach and reasoning on the general issue of how to evaluate aids, and illustrates this approach with reference to the evaluation of a specific device, the Sonic Pathfinder.

A serious problem, largely ignored in sensory aid research to the present time, is the nature of the training process employed with blind travelers. The use of a sensory aid represents a complex process of perceptual learning, and the means by which this is achieved are by no means well understood. The paper by Warren and Strelow is illustrative of the use of an aid, Kay's Binaural Sensory Aid, and its successor the Trisensor (see Kay, this volume) to address research questions relevant to their use by the blind but whose implications range beyond issues of aid use by the blind, in this case the classic questions of perceptual learning. To understand their approach it is necessary to realize that a spatial sensor provides a lawful but novel representation of the physical environment. The potential user must come to understand both that the display varies along several stimulus dimensions (most notably volume, frequency, timbre, and interaural intensity in the binaural/trisensor devices) and that instances of this variation describe aspects of the physical environment.

One question which Warren and Strelow address is how the user of a sensory aid develops an understanding of the correspondence between physical reality and the artificial sensory stimulation provided by the device. The general alternatives they consider are (a) that an understanding the dimensions of the sensor is acquired from discrete instances of correspondence of individual stimulus experiences with specific spatial locations, and (b) that the user begins with a sense of the spatial dimension, and its electronic correspondence, and differentiates individual experiences out of an initially confusing array of instances. Questions of generalization of perceptual learning and the role of feedback in perceptual learning are also addressed. The sensory aids are significant in this instance as research tools allowing the experimental presentation of novel but lawfully-structured spatial stimuli. It is otherwise very difficult to study this type of problem in adults.

Warren and Strelow also deal with the issue of training for the purpose of aid use in the blind, in that their concerns for establishing the parameters of perceptual learning with sensory aids should lead toward the design of more effective training programs for aid use.

Veraart and Wanet present a model of the sensory substitution process that also has physiological overtones, and a research report that evaluates the effectiveness of a sonar-based binaural aid to mediate perception of objects in near space relationships, as well as obstacle avoidance in locomotor space.

The papers by Easton and by Hornby, Kay, Satherley, and Kay are also oriented to the question of how to go about using the Kay devices to accomplish perceptual and conceptual learning in the blind, specifically in blind children. Easton's study is oriented to near space, and compares two training approaches, one using haptic information and the other using the Kay Trisensor. The tasks are simple ones as well as ones involving more complex mental rotations. While the pattern of results is complicated, it is clear that the Trisensor experience was valuable for these totally blind school-age children.

The Hornby et al. approach involves the design of an integrated and sequential set of training exercises with the sonar aid, first in a tabletop setting and then in a larger locomotor setting. Considerable facilitative transfer occurred from the tabletop to the environmental setting.

Strelow and Warren discuss some of the spatial problems of blind children and also briefly describe projects with school age children which attempt to move in the training program from simpler concepts (and exercises) to more complex ones.

Muir, Humphrey, Dodwell, and Humphrey address issues of the use of the Kay binaural devices by infants and younger children. They provide a useful review of existing work, including general issues of auditory perception in infancy, and conclude that there is no general rule, such as an age progression, that can explain the variety of reported successes and failures. Instead, individual characteristics of subjects apparently determine outcomes. Their own work shows similar subject variability.

The implications of potential aid use by very young blind human infants are significant. The ability to understand and move about through space is one of the most threatened functions under conditions of blindness, and the evidence is that the earlier blindness occurs, the more significant are the consequences for spatial perception. Accordingly, sensory aids may be useful for very young infants, in that they may provide spatial information to the infant at the time when such information is particularly important to enable later spatial understanding.

As Muir et al. note, the available studies have not been strikingly successful. However, studies with human infants have not, to date, been able to apply sensory aids (almost all of this work has been conducted with Kay Binaural Aids) for a concentrated or long enough period of time and this may explain the weakness of some of the reported studies. In any case, no study has been reported using human infants younger than four months. But there is good reason for caution in such research. The blind infant is already at risk of developmental delay and it is well known that the central nervous system (CNS) is very plastic during the early months of life. Irregular forms of sensory stimulation could lead to non-normal behavioral and neural development. Before undertaking such work with human infants, therefore, it is necessary from both a practical and an ethical point of view to conduct trials with animals, both to ascertain that there are potential benefits from such experience and to determine whether there are potential adverse consequences.

Strelow and Warren report preliminary evidence from their study of the use of the Kay Trisensor with infant monkeys. The early results are very promising, but there is much yet to be done before trials can be undertaken confidently with human infants.

The issue of plasticity of the CNS, noted above, deserves further mention. There are many unanswered questions about the effects of substitute sensory stimulation and the questions about potential impact on the CNS deserve special scrutiny. The same plasticity of the developing CNS that makes it potentially advantageous to begin aid use early in life could, however, potentially

result in maladaptive brain development. At this point we simply
do not know enough about plasticity in the nervous system.
Sonnier and Riesen, who are colleagues of Strelow and Warren in
the work with infant monkeys, review several factors of CNS
development and draw general implications for the relationships
between behavioral and physiological research. Sonnier considers
more speculatively the implications of sensory substitution procedures as research tools for the study of neural and behavioral
work in her Comment which follows the Sonnier and Riesen paper.

The Editors

EVALUATING MOBILITY AIDS: AN EVOLVING METHODOLOGY

Allan G. Dodds

University of Nottingham

The current evaluative work carried out by the Blind Mobility
Research Unit owes its existence to the pioneering work of Dr. J.
Alfred Leonard and his collaborator Dr. John D. Armstrong. I wish
to make it clear from the outset that my involvement in electronic
aid evaluation does not reflect my main research interest, and
that any contribution I may have made to the Nottingham evaluation
procedure effectively amounts to a refinement of the original procedure. However, my experiences with it have been most instructive, and indeed they have convinced me that the job of the
evaluator is not an enviable one. I shall elaborate upon that
assertion later; suffice it for the moment, for those who are not
aware of the most recent developments in the Nottingham procedure,
to give an account of the evaluative procedure as it existed a
few years ago in comparison to its current status.

When I first inherited the evaluation procedure on the resig-
nation of Dr. John Armstrong in 1979, it was committed to a type
of evaluation in which a person's mobility could be rated on
three criteria, viz. safety, efficiency, and stress. Under these
three categories, a number of behavioral events were further
enumerated.

The criteria upon which those measures were based are similar
to those of Foulke (4) who defined mobility as: "The ability
to travel safely, comfortably, gracefully, and independently"
(p. 1). Had they been based upon a different definition of
mobility, for example that successful mobility involves knowing
exactly where you are on a moment to moment basis, then presumably
the measures chosen by Armstrong would have been different. Also,

SAFETY	EFFICIENCY	STRESS
a) Body contacts with obstacles	a) Continuousness of walking (PWI)	a) Heartrate
b) Body contacts with ISL	b) Cane contacts with ISL	b) Stride length
c) Kerb incidents	c) Cane contacts with OSL	

Figure 1.   Categories of mobility evaluation.

although Foulke's working definition did lead to a task-analysis of mobility, the purely behavioral approach adopted subsequently does not address even indirectly the various psychological processes involved. This may still be seen as a weakness of the Nottingham approach, but we are aware of it and have gone some way towards rectifying this omission.

Rather than enter into an analysis of how the evaluation procedure could have developed given a different definitional underpinning, I propose to present my experiences with it, together with the modifications which I felt had to be introduced in order for it to be both reliable and valid and more comprehensive. By valid I mean valid as a tool for differentiating between the use of a sensor as a primary or secondary aid to mobility: I am not talking about validity in the wider sense of being able to predict how often a blind traveler will go out on a day to day basis after being provided with a secondary aid.

The first time that Armstrong (1) used the procedure in its original form was when he evaluated the Binaural Sensor in 1972. The results demonstrated that only one of his measures showed a significant difference between the Sensor aided trial and the long cane only trial, and that this was only true for one subject. Yet in spite of the absence of statistical significance he concluded that: "There is little doubt that the use of the Binaural Sensor leads to a considerable improvement in mobility performance" (p. 29). Whether Armstrong was basing his judgment on some implicit criteria which did not appear in the methodology, or was simply not prepared to say that the aid made no observable change in mobility, one can only conjecture. Suffice it to say that in spite of the attractiveness of the procedure, it did not enable one to determine if the secondary aid under evaluation would produce a change in performance.

This major setback was very quickly followed by another, but fortunately it led to an understanding of the first. Because the Sonic Pathfinder was ready for a first evaluation, I had been familiarizing myself with the Armstrong procedure in order to be able to carry this out. However, it became immediately apparent that there were two fundamental problems inherent in the procedure. In the first place, a number of the measures suffered from either floor or ceiling effects. For example, the productive walking index (PWI), a measure of continuousness of walking, is always near unity. This is because clients who agree to use a secondary aid for a period of time and who are prepared to subject themselves to the rigors of an evaluation are already very competent long cane travelers, and they do not make frequent stops as they walk. Similarly, and by the same token, bodily contacts with obstacles on a long cane only trial are extremely rare occurrences, as are bodily contacts with the environment. Most evaluees already score high on safety and efficiency, and the provision of a secondary aid is unlikely to change these scores significantly.

Secondly, there was the problem of unreliability of data between trials. As we collected experimental data on the test route it became clear that although the bind person's mobility looked different with the secondary aid, this could not later be captured with statistical significance once the video tapes had been analyzed. Close examination of successive passes over the route revealed that although the same physical environment was used on each occasion, the actual path taken by the blind person differed, although not by much, from trial to trial. This small discrepancy, however, had a major influence on whether a particular obstacle or environmental feature was encountered by the long cane or whether it fell within or without the range of the secondary aid. Whether or not one obtained a score on a number of the measures was very much a matter of chance. Furthermore, this degree of variability was greater than the amount of behavioral change produced by the secondary aid. In other words, there was a low signal to noise ratio in the system.

Further scrutiny of video tapes showed that the Armstrong test route contained long sections where there were few environmental features save for an uninterrupted shoreline, and that there were sections containing very wide pavements with few obstacles in the traveler's path. Taken together, these accounted for most of the unreliability and ceiling and floor effects. We therefore decided to abandon the original route and look for one in which the blind traveler would be forced to encounter a larger number of obstacles and be constrained more in his line of travel. This meant finding a route which had narrower pavements and a greater amount of clutter. We also decided that the route should be much shorter, since the original route length of 1200 meters had proved to be too demanding for some subjects.

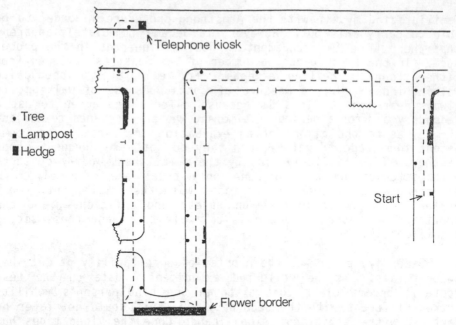

Figure 2.   Schematic design of the test route.

Having selected the route, we then took three blind long cane users and three blindfolded mobility instructors and put them over it three times.   During subsequent video analysis we collected data on the Armstrong measures and correlated the second and third trials for each measure.

Seven of the 10 measures showed significant correlation on the last two trials.   Regarding the three which did not reach statistical significance, Total Time Taken, although unreliable in itself, is used to derive PWI, which is reliable, so that this measure was retained.   Body contacts with obstacles still suffered from a floor effect, so that they were combined with curb incidents.   This measure we called Major Safety Errors, which had an acceptable reliability. Steps Taken, the measure used by Armstrong to derive average stride length, was dropped due to its unreliability.   All but one of the existing measures are considered to be sufficiently reliable to be retained in any further evaluation.

However, we had always been unhappy that the two measures, Cane Contacts with inner shoreline (ISL) and outer shoreline (OSL), had been rather indirect and hence insensitive measures of pavement position.   Armstrong himself had realized this and had tried various ways of tracking the subject's path on the video screen using superimposed lines, without success.   We decided

Measure	Correlation
1. Total time taken	$r = .79, p > .05$, N.S.
2. Time spent walking	$r = .87, p < .05$ [a]
3. Productive walking index (PWI)	$r = .86, p < .05$ [a]
4. Cane contacts (obstacles)	$r = .91, p < .02$ [a]
5. Cane contacts (inner shoreline)	$r = .89, p < .02$ [a]
6. Cane contacts (outer shoreline)	$r = .89, p < .02$ [a]
7. Body contacts (obstacles)	$r = .71, p > .05$, N.S
8. Body contacts (inner shoreline)	$r = .96, p < .01$ [b]
9. Steps taken	$r = .72, p > .05$, N.S.
10. Curb incidents (up, down, and side)	$r = .88, p < .02$ [a]

[a] $p \leqslant 0.05$
[b] $p \leqslant 0.01$

Table 1. Test-retest reliability coefficients.

that the simplest way to do it was to get observers to estimate
pavement position in terms of five imaginary zones, and to log
their estimations via a five-channel keyboard, each of whose
keys was connected to an electronic clock. As long as the
subject is in a particular zone, the observer keeps a key depressed, and when the subject moves into a new zone, the observer
releases the current key and presses the adjacent one. Total
time spent in each zone is then expressed as a proportion of the

Observer	Viewing Condition	Route Section						
		1	2	3	4	5	6	7
					Means			
A	1	3.194	3.816	4.149	2.362	3.261	3.380	3.344
	2	3.300	3.832	4.152	2.374	3.152	3.416	3.495
B	1	3.083	3.722	4.317	2.126	2.981	3.123	3.513
	2	3.305	3.832	4.331	2.123	3.156	3.052	3.649
C	1	2.936	3.842	4.352	2.204	3.113	3.131	3.311
	2	3.090	3.883	4.263	2.184	3.155	3.120	3.680
					Standard Deviations			
A	1	0.753	0.396	0.427	0.555	0.683	0.654	0.476
	2	0.859	0.399	0.416	0.505	0.692	0.610	0.501
B	1	0.788	0.479	0.465	0.425	0.788	0.903	0.501
	2	0.716	0.443	0.471	0.412	0.938	0.883	0.504
C	1	0.691	0.443	0.567	0.553	0.792	0.478	0.464
	2	0.740	0.371	0.565	0.508	0.813	0.549	0.543

Table 2. Means and standard deviations obtained from three
observers over two viewing repetitions.

total time taken, and means and standard deviations of pavement position may then be calculated for each route section. Intra- and inter-observer reliability coefficients were calculated and were found to be acceptable at the 95% level (2,3). Thus al- though the scoring procedure involves a subjective element, this is not a problem in practice.

We had now reached the stage where we felt competent to carry out the Pathfinder evaluation. However, a third hurdle presented itself. In a letter to JVIB Leslie Kay claimed that the Notting- ham procedure was unable to measure the enhancement in mobility afforded by the Sonicguide (8), because it was something which could not be measured objectively (9). I decided that Kay might be talking about something important; therefore, I took the liberty of supplying an operational definition of enhancement, viz. an increase in perceptual awareness which need not be reflected in behavior, but which might be valued by the blind traveler. Having done this, the next problem was to find a way of measuring it.

Unfortunately, there is no direct access to the immediate experiences of others, but verbal reports have been used success- fully in areas such as advanced driving instruction and pilot training (5,10). It seemed that this might be a useful way of obtaining data relevant to enhanced perceptual experience, if it could be categorized reliably.

The procedure we finally adopted after a number of false starts was to play a tape recording to the blind person, prior to commencing the route, of someone (myself) traveling the route under blindfold and commenting upon as many environmental features as possible. Subjects were then provided with a pair of Sennheiser microphones which fitted loosely in the ears, and were asked to make a similar sort of running commentary, which was telemetered onto the video tape. These commentaries were subsequently ana- lyzed and an attempt made to categorize statements. Again, intra- and inter-rater reliability coefficients were calculated and found to be acceptably high. This complementary procedure was subsequently employed in the Pathfinder evaluation.

The Pathfinder evaluation provides an opportunity to validate a procedure whose reliability has been established. But one must be cautious. If the evaluation should fail to differentiate primary from secondary aided performance, can one conclude that it is an invalid procedure? One could equally conclude that the secondary aid did not change mobility to any great extent (7). At this stage the evaluator has only further recourse to face and content validity plus, possibly, concurrent validity, and I don't think that one can expect better than this.

			With Pathfinder	Without Pathfinder	P
1	Productive Walking Index (time taken divided by time spent walking)		0.947	0.964	N.S.
2	Cane contacts with obstacles ($\bar{x}$)	All	6.33	8.83	<0.05
		Accidental	3.16	5.67	<0.025
3	Cane contacts with ISL ($\bar{x}$)		9.17	51.16	<0.05
4	Cane contacts with OSL ($\bar{x}$)		26.16	19.00	N.S.
5	Pavement Position	$\bar{x}$	2.61	2.32	<0.05
		S.D.	0.751	0.759	N.S.
6	Body contacts with shoreline ($\bar{x}$)		1.16	4.33	<0.025
7	Major Safety Errors ($\bar{x}$) (tripping, bodily contacts with obstacles)		1.83	2.66	N.S.

Table 3. Objective measures of mobility performance.

So how did the Pathfinder fare on the evaluation? Or perhaps I should put it the other way round how did the evaluation fare with the Pathfinder? In order to answer these questions, we took six competent long cane travelers and placed Pathfinders with them for a period of around six weeks. Some were supervised by Mobility Instructors who were made familiar with the device, others were trained under the supervision of Dr. Anthony D. Heyes. When each felt ready for evaluation, he was put over the standard test route using either long cane alone or long cane plus aid. In Table 3 it can be seen that on quite a number of the objective measures, mobility performance with the Pathfinder changes. For example, objects previously encountered with the cane are now avoided by use of the Pathfinder. Similarly, the number of cane contacts with the ISL is markedly reduced using the Pathfinder, and pavement position generally becomes more central, although veer does not change. As a consequence, the Pathfinder reduces accidental brushing of the ISL with the body.

Turning to the verbal commentary, it may be seen that only two categories of statement changes significantly, viz. there is an increased awareness of obstacles and a decreased awareness of environmental sounds. This means, taking the objective measures and the verbal report together, that the Pathfinder makes subjects more aware of immediate obstacles and at the same time reduces physical contact with them. Also, absence of change as observed in the case of awareness of surfaces indicates that the Pathfinder information can be used without loss of attention to information coming through another channel. However, intramodal competition for information is apparent in the reduction in the number of reports on environmental sounds.

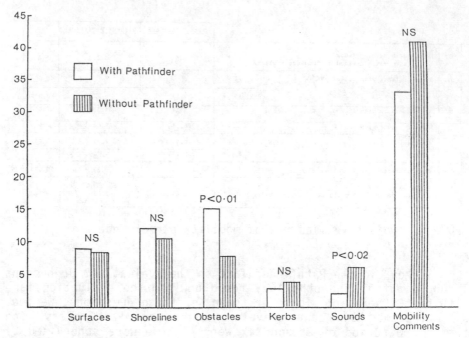

Figure 3.   Comparison of performance with and without Pathfinder.

In summary, the development of a reliable and valid evaluation procedure has taken longer than was envisaged, but by using
a number of techniques I feel that the present system can be
confidently applied to any sort of mobility aid which might be
developed in the future--even surrogate vision.   But although the
changes which I have introduced into the Nottingham procedure do
not amount to much in themselves, I have implicitly abandoned the
evaluation of blind mobility with reference to the criteria of
safety, efficiency, and stress.   I think that Armstrong himself
would have moved to the same position, since safety and efficiency for the reasons previously stated, do not change significantly
with the use of secondary aids, and since no one has yet managed
to measure moment-to-moment stress satisfactorily.

So, it appears that I have unwittingly shifted our philosophy
of evaluation from the goal-based Armstrong approach in which a
device is evaluated with reference to previously stated criteria,
to what House (6) has called a goal-free approach in which the
evaluator is looking for all outcomes.   Each of these approaches
presents its own set of problems, and I may simply be replacing
one set of problems for another.   As far as informing the aid
designer of the adequacy of the original conceptualization or
informing the blind person of the desirability of any particular

device are concerned, I would argue that the results of such an evaluation can tell an aid designer and a potential purchaser a lot, even if it is only that the aid does not change mobility appreciably. I would like to encourage aid designers to take on board the sort of evaluative approach that I have outlined, if they can only live with the results.

I should like to make one final suggestion, and that is that I think that the evaluator should be not so much the final arbiter of whether an aid is good or bad, but more the dispassionate technician who may be "employed" by either the aid designer, the potential consumer or whomever, to demonstrate what changes really do occur when new mobility aids are used, irrespective of the designer's intentions or the consumer's needs. What these various interested parties conclude from such an evaluation may be very different, and if the evaluator does have a further role to play, it may be to act as mediator between parties who may come to opposite conclusions once they have seen his data. Given that the evaluator, unlike the aid designer or the potential consumer, has less vested interest in the outcome of his work, he should be in a better position to evaluate the criteria adopted by other parties, and where they differ to offer a means of reconciliation. However, such neutrality means that the evaluator is unlikely to be appreciated either by the aid designer who thinks his aid is superb and expects the evaluator to endorse his sentiments irrespective of the results of the evaluation, or by the blind person who simply wants to be advised about which aid to buy and expects the evaluator to be able to tell him. But unpopularity is surely a small price to pay for truth.

ACKNOWLEDGEMENTS

The research described in this paper was funded by the Department of Health & Social Security and carried out under the direction of Professor C. I. Howarth.

REFERENCES

1. Armstrong, J. D. (1972). An independent evaluation of the
   Kay binaural sensor. Internal Report, Blind Mobility Research Unit, University of Nottingham.

2. Dodds, A. G., Carter, D. D. C., & Howarth, C. I. (1983).
   Improving objective measures of mobility. Journal of Visual
   Impairment & Blindness, 77, 438-442.

3. Dodds, A. G., Carter, D. D. C., & Howarth, C. I. (1984).
   The Sonic Pathfinder: An evaluation. Journal of Visual
   Impairment & Blindness, 78, 203-206.

4. Foulke, E. (1971). The perceptual basis for mobility. AFB
   Research Bulletin, No. 23, 1-8.

5. Ganton, N. & Wilde, G. J. S. (1971). Verbal ratings of estimated danger by drivers and passengers as a function of
   driver experience. Queen's University, Studies of Safety in
   Transport.

6. House, E. R. (1980). Evaluating With Validity. Sage Publi-
   cations, Beverly Hills, London.

7. Jansson, G. (1984). The development & evaluation of mobil-
   ity aids for the visually impaired. Paper presented at the
   Workshop on the Rehabilitation of the Visually Impaired,
   Florence.

8. Kay, L. (1980). Reply to article by W. H. Jacobson. Journal of Visual Impairment & Blindness, 74, 277-279.

9. Kay, L. (1981). Response to letter entitled "Criteria for
   enhanced mobility." Journal of Visual Impairment & Blindness
   75, 184-185.

10. Laidlaw, J. (1978). Hazard awareness, driver performance
    and training. Unpublished Doctoral Dissertation, University
    of Nottingham.

TRAINING THE USE OF ARTIFICIAL SPATIAL DISPLAYS

David H. Warren and Edward R. Strelow

University of California, Riverside

There are two major points that we want to stress. One has to do with the relationships both actual and potential between perceptual theory and research on sensory aids. The other has to do with research, particularly the need for carefully constructed empirical studies of issues in the area of sensory aids. The two points are closely connected.

This paper is primarily concerned with training the use of sensory aids. Such questions are of fundamental applied importance to the use of sensory aids but have been largely overlooked in research to the present time. As well, examination of the sensory aid training problem raises important general questions about perception, particularly in the field of perceptual learning. We hope to show that research, guided by perceptual theory, can not only shed light on some of the most important problems facing the sensory aids field, but can in fact help to define what the most important problems are. In the process, we will describe part of our laboratory program with sensory aids and some of our findings to date.

Our goal, in setting out to construct a laboratory program of studies of sensory aids for spatial perception, was to unite theory and research, to explore the points of intersection between perceptual theory and sensory aids, and to conduct research designed to address the issues thus identified. I (DHW) confess personally that despite training in perception and developmental psychology, and despite a serious professional interest in problems of blind mobility and spatial perception, I did not for a long time see why I should incorporate a sensory aid into my laboratory. What, aside from purely evaluative research, would I do with a device such as the Sonicguide?

Ultimately, I realized that aside from a couple of highly unlikely cases where young infants were reported to function spatially with the Sonicguide virtually upon first exposure to it, the rest of humanity had to go through a learning process to use such aids effectively for the perception of space. Thus it is indeed a legitimate problem of perceptual learning.

PERCEPTUAL LEARNING

The term perceptual learning was popularized by Gibson (1) and refers to the refinement of perceptual ability as a result of experience. There are many examples from real-world situations of persons who develop special perceptual skills. Thus a wine-, cheese-, or other food-taster has developed refined skills of smell and taste; a microscopist may have skills of visual identification which allow him or her to identify an obscure blob of cells on a slide as the potential body structures of an embryo.

Perceptual learning is not restricted to persons in unusual occupations. We all have skills which are a result of the refinement of perception. Most obviously, reading involves a range of visual and other skills. We may overlook the learning which underlies reading because of the pervasiveness and rapidity of this activity. Yet there is nothing natural about interpreting audible language from a written form. This is most evident when we consider the differences in writing across different cultures (7,8). Spoken languages themselves vary widely, but in all cases they consist of a sequential series of vocal utterances. However, there is no universal agreement about how these sequences are best represented graphically, in another modality. In western cultures, writing involves the use of an alphabet, while in others such as Chinese, pictographs are used. Some languages read from left to right, others from right to left, still others up and down.

The issues in reading and language representation are not unlike those found in sensory prostheses. Both areas deal with cross-modality information matching. In language, we represent sounds by visual forms; with a sensory prosthesis, objects normally perceived visually are represented by sound, in the case of the devices of Kay (e.g. 4), or by tactile information in the Collins/Bach-y-Rita TVSS devices (see chapters by Collins and by Bach-y-Rita and Hughes, this volume). While we all accept the need for learning the written form of language, the learning processes which underlie the use of a substitute visual sense have been given comparatively short shrift. This inattention is at least partly due to an emphasis on the perceptual aspects of the display of sensory aid information. In several instances the design of spatial sensors has attempted to provide 'natural' spatial information. Thus the Kay systems use a natural auditory cue for direction, and the TVSS is built on the premise that visual-type information can be presented to the skin in such a way that the tactile outline is like the outline of a visual image. By these means it is hoped that use of the sensor will occur in a more or less natural fashion and that the learning problem will be minimized. In effect, research in this field has been asking a modern version of the Molyneux question (5,11), but whereas the original question asked whether or not a blind person would be able to use visual information upon first regaining sight, the modern version instead asks about the ease of use of quasi-visual information presented to another sense modality.

However, it is not clear that the attempt to find a good match to vision actually works in practice. There is no obvious correspondence between a projected image on the skin and the physical object of haptic touch, and as will be seen in our investigation of the Kay system, the more natural direction code appears to require more learning than the unnatural distance code. In any case, neither Locke nor his more modern counterparts (2,9, 10) found evidence for a natural and immediate ability of a congenitally blind person to interpret visual information. The importance of this result has been generally overlooked in the area of sensory prostheses. If a sight-restored human cannot easily utilize natural visual information, how effective will be the use of any artifical representation of visual-type information? While there may be some advantages to one form of coding or another, our collective experience with the diversity of human written language should make us aware that a problem of cross-modal representation can be solved by a variety of means, and that all such means require learning.

For these reasons, we argue that the questions of perceptual learning are at least as important to the effective use of sensory aids as the choice of perceptual parameters. In fact, sensory aids may provide perceptual psychologists with a tool to help answer some of their most basic questions about perceptual learning and cross-modal processes. It is this theme that we want to elaborate and illustrate.

The best example of this potential theory-practice-research interplay lies squarely in the field of perceptual learning, where a number of classic problems remain incompletely answered. One of the most classic is the issue of dimensional learning.

When presented with an apparent hodgepodge of stimuli that in
fact fall along a lawful continuum, a dimension, does the human
perceptual learner establish the dimension first and then gradually differentiate the values along it, or does he or she learn
discrete values and from these gradually construct the dimension?
This question remains fundamentally unanswered because it is so
difficult to study.

It is often studied with children, on the grounds that since
they are developing organisms, they should show the processes
of perceptual learning more clearly than adults. But children
are not always such good experimental subjects, since their
behavioral and verbal repertoires are not as well developed as
those of adults. The dimensional learning problem is also studied
with adults, who have the advantage of being tractible and informative subjects, but at the same time the distinct disadvantage,
in this problem area, of having had experience with most perceptual dimensions. It is extremely difficult to study dimensional
learning in a mature observer. Thus the common use of "nonsense"
stimuli in studies of perceptual learning.

The area of mobility aids for the blind, and more broadly
the whole area of sensory substitution, not only needs the answers
to these basic questions of perceptual learning, since much of
what has to be accomplished in coming to use an aid effectively
involves perceptual learning of display stimuli whose parameters
vary along dimensions, but in fact this area may serve as a fer-
tile ground for the examination of these basic issues. Consider:
we can present to a mature observer a collection of stimuli that
co-vary lawfully with respect to some dimension (such as a spatial
dimension) that has functional importance for the observer, and
we can examine the course of learning. He or she is initially
naive with respect to the relationships between the stimulus
array presented by the device and the physical dimension which it
represents, and so we can study dimensional learning as if with
a neonate. At the same time, the perceptual learning mechanisms
are mature. Furthermore, the subject can let us know the results
of learning verbally or by means of other functional behavior far
more effectively than a neonate can.

We are studying some of these basic perceptual learning
issues in one of our research programs. We will briefly describe
our laboratory program with the binaural sensory aid and some of
our findings. Wearing the binaural aid, the user hears a signal
which rises from 0 to about 6 kHz as a target recedes from the
observer, and which appears to move left and right in auditory
space with changes in target direction.[2]

PROTOTYPE EXPERIMENT ON PERCEPTUAL LEARNING

     The first experiment is a simple localization experiment, in
which we train the subject, with feedback, to locate targets that
vary in both direction and distance. A set of 72 training trials
is followed by a set of 25 test trials, conducted without feedback. The subjects are sighted but blindfolded college students.

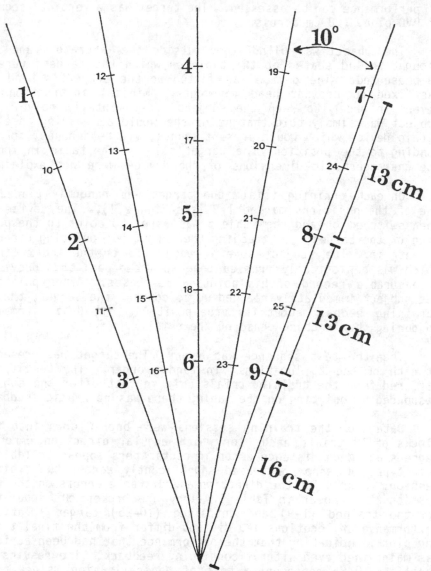

Figure 1. The array of target locations. Numbers in boldface
are training targets; these plus the smaller numbers are test
targets.

Figure 1 shows the array of target locations used in the training and test trials. Locations 1 through 9 were used in training, and these together with the remaining locations 10 through 25 were used in the test. The arrangement of test and training locations was designed to allow the separate testing of the two spatial dimensions, and to allow testing to occur both at trained locations and at other locations, so that generalization of performance can be assessed. The target was a vertical segment of PVC pipe, 1.8 cm across.

The subject was blindfolded outside the laboratory and then brought in and seated at the table on which the targets were to be presented. The device was fitted to the subject's head and was fixed to prevent head movements. Minimal instruction was given, in order to keep the subject experimentally naive. The subject was simply told that he or she would be wearing an electronic device which would present sounds, via headphones, corresponding to the position of a target pole on the table in front. The characteristic dimensions of the device were not explained.

On each training trial, the target was randomly placed at one of the positions marked 1-9 (see Figure 1). The device was then switched on and the subject was asked to point to the position of the target, not touching the target but pointing directly beneath it. The subject wore a rubber tip on the index finger which was periodically pressed onto an inked pad, thus providing a measurable record of his pointing responses. After pointing, the subject immediately reached up to contact the target, thereby obtaining feedback about its true position. The device remained on during the feedback phase of the trial.

Then the test sequence was begun. The target was presented at each of the 25 locations, in random order. The test trials differed from the training trials only in that after the subject responded by pointing on the table, there was no haptic feedback.

Data from the training sessions were broken down into four blocks of 18 trials each, for which angular direction error in degrees and mean distance error in centimeters appear in Table 1. Both types of error decreased significantly across the training session. Scores for the direction and distance errors on the test session also appear in Table 1. They are broken out separately for the trained (1-9) and untrained (10-25) target locations. Performance on locations 1-9 did not differ from the final training block, indicating that the performance that had been achieved was maintained even without continuing feedback. The results for locations 10-25 represent a test of generalization, since these locations had not been trained with feedback. There was not a significant generalization decrement for the distance errors, t

A. Single-session group (n=18)

	Training Block				Test Positions		
	1	2	3	4	1-9	10-25	1-25
Direction error	15.2	12.7	11.5	12.1	11.0	13.9	12.9 (4.6)
Distance error	6.4	5.2	5.7	4.8	5.2	5.6	5.5 (1.4)

B. Three-session group (n=6)

	Session 1 Test	Session 2 Test	Session 3 Test
	Positions 1-25	Positions 1-25	Positions 1-25
Direction error	14.9 (5.8)	10.5 (5.7)	10.6 (4.7)
Distance error	5.1 (1.3)	5.6 (1.6)	5.2 (0.8)

Table 1. Training and test results for prototype experiment. Positions 1-9 were training targets, and 10-25 were untrained locations. Direction errors are in deg, distance errors are in cm, all are absolute errors. Standard deviations in parentheses.

(17) < 1.0. For direction there was a significant decrement, t (17) = 2.56; p < .02, indicating some generalization decrement. Nonetheless, the generalization performance was far better than chance.

Six of the 18 subjects were run for two additional identical sessions on subsequent days. Their results also appear in Table 1. Performance on the direction dimension continued to improve significantly in the additional sessions, F (2,10) = 13.8 p < .01, while the distance error did not change, F < 1.0. This result shows, as was suggested earlier, that the pitch-distance code is easier to learn and improves to asymptotic performance more quickly than direction. We will return to this issue later.

Just how good are these levels of performance? We offer three points of comparison. First, we calculated what purely random responding would be by taking a subset of six subjects, detaching each test response from its target, and reattaching the response to another target location taken at random. We then calculated distance and direction errors as though the responses had been to those (randomly assigned) target locations. These calculations yielded a mean distance error of 13.1 cm and a mean

direction error of 22.8 deg. It is clear that performance with
the aid was far better than would be expected by chance. Next,
we trained and tested a new set of six blindfolded subjects with
real auditory targets, unmediated by the aid. The subject localized, by pointing, a 500-Hz click presented at 65 dBA at eye
level. Four blocks of training trials with feedback were followed
by 25 test trials without feedback. Performance on the test
yielded mean error scores of 11.3 deg for direction and 6.9 cm for
distance. These scores are quite comparable to the aid-mediated
performance of 11.9 deg and 5.7 cm. Third, we trained and tested
six new subjects with visual targets, seen through a shutter
which prevented the subject's view of his hand. Mean errors for
direction and distance were, respectively, 2.7 cm and 5.1 deg.
As expected, localization of visual targets was better than that
of aid-mediated targets.

This, then, is the prototype experiment on which most of the
subsequent experiments were modeled. It shows that the dimensions
can be learned, that very good generalization to untrained targets
occurs, and that trained performance is comparable to localization
of normal auditory targets but is not as good as localization of
visual targets.

EFFECTS OF SPATIAL REGULARITY

In the second and third experiments, we were concerned with
the issue of the regularity of target presentation during training. Specifically, would regularity of presentation of the
dimensions improve learning, compared to the randomly ordered
target presentation of the prototype experiment? In the second
experiment, we used three kinds of regularity:

(a) direction constant with regular variation in distance.
The order of target presentation (refer to Figure 1) was 123456789
123456789;

(b) distance constant with regular variation in direction.
The order of target presentation was 147258369 147258369;

(c) direction and distance varying regularly. The order of
target presentation was 147123 258456 369789.

A group of six subjects was trained with each of these for-
mats and then was tested with randomly ordered test locations
1-25. The results appear in Table 2. The results were analyzed
in comparison to the purely random ordering of training locations
in the prototype experiment. There were no differences between
groups. These kinds of regularity in target sequencing during
training did not aid the course of learning.

	Training Block				Test Positions		
	1	2	3	4	1-9	10-25	1-25
Random (Exp. 1)							
Direction	15.2	12.7	11.5	12.1	11.0	13.9	12.9
Distance	6.4	5.2	5.7	4.8	5.2	5.6	5.5
Distance Constant							
Direction	11.1	10.8	12.4	9.0	10.5	14.8	13.1
Distance	7.3	6.6	7.9	7.2	8.1	8.9	8.6
Direction Constant							
Direction	8.5	10.6	9.4	8.1	11.4	15.4	14.0
Distance	6.3	5.4	6.3	5.1	6.4	5.6	5.9
Direction/Distance							
Direction	15.8	10.4	11.6	8.6	12.4	16.8	15.1
Distance	7.1	5.4	5.4	4.8	6.1	6.2	6.1

Table 2. Mean direction (deg) and distance (cm) errors for various target sequence groups.

	Test Block 1 (5 positions)	Test Block 2 (25 positions)	Prototype Exp. (25 positions)
Direction training	13.8	20.5	12.9
Distance training	5.0	6.4	5.5

Table 3. One-dimensional training: mean distance error (cm) and direction error (deg). Data are also shown from corresponding tests in prototype experiment.

In the third experiment, we pushed the regularity to an extreme, training one group with only distance variation and with direction held constant (at the straight ahead radial) and a second group with only direction variation and with distance held constant (at the middle distance). Thus the first group was trained with locations 4, 5, and 6, whereas the second group was trained with locations 2, 5, and 8. The initial 25-trial test for the first (distance variation) group used only the five locations on the trained radial (4, 17, 5, 18, 6), and that for the second (direction variation) group used only the five locations at the trained distance (2, 14, 5, 21, 8). The results appear in Table 3. Neither dimension proved to be better learned than in the prototype experiment in which both dimensions had been varied during training. Thus isolating a single dimension for training did not improve acquisition.

In a second block of 25 test trials, which followed the first block immediately, we used all 25 locations, as in previous experiments. We were interested in whether introducing variation in the untrained dimension would cause performance on the trained dimension to deteriorate. It did, particularly for direction, where the mean angular error for the direction-trained group deteriorated from 13.8 deg in the first test block to 20.5 deg in the block where all 25 locations were used. For the group trained on distance variation, the deterioration, although significant, was not extreme, going from a mean of 5.0 cm to a mean of 6.4 cm when direction was allowed to vary in addition to distance. Again, then, we find evidence that distance for some reason shows better or more robust acquisition.

Why should this be? In fact, the finding seems counterintuitive, in that the direction code of the aid uses the interaural difference (IAD) as a basis, and IAD is a natural cue for auditory direction for humans. The distance cue has no such built-in "natural" correspondence, so it is logical to expect that it would be more difficult to learn. Yet distance is quicker to be learned to asymptote, it shows better generalization, and it deteriorates less with variation introduced in the other dimension.

One possibility is that the IAD dimension used in the aid to code direction is less discriminable than that (pitch) used to code distance. This is a purely psychophysical question, and an important one for aid design and evaluation. We did a brief experiment to evaluate the JND for the two dimensions as they are presented by the binaural sensory aid. A motor-driven carriage was arranged to move the target, starting from the center position numbered 5, either toward or away from the subject or to his left or right. The subject simply identified, as quickly as possible, the direction of travel of the target, and from these responses we calculated the JND. The mean displacement required for a correct distance judgment was 1.1 cm, whereas the mean displacement required for a correct direction judgment was 2.7 cm. These results suggest that the lateral sensing field of the device may be divided into roughly 10 useful units, whereas distance is divisible into roughly 40 discriminable units. This difference may contain the explanation for the apparent greater ease of learning and robustness of the distance cue than the direction cue. In any case, the need for psychophysical evaluation is evident.

HEAD MOVEMENTS

Another of the classical issues in perceptual learning is that of the observer's motor activity in engaging the stimulus situation. Active exploration, for example, typically leads to better learning than passive exposure (12). Along these same lines, we were interested in the role that head movements might play in the learning of the distance and direction codes. Up to this point, the training and test conditions all involved a fixed head. In this experiment, we allowed the head to move in some conditions, and indeed encouraged the subject to make target-directed head movements. The four conditions were as follows: head fixed in both training and test, head free in both training and test, head fixed in training but free in test, and head free in training but fixed in test. The results appear in Table 4.

The best performance apparently occurred in the condition where the head was free in both training and test. However, the results of the condition where the head was free in training but fixed in the test lead us to question whether learning of the direction code actually occurs when the head is free: In this condition direction performance was virtually random. Subjects with head free in training may have localized in training simply by pointing the head toward the target on the basis of maximizing the signal intensity, thereby avoiding the necessity of learning the IAD code. Subjects with head free in the test could continue the same strategy and perform well, but those with head fixed in the test reveal the lack of learning of the direction code. This result seemed counterintuitive at first glance, but it is a very clear outcome and upon reflection the explanation seems sound. In any case, we give this as evidence for the need to bring intuition under experimental scrutiny in the design of training experience for sensory aid use.

Head condition		Direction error (deg)	Distance error (cm)
Training	Test		
Fixed	Fixed	12.5	6.0
Free	Free	6.0	6.3
Free	Fixed	19.0	6.0
Fixed	Free	9.5	7.2

Table 4.   Results of fixed-head and free-head conditions.

FEEDBACK VARIABLES

Another issue of fundamental importance in perceptual learning has to do with the role that feedback plays in learning. We have only begun to explore this area in our research, but we have several provocative findings, of which we will report two very briefly.

The first has to do with delay of feedback. In our prototype experiment, and in all others reported to this point, we gave feedback during training by having the subject, immediately after responding, raise his or her hand to encounter the target at its true location. In the next experiment, we varied the timing of that feedback. One condition involved even more immediate feedback than the prototype in that the target sat on the table, not above it, so that it would be immediately contacted by hand movements. A second condition involved a 10-sec delay, a third involved a 30-sec delay, and in a fourth the subject received no feedback at all during training. The head was fixed in both training and test phases.

The results appear in Table 5. In the no-feedback condition, performance was virtually random, as expected. In the other conditions, increasing delay created a gradual decrease in learning performance for the direction dimension, but no such decrease for distance. Again the distance-direction difference emerges, with distance again the more robust dimension. In significant respects, the outcome of this experiment is in accord with the literature which generally reports that performance deteriorates with increasing interposed delay between response and feedback (e.g., 3,12).

Feedback condition	Direction (deg)	Distance (cm)
No delay	12.9	5.8
10 sec delay	16.4	7.2
30 sec delay	17.6	4.5
No feedback	23.8	11.1

Table 5. Experiment on delay of tactual feedback. Head fixed throughout. Error measures.

	Direction (deg)	Distance (cm)
Stationary target	25.8	12.3
Moving target	10.8	8.7

Table 6. Experiment with moving target, head free throughout. No tactual or other feedback. Error measures.

In the second experiment, we explored the apparently uninteresting no-feedback situation a bit further. There were two conditions. In one, the target was stationary as in the previous experiments. Performance was very bad on both dimensions, as can be seen in Table 6, even though in this experiment the head was free to move in both training and test. There was clearly no learning occurring, since the results were virtually the same as those expected at random. In the other condition, there was again no feedback, but the target was made to move, and again the subject's head was free in both training and test. The stimulus was moved in an irregular pattern on each trial for approximately 15 sec, the typical time for which a stationary target had been exposed in the previous conditions. Despite the absence of feedback, performance was relatively good. Thus stimulus movement which the subject was free to track by head movements produced fairly good performance, even without haptic feedback.

There are many questions about feedback that will need firm answers before an optimal training program may be designed, and we expect this area to occupy our attention in the laboratory program for some time to come.

CONCLUSION

Our goal was to illustrate the importance of the interplay between perceptual theory and research in the area of sensory aids. A number of the current findings have a bearing on applied questions of sensory aid work. For example, we have found a notable difference between the two spatial codes of the binaural sensor; even more surprising is that the more natural direction code was more difficult to learn than the wholly artificial distance code. However, this result appears to be related to the perceptual discriminability of the stimulus dimensions employed. As well, we have identified at least two distinct processes of feedback in the perceptual learning of the dimensions of a sensory aid. Haptic grasping of a target as it is sensed can provide one avenue of dimensional learning. In other situations learning can still take place in the absence of such tactile feedback, if the observer can actively turn his head to follow targets moving in both dimensions. However, this latter type of skill does not appear to produce much actual learning of the static direction code. Instead, the observer simply learns how to turn his head to face a target.

These results indicate something of the complexity of the psychological issues of perceptual learning that are raised by sensory aid research. The counter-intuitive nature of several of the findings indicates that simple assumptions about training programs are not likely to provide effective results.

The field not only needs and can benefit from good experimental research, but this research needs to be grounded in perceptual theory, particularly perceptual learning theory. Moreover, there are also some basic issues of traditional perceptual learning that can be fruitfully explored using sensory aids as a fundamental research tool. We believe that this point applies no less to the future generations of sensory aids than to the current types -- the principles of interplay among theory, research, and sensory aids will apply just as much 10 years from now, with as-yet unimagined aids, as they do today.

NOTES

[1] This research was partially supported by a University of California Intramural Research Grant to the first author, and by BRSG2-507-RR07010-16 awarded by the Biomedical Research Support Grant Program, Division of Research Resources, National Institutes of Health.

Thanks are due Prof. L. Kay for his assistance in providing the sensory aid used in the research, and Dana Plumley for assistance in conducting the experimental sessions.

[2] The sensor used in these experiments was an experimental version of the BSA, using an ultrasonic transmitter and two receivers. The transmitter emits linear, frequency-modulated sweeps of ultrasound, between 100 kHz and 50 kHz, at rates between 4 and 15 times per second depending on the maximum range selected by the experimenter. For each sweep, the returning echo is mixed with part of the transmitted signal to yield an audible frequency varying (linearly with distance) between 0 and about 6 kHz. The settings resulted in a maximum range for these experiments of about .6 m.

The direction code is provided by splaying the two receiving transducers so that each looks slightly to one side. Targets off from center therefore give slightly stronger echoes in one channel or the other, producing an IAD characteristic which is the basis for the direction code. The IAD variation was .7 db/deg, a value consistent with settings reported by Kay (14) for the BSA and representing what the majority of users require to sense that a target is off to one side (6).

The field of view corresponds to a flattened cone about 40 deg wide and 30 deg high. Audible signals are received from all targets within this field, as long as one dimension of the target exceeds about .5 cm. The overall loudness of the left plus right channels combined falls off about 6 db at the 20-deg lateral positions compared to the center of the field. The volume was set to give a signal of 65 dBA for a target at location 5 (Figure 1).

REFERENCES

1. Gibson, E. J. (1969). Principles of Perceptual Learning and Development. New York: Appleton-Century-Crofts.

2. Gregory, R. L. & Wallace, J. G., Jr. (1963). Recovery From Early Blindness. EPS Monograph No. 2 Cambridge: Heffer.

3. Held, R. L., Efstathiou, A. & Green, M. (1966). Adaptation to displaced and delayed visual feedback from the hand. Journal of Experimental Psychology, 72, 887-891.

4. Kay, L. (1974). A sonar aid to enhance spatial perception of the blind: Engineering design and evaluation. The Radio and Electronic Engineer, 44, 40-62.

5. Morgan, M. J. (1978). Molyneux's Question. Cambridge: Cambridge University Press.

6. Rowell, D. (1970). Auditory display of spatial information. Unpublished doctoral dissertation, University of Canterbury, Christchurch, New Zealand.

7. Taylor, I. & Taylor, M. M. (1983). The Psychology of Reading. New York: Academic Press.

8. Tzeng, O. J. L. & Hung, D. (1981). Orthographic variations and visual information processing. Psychological Bulletin, 90, 377-414.

9. Valvo, A. (1971). Sight Restoration After Long-Term Blindness. New York: American Foundation for the Blind.

10. von Senden, M. (1960). Space and Sight: The Perception of Space and Shape in the Congenitally Blind Before and After Operation. Glencoe, IL: The Free Press.

11. Warren, D. H. & Strelow, E. R. (1984). Learning spatial dimensions with a visual sensory aid: Molyneux revisited. Perception, 13, 331-350.

12. Welch, R. (1978). Perceptual Modification: Adapting to Altered Sensory Environments. New York: Academic Press.

SENSORY SUBSTITUTION OF VISION BY AUDITION

C. Veraart and M.-C. Wanet

Universite Catholique de Louvain

For many years, attempts have been made to compensate for the impairment of blindness. Recently, these efforts have been oriented toward the design of sophisticated sensory aids. A visual prosthesis is an artificial system controlled by blind subjects enabling them to interact with spatial aspects of the environment that are normally visually perceived. Among the possible solutions for these artificial systems, direct input of the prosthesis to some part of the visual modality has been studied (3,6). The main drawback of this method is that it is invasive. In other approaches, visual prostheses stimulate an intact sensory modality like touch or audition, thus avoiding problems of long-term compatibility with implanted biomaterials. Visual information has to be detected by an artificial system, decoded, and transmitted in the form of vibrations or sounds to the substitutive organ; moreover, this tactile or auditory stimulation has to be interpreted correctly by the subjects, leading to problems of learning and of plasticity of nervous structures. Comparable considerations led Bach-y-Rita (1) to propose a theory of sensory substitution.

How can we precisely define the problems raised by sensory substitution? Firstly, let us consider its psychophysiological implications. The processing of substitute auditory information would be made by the auditory modality until the perceptual level. In order to be interpreted as rapidly and efficiently as possible, this information flow in the nervous structures may be reoriented from a certain level in the auditory to the visual modality. If this diverted flow becomes established by training, intensive use of visual prosthesis, inducing sensory-motor interactions, will certainly reinforce this flow, thanks to neuronal plasticity. The nervous mechanisms involved in this model of sensory substitution would occur at levels where the convergence between the different sensory modalities normally appears, i.e. in associative structures, at the level of an amodal perception. A second problem concerns the fact that the visual sense, as emphasized by recent neurophysiological findings (20), is a plurimodal system. Processing of visual information involves action of functions as different as pattern recognition, color vision, movement detection, and spatial localization. The designer of a visual prosthesis might focus on the visual function which is to be artificially restituted, but perhaps such an approach would be too restrictive. Alternatively the problem is to design a prosthesis to represent more than one visual function. Other considerations are information capacity and the sensory functions of the substitutive modality. Like vision, other sensory modalities are plurimodal. Audition and touch, for example, are concerned both with pattern recognition and spatial localization. Channel capacity is also dependent on the sensory modality involved. Finally, the optimal design of a visual prosthesis is highly involved with the ease of training the prosthesis user. Thus, the general problem is one of compatibility: How can one make the visual substitutive information acceptable for the brain, whatever the technological solution employed?

We are involved in a program devoted to the study of sensory substitution. Our research goals are to evaluate this theory, by physiological means, on humans and animals. To achieve that, we are following two main paths. Firstly, we are conducting behavioral studies to study the enhancement of space perception obtained by using an ultrasonic binaural sensory aid. Then, we plan to detect possible sensory substitutions; for this purpose, an autoradiographic method will be used to map brain metabolic activities and electrophysiological investigations will be performed. Secondly, we focus on designing more sophisticated visual prostheses, involving the pattern recognition function in addition to spatial localization. We plan to pursue these design efforts, keeping in mind efficient real time functioning as well as training optimization.

The aim of the present paper is to report preliminary results of this approach and to propose a conceptual model of sensory substitution prostheses. Spatial behavior is usually described as being impaired by blindness (17,23). The accuracy of spatial representation seems to depend on the amount of visual experience, early blind subjects having poorer performance for spatial tasks than late blind subjects. We quantitatively compared blind subjects' performance in spatial tasks to that of blindfolded sighted subjects and measured improvements in these spatial tasks, when performed by blind subjects trained to use the ultrasonic prosthesis. This was achieved, in a first experiment performed in the near space, by positioning either a sound source or a target to be detected by the ultrasonic prosthesis. In both conditions, we collected pointing and verbal responses, direction and distance aspects of these responses being separately measured. A second experiment was performed involving locomotion in a large area explored with or without the help of the ultrasonic prosthesis. Tasks assessed the perceived location in direction and distance of landmarks in the explored area, or how efficiently an obstacle field was crossed. Part of these results have been the subject of a previous note (22). Experiments with cats wearing a special version of the ultrasonic prosthesis are in progress.

GENERAL METHOD

An ultrasonic prosthesis (5) was devised, roughly similar to the binaural sensory aid designed by Kay (12). The prosthesis consisted of a pair of spectacles containing an echolocating device and a pair of small earphones, and connected to an electronic case powered with batteries. The echolocating device emitted ultrasound in a cone of about 70°. Like in the Sonicguide, an ultrasonic carrier wave was frequency modulated by a saw-tooth wave. Echoes were received by two microphones; these signals were processed by the electronic box, decoded in audible sound, and sent to the user's earphones. The distance of obstacles was coded proportionally to the pitch of the sounds (slope: 900 Hz/m), and their direction by binaural intensity balance. A pole (diameter: 9 cm; length: 2 m) could be detected inside a roughly oval perimeter whose large diameter was about 3 m and the small one about 2 m. A broad obstacle like a wall could be detected up to about 6 m (the related frequency being about 10.8 kHz).

The learning program intended for training the blind subjects to use the prosthesis consisted of a minimum of six 50-minute sessions. Firstly, subjects were trained to detect easily detectable objects nearby. Then they learned to adapt their locomotion to the new spatial information received and to take advantage of the scanning possibilities of the prosthesis. During the last session, training was performed outside, in a residential area.

Experiment 1: Human Subjects' Performance in the Near Space

Procedure. This task tested the subjects' abilities to localize a target positioned in near space. During the experiment, the subject sat in front of a horizontal field provided with an

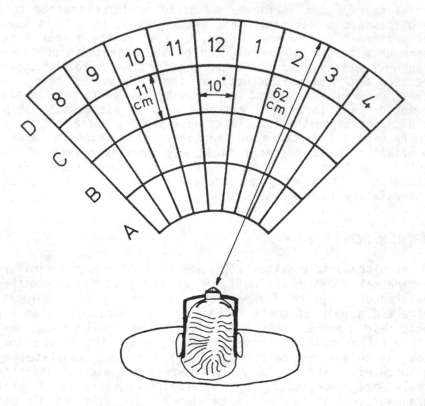

Figure 1. Outline of the experimental set-up designed for tests in the near space. Targets were positioned above the 28 middle compartments (4 distances and 7 directions from 9 o'clock to 3 o'clock). Pointing was recorded in all the 36 compartments.

obvious co-ordinate system. A sector of 90° was divided into 36 tactually discriminable compartments arranged in 4 ranges of distance and 9 ranges of direction (Figure 1). Increasing ranges of distance were respectively labeled A, B, C and D; direction ranges were identified according to a clockwise code (noon in front, 8 o'clock to 11 on the left and 1 o'clock to 4 on the right). In one condition, the target to be located was a sound source; in a second condition, the target was silent but the subject used the prosthesis to localize it. This last condition was presented before and again after training with the prosthesis. The sound source consisted of a small loudspeaker emitting a succession of short tones (300 ms) of fixed frequency (800 Hz) until the response was given. This loudspeaker was mounted in a cylinder which also constituted the silent target to be detected when the prosthesis was used. The target was positioned along a plexiglas

horizontal plate, situated 30 cm above the pointing field. In a
typical session, this target was randomly located on the plexiglas
plate, just above each of the 28 compartments (distributed in the
four distances and the seven central directions, from 9 o'clock
on the left to 3 o'clock on the right). After each response, the
target was silently moved toward a new location. The position of
the subject was controlled. Before each response, both forefingers
were placed on a tactile reference (a small piece of foam-rubber
at the origin of the co-ordinate system). The subject was asked
to keep his face above the piece of foam-rubber. In addition,
sighted subjects were blindfolded.

     Two kinds of response could be given. The verbal response
consisted of the naming of the co-ordinates (e.g., B-10 or D-2)
of the estimated position of the sound source. In the open-loop
motor response, the dominant forefinger was moved from the foam-
rubber and pointed directly to the chosen compartment. In each
experimental condition the subject was asked to respond to a random presentation of the sound source in each of the 28 possible
locations. In order to avoid any kind of learning, error feedback was not given.

     Data were processed in the following way. To each response
were assigned two error values (direction and distance), defined
as the number of compartments between the co-ordinates of the
stimulus and those of the response. Errors in direction and in
distance, from the 28 responses for a given subject in a given
experimental condition, were cumulated in two mean errors.

     Six early blinded and five late blinded subjects were com-
pared to 10 sighted subjects (male and female, aged from 21 to
54). Of the blind subjects, four late and three early blind
subjects completed the training program with the prosthesis.

     Results. In the first condition, when the target was a
sound source, the three groups of subjects differed in their
performances as shown in Figure 2. In this figure, the horizontal axis shows the group mean error in direction and the
vertical axis shows the group mean error in distance.

     We performed two one-dimension analyses of variance for
direction and distance, on the three groups of subjects. There
was no significant difference between the groups for direction
for either the verbal or the motor response. For distance, on
the contrary, the analysis of variance was nearly significant
($p < 0.10$) and thus a Student's t-test was carried out to see
which group errors were different from the others. In a first
hypothesis, we proposed that early blind subjects' errors would be
larger than those of sighted subjects. This was always verified

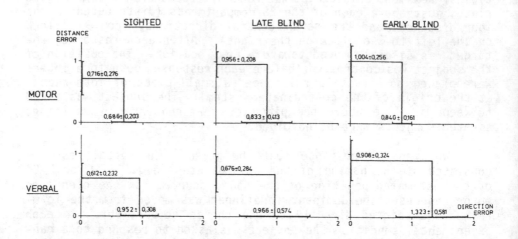

Figure 2. Motor and verbal response errors, recorded in distance and in direction, for three groups of subjects during sound source localizations performed in the near space. Errors are scaled in number of compartments. Mean and standard deviation are indicated graphically and numerically for each measure.

($\underline{p}$ < 0.05). In a second hypothesis, we proposed that the early blind subjects would show larger errors than the late blind: this was never verified. Lastly, we hypothesized that errors of the late blind and the sighted subjects would not differ significantly. This was always verified. Considering motor vs verbal performances, we hypothesized that the verbal response would be more accurate than the motor one. This hypothesis was supported for distance assessments: As shown in Figure 2, distance errors with verbal response were always smaller than with motor response, whatever group was considered. These differences were checked by $\underline{t}$-test for matched pairs and were found to be significant for the whole blind group ($\underline{p}$ < 0.02). On the contrary, direction assessments tended to follow a reverse relation: direction errors in motor responses were always smaller than verbal ones. These differences were significant for the sighted group ($\underline{p}$ < 0.05) and nearly so for the whole blind group ($\underline{p}$ < 0.06).

When the silent target was localized with the help of the prosthesis, performance was separately analyzed for verbal and motor responses. With verbal responses, the three kinds of performance (sound localization, localization with the prosthesis before and after learning) differed as indicated in Figure 3.

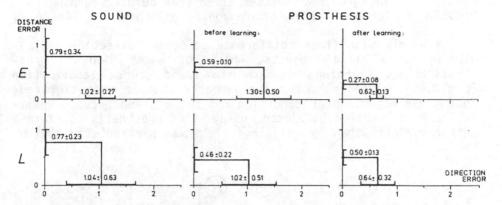

Figure 3.   Verbal response errors in distance and in direction, recorded for early (E) and late (L) blind subjects during silent target localization performed in the near space, with the help of the ultrasonic prosthesis.   Errors performed before (middle column) and after (right column) completion of a training program are compared to one another and with regard to verbal response errors in sound source localization (left column).   Other conventions as in Figure 2.

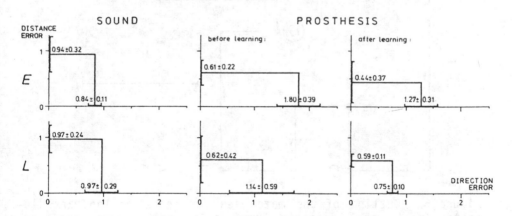

Figure 4.   Motor response errors in distance and in direction for target localizations performed in the near space, by blind subjects using the prosthesis.   Data presentation and conventions as in Figures 2 and 3.

From a quantitative point of view, distance estimation for the early blind group was better after than before learning ($p <$ 0.005). Performance in motor responses is shown in Figure 4.

The only significant difference concerned direction estimation by early blind subjects, which was worse with the prosthesis before learning, compared to sound source localization ($p < 0.05$). Finally, motor and verbal responses were compared, in a given experimental condition and for a given group. Qualitatively, all blind subjects using the prosthesis performed better verbally than by pointing: This was particularly obvious

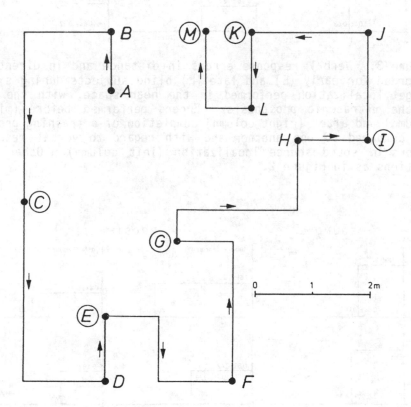

Figure 5. Outline of the maze used for tests of landmarks localization in the locomotor space. Six routes were designed, each one comprising 2 landmarks and a viewpoint. The landmarks are labeled by letters; in addition, the six viewpoints are circled. Routes were explored in directions shown. As an example, in route A B C, A and B were the landmarks to be localized from the viewpoint C; in route C D E, C and D were landmarks and E viewpoint, etc.

for the early blind subjects in direction estimation. Quantitatively, this last difference was only significant before
learning ($p < 0.04$).

Experiment 2:   Human Subjects' Abilities to Localize Landmarks within Space of Locomotion

   Procedure. Inside an area of 40 m^2, easily identifiáble
landmarks were set out and six routes were designed in such a
manner that each one contained three landmarks, such that the
start and end points of the route corresponded respectively to
the first and the third landmarks (Figure 5).   During a first
experimental condition, blind or blindfolded-sighted subjects
were guided along a given route to explore.   For the second
experimental condition, only the blind group was employed and
it used the ultrasonic prosthesis when exploring the routes.   In
all conditions, each route was traveled twice before the assessment of the landmark positions.   Assessment occurred as follows:
Subjects positioned at the third landmark level (e.g., at C in
Figure 5) judged the relative distances of the first and the
second landmarks encountered (A and B in Figure 5), and they gave
their direction estimation by successively turning their body
toward each landmark.   The angular direction of the body was
recorded.

   Data were processed as follows. In relative distance evaluation, a correct response was scored as 0 and an error as 1.
For direction estimations, angular differences between real and
evaluated directions were measured for both landmarks.   This
constituted our so-called "absolute error."   Furthermore, an
"angular separation error" was defined as the difference between
evaluated and real angular separations of the two landmarks.

   This test involved three early and three late blind trained
subjects and the 10 sighted subjects taken from the same sample
as in Experiment 1.

   Results. In the first experimental condition, where subjects were guided along a given route to explore, the three
groups of subjects performed as indicated in Figure 6.   A one-
dimension analysis of variance was performed on the three groups
of subjects, for distance and for direction scores.   The three
groups differed nearly significantly, as well in distance as in
direction estimations ($p < 0.06$ in both cases).   A t-test of
Student was then carried out.   The hypothesis that the early
blind performed less accurately than the sighted subjects was
verified in distance evaluations ($p < 0.025$) and also in direction estimations computed with the absolute error ($p < 0.025$).   A
second hypothesis was tested: It was verified that the early

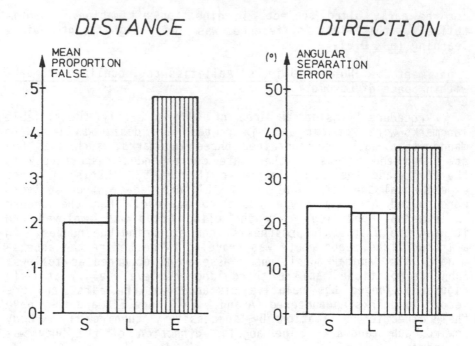

Figure 6. Mean errors in distance and in direction performed in landmark localizations, as estimated by three groups of subjects guided in the locomotor space. S: sighted subjects; L: late blind subjects; E: early blind subjects.

blind indeed performed significantly poorer than the late blind in direction estimations computed with the absolute error ($\underline{p} <$ 0.025), but not in distance.

Performance of the two groups of subjects (blind subjects with and without the ultrasonic prosthesis) is displayed in Figure 7. Results were compared by means of a $\underline{t}$-test for matched pairs in distance and in direction for both groups of subjects. No significant differences were found in direction assessments. In distance estimation, performance with the prosthesis was significantly better than that obtained without it, but for the early blind only ($\underline{p} <$0.04). Meanwhile, if responses of the whole blind group were considered, significant differences appeared between results obtained with and without the prosthesis, as well in distance ($\underline{p} <$0.006) as in direction ($\underline{p} <$0.04). Finally, when estimations made with the help of the prosthesis by the two groups of blind subjects were compared, results in distance differed significantly, the late blind remaining more accurate ($\underline{p} <$0.05).

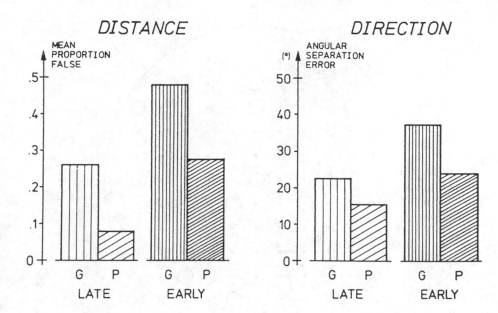

Figure 7. Mean errors in distance and direction, during land-marks localizations performed in the locomotor space by two groups of blind subjects using the ultrasonic prosthesis, by comparison with results obtained when these subjects were guided along the maze. G: guided subjects' errors. P: errors made with the help of the prosthesis.

Experiment 3: Human Subjects' Acquisition of Obstacle-Avoidance with the Ultrasonic Prosthesis

Procedure. The tests occurred during three different ses-sions taking place during or just after training. As shown in Figure 8, a large circular field of about 80 m^2 was occupied by 16 randomly positioned poles (+ 2 m high and 9 cm in diameter). During each session, subjects were asked to cross the field eight times, once from each of the eight different starting points, toward a sound source (800 Hz tones of 300 ms duration each second) located on the opposite side of the obstacle field. Time spent for crossing as well as number of fallen and grazed poles was recorded. In this test, 13 blind subjects were included (six early and seven late blind, male and female, aged from 12 to 54).

Results. To measure subjects' performance in this test, a score index was defined as the total number of positioned poles minus the number of fallen poles and minus half the number of

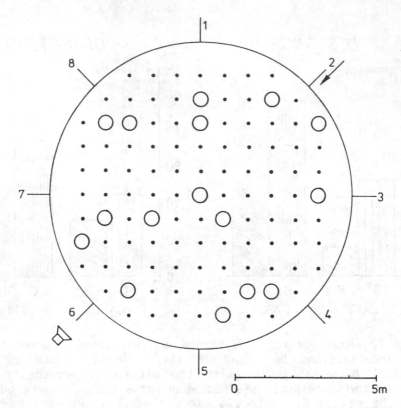

Figure 8.   Outline of the obstacle field.   The large circle indicates its boundaries.   The 8 starts are labeled by numbers;
corresponding goals, provided with a sound emitter, are at the
opposite end of a diameter.   Poles (2 m length and 9 cm diameter)
were randomly raised at 16 positions, marked by small circles,
among 109 possible locations indicated by dots.   Crossing duration corresponded to the time spent inside boundaries of the
obstacle-field.

grazed poles during the crossing, divided by the crossing duration measured in seconds.   Results are shown in Figure 9, in
which the mean score reached in each session by each group of
blind subjects is plotted against session number.   In both groups,
score value increased from earlier to later sessions.   Late blind
subjects' mean scores remained always above those of early blind,
but this difference tended to decrease with time.

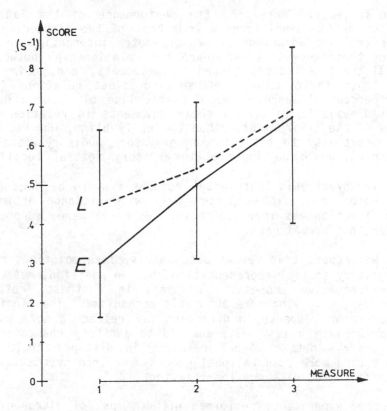

Figure 9. Mean scores obtained by early (E) and late (L) blind subjects during obstacle field crossings measured during three consecutive moments taking place during or just after training to the use of the ultrasonic prosthesis. One standard deviation is figured in relation to each score.

DISCUSSION

     In this research, factors have been studied that may influence spatial localization by human subjects without vision. Among these, spatial extent (near space, locomotor space), amount of early visual experience, use of an ultrasonic prosthesis, influence of training with the prosthesis, and response modalities (verbal or motor, direction or distance evaluation) were considered.

     Firstly, auditory spatial localization in direction and in distance has been investigated, in the near space, as a function of amount of visual experience and type of response. Early blind subjects performed less accurately than sighted subjects or late blind subjects.   Moreover, the performance of the late blind did not differ significantly from that of the sighted.   Sighted observers take advantage of sensory-motor interactions occurring during their movements and learn the relationships between non-visual characteristics, linked to movements, and their visible effects on their network of self-to-object relations (17,23). This perceptual learning would enable late blind or blindfolded sighted subjects to update their movements in relation to features of the environment.   Thus the early blind, who had not had the opportunity to establish intersensory auditory-visual relationships, would be impaired in auditory spatial localization.

The hypothesis that verbal responses would be more accurate than motor ones was supported only with distance estimations. When direction was involved, motor responses were, surprisingly, better than verbal ones.

We propose that verbal assessments, like pointing, refer to an auditory spatial representation, but in addition, reflect some higher cognitive process.   Pointing, in contrast, reflects a motor map, involving more automatic mechanisms.   The finding of a better motor response in direction may reflect a more automatic performance in a task well adapted to auditory characteristics. Similarly, a better verbal response in distance could be the result of a more computational process required by the inadequacy of audition for distance localization.

When experiments performed with the use of ultrasonic prosthesis are considered, one question is whether such patterns of auditory spatial localization are preserved, or even enhanced, if silent targets are artificially "sonarized" by the prosthesis.

In our results, distance evaluation by verbal and motor responses was better with the prosthesis than with the sound source even before training.   This is not surprising considering the choice of distance coding of the prosthesis.   If we consider direction estimations, verbally recorded results lead to different conclusions than pointing results.   Indeed, motor performance obtained with the prosthesis before learning was always poorer than that for sound localizations and remained poorer or became similar to sound localization after training.   For verbal responses, on the contrary, performance with the prosthesis was worse than for sound localization before learning but after, became better than performance in sound localization for both groups of subjects.   These differences, related to the kind of response, encourage us to speculate that such improvements in verbal performances could extend, by further extensive use, to similar improvements in motor performance.

The last two tasks concerned locomotor space. The first of these tasks consisted of landmark localization. In contrast to the test in near space, where distance and direction parameters could be separately evaluated by verbal and by motor responses, clear dichotomy between direction and distance could not be made. Hence, we chose to ask our subjects to orient the body (motor action) to face the estimated landmark position. This body orientation does not constitute the complete motor response in direction but only its first component (15) which would be followed by a locomotion phase.

The main result consisted of the poor spatial representation of early blind subjects by comparison with sighted and late blind subjects, whose performance was more or less similar. Such deficits in early blind space perception have been previously reported by others (4,7,9,17,23). When blind subjects used the ultrasonic prosthesis in this task, their performance improved. It must be emphasized that here, in contrast to tests in near space, the task did not consist of localizing a silent landmark "sonarized" by the prosthesis, but rather of gaining spatial information about landmarks lying along a route. As a result, knowledge of spatial organization of this route should be improved, since during exploration of routes using the ultrasonic prosthesis, subjects could get some external feedback of the effects of their movement. This feedback could result from frequent opportunities to update their position with respect to various particularities of the explored space (presence of a wall, approaching of a landmark, etc.). Blind people in natural conditions lack such external references, and accordingly rely on self-references or movement memory, as stressed by Millar (14).

In our opinion, this first task in the space of locomotion mainly involved spatial representation. In the second task, crossing of the obstacle field involved the concrete utilization of these spatial representations in a motor performance. Results recorded during this second task in locomotor space indicated that late blind subjects seem to calibrate their locomotion more quickly with respect to the new information given by the prosthesis. Projecting the score increase along time, we could suppose that an extensive use of this sensory aid would eventually abolish the discrepancy between the two groups of blind subjects.

A MODEL OF SENSORY SUBSTITUTION

This sensory aid detects some kind of "visual" information (mainly related to spatial localization) and, thanks to a suitable coding, transmits it to the auditory system of blind subjects.

Thus, missing visual information is substituted by auditory information. Accordingly, we generally consider the ultrasonic prosthesis to be a sensory substitution system of vision by audition.

Since sensory substitution systems may improve spatial localization by the blind, how could one optimally design these systems in order to 1) further improve spatial localization; 2) improve performance related to other visual tasks, e.g. pattern recognition; and 3) in spite of resulting design sophistications, keep learning to a minimum of length and difficulty? To address these questions, we propose the following model for sensory substitution systems.

Let us first consider the organization of sensory modalities.

Although each sensory modality has its own specific features, due to the different energies to be transduced, one is struck by the similarities in functioning and organization principles of the more central parts of these modalities, for example lateral inhibition, topographic organization, and multiple cortical representations. As an example, the visual modality is organized both serially and in parallel (see Figure 10). At the first level,

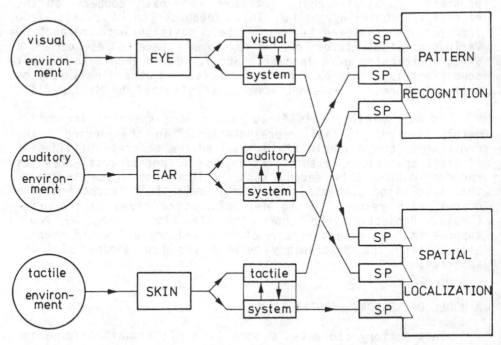

Figure 10. Three functioning levels of sensory channels. SP: channel specific parts of the perceptual modality.

light is transduced into neuronal action potentials by the retina. These signals are processed by the visual system, including the pathways between the retina and the primary visual cortex (area 17) as well as a number of visual cortical areas surrounding the primary visual cortex. It has been proposed (13) that the visual information flowing through the visual cortical areas splits into two main directions: infero-temporal and parietal cortex, supposedly corresponding to the two main perceptual functions of the visual sense, pattern recognition (what?) and spatial localization (where?).

The auditory and tactile senses seem to be organized in a similar fashion, wherein transduction and processing lead to both pattern recognition and spatial localization. We suggest that these two perceptual functions comprise first a modality-specific process, followed by an amodal symbolic level.

Keeping in mind this functional organization of sensory systems, we will precis our views concerning sensory substitution systems. Our definition of sensory substitution is more restricted than that initially proposed by Bach-y-Rita (1). Contrary to Bach-y-Rita, we propose that the neuronal mechanisms involved in sensory substitution are restricted to levels where the convergence between the different sensory systems occurs normally, i.e., at the level of the amodal perceptual systems. There is very little evidence for connections between different sensory modalities at lower levels, other than those carrying nonspecific arousal types of signals. In addition, adult plasticity at the cortical level is limited (11) to the compensation of small defects within the modality and it seems unlikely that in an adult organism one modality could massively take over afferents of another one.

A sensory substitution system (SSS) for the blind would contain an artificial visual system devoted to processing of visual information. The three levels of hierarchy (Figure 10) in the sensory modalities suggest a similar architecture for such an artificial visual system: a transducer corresponding to the eye, a decoder corresponding to the sensory processing system, and finally an interpreter corresponding to perceptual functions. Since, in our hypothesis, the neuronal convergence underlying substitution occurs at the amodal perceptual level, an optimally designed SSS should deliver at that level, but through the substitutive sensory modality (i.e., the auditory system, E in Figure 11), the same information as normally delivered by a non-impaired visual modality (D in Figure 11). In order to do so the SSS first has to generate a signal carrying this information. This is achieved by modeling as closely as possible the natural visual system. The resulting information is processed by a de-

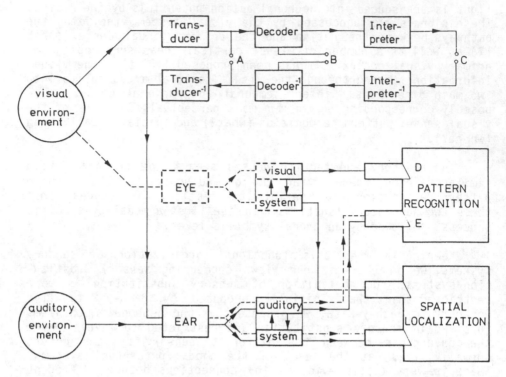

Figure 11. Model for an optimized prosthesis allowing sensory
substitution of vision by audition.

coder modeling the visual system and an interpreter modeling the
specific stage of the perceptual functions, yielding the required
signal (C in Figure 11). The second step is to carry this signal
to the amodal perceptual system through a given substitutive
modality, e.g. the auditory system. This involves modeling the
substitutive system and inverting the information flow. In this
part of the SSS, signals provided by an inverse interpreter would
be coded by an inverse decoder to be transduced into an auditory
signal, then delivered to and processed by the auditory system.
This processing will then result in detection by the ear, decoding by the auditory system, and perception according to the
modeled sensory modality. It must be emphasized that, after
each of these three processing levels, the auditory system would
reconstruct signals similar to those feeding respectively the
inverse transducer, the inverse decoder, and the inverse interpreter; i.e., finally a signal of a same level of complexity
as C in Figure 11 would be generated. As a result, the visual
prosthesis will be completely symmetrical: a model of the
impaired system is connected to an inverse model of the substitutive modality (16,21).

Such an ideal system has still to be developed. Two of the presently available aids, however, follow this symmetry principle, but with only a limited amount of modeling. In the Tactile Vision Substitution System (2), the video signal supplied by a television camera is converted into mechanical or electrical stimulation of the skin. The resolution of this system depends on the number of elements in the stimulation matrix. The connection between the two symmetrical parts of the prosthesis is at the output of the transducer (A in Figure 11). Since the visual signal is not processed in the TVSS, it is not committed to either of the two perceptual functions, and depending on the choice of the matrix it can be used either in pattern recognition tasks (1) or as a mobility aid (10). In the optophone (8) and its more recent version the stereotoner (19), the visual information is processed to a limited extent: the inclination of the line segments of letters is translated into pitch variations of sounds delivered to the auditory system. By the choice of the decoding parameter this system is committed to text reading, a limited aspect of object recognition. In this system the link between both symmetrical parts of the prosthesis is at the level of the decoder (B in Figure 11).

The ultrasonic prosthesis used to collect the observations - reported here could be assimilated to these requirements of the SSS model, even if its initial stage does not model visual information processing.

In conclusion, sensory substitution systems are potentially useful aids for blind persons: they are non-invasive, they process information on-line, they allow sensorimotor interaction with the environment and, because of their similarity to the natural sensory systems, they require minimal training. To optimize their design one should model as closely as possible the two concerned sensory systems. The more specifically this modeling is intended, the more one should distinguish between the two main functional roles of sensory systems: spatial localization and pattern recognition. With further technological developments one can hope to incorporate both functions into one prosthesis.

Of course, these long-term perspectives could be considered utopian, in view of the amount of technological, neurophysiological, and psychological research progress to be achieved before a concrete design could be made. Nevertheless, this challenge deserves to be accepted with regard to the various deprivations suffered by blind persons.

ACKNOWLEDGEMENTS

Thanks are due to Ms. C. Mehauden and to Mr. A. Buisseret, V. Ciselet, B. Englebienne, M. Michiels, F. Pequet and C. Vanbaelen who participated either in prosthesis design or in the experiments. We are very indebted to people involved in Societies for blind assistance and education. These include: Mr. C. Schepens (Ligue Braille, Belgium), Mrs. C. Hanssens, Ms. A. Evrard and C. de Mesmacker, and Mr. Van Lembergen and M. Votion (IRSA - Uccle and Woluwe, Belgium). The authors wish particularly to thank all blind persons who took part in the experiments. We are indebted to I. Richard, to Dr. J. Crémieux and Dr. E. Strelow, and to Prof. C. Eugène and G. A. Orban for fruitful discussions. We are grateful to Prof. M. Meulders, Scientific Councillor at the University of Louvain, for continuous encouragements. Thanks are also due to Mrs. L. Gomes da Silva and C. Klepper for secretarial assistance, to Mr. P. de Tiège, P. Dubrulle and J. Schouppe for technical assistance and to the staff of the Laboratory. This study was partially supported by a grant from the Ministère de la Communauté Francaise, Affaires sociales, Belgique.

REFERENCES

1. Bach-y-Rita, P. (1972). Brain Mechanisms in Sensory Substi-
    tution. New York & London: Academic Press.

2. Bach-y-Rita P., Collins, C. C., Saunders, F., White, R., &
    Scadden, L. (1969). Vision substitution by tactile image pro-
    jection. Nature, 221, 963-964.

3. Brindley, G. S. & Lewin, W. S. (1968). The sensations pro-
    duced by electrical stimulation of the visual cortex. Journal
    of Physiology (London), 196, 479-493.

4. Byrne, R. W. & Salter, E. (1983). Distances and directions in
    the cognitive maps of the blind. Canadian Journal of Psycho-
    logy, 37, 293-299.

5. Ciselet, V., Pequet, E.,Richard, I., Veraart, C., et Meulders,
    M. (1982). Substitution sensorielle de la vision par l'audi-
    tion, au moyen de capteurs d'information spatiale. Arch. int.
    Physiol. Bioch., 90, 47.

6. Dobelle, W. H., Quest, D. O., Antunes, J. L., Roberts, T. S.,
    & Girvin, J. P. (1979). Artificial vision for the blind by
    electrical stimulation of the visual cortex. Neurosurgery,
    5, 521-527.

7. Dodds, A. G., Howarth, C. I., & Carter, D. C. (1982). The
    mental maps of the blind: The role of previous visual experi-
    ence. Journal of Visual Impairment & Blindness, 76, 5-12.

8. Fournier d'Albe, E. E. (1920). The Optophone: An instrument
    for reading by ear. Nature, 105, 295-296.

9. Herman, J. F., Chatman, S. P., & Roth, S. F. (1983). Cogni-
    tive mapping in blind people: Acquisition of spatial rela-
    tionships in a large-scale environment. Journal of Visual
    Impairment & Blindness, 77, 161-166.

10. Jansson, G. (1983). Tactile guidance of movement. Interna-
    tional Journal of Neurosciences, 19, 37-46.

11. Kaas, J. H., Merzenich, M. M., & Killackey, H. P. (1983). The
    reorganization of somatosensory cortex following peripheral
    nerve damage in adult and developing mammals. Annual Review
    of Neuroscience, 6, 325-356.

12. Kay, L. (1974). A sonar aid to enhance spatial perception of the blind: Engineering design and evaluation. The Radio and Electronic Engineer, 44, 605-627.

13. Macko, K. A., Jarvis, C. D., Kennedy, C., Miyaoka, M., Shinohara, M., Sokoloff, L., & Mishkin, M. (1982). Mapping the primate visual system with [2-14] deoxyglucose. Science, 218, 394-396.

14. Millar S. (1981). Crossmodal and intersensory perception and the blind. In H. L. Pick, Jr. & R. D. Walk (Eds.), Intersensory Perception and Sensory Integration. New York: Plenum.

15. Paillard J. (1974) Le traitement des informations spatiales. In De l'espace corporel à l'espace écologique. Presses Universitaires de France.

16. Richard I., Veraart C., & Wanet M.-C. (1983). Space perception by blind subjects using an ultrasonic echo-locating prosthesis. Journal of Physiology (London), 345, 126.

17. Rieser, J. J., Lockman, J. J., & Pick, H. L., Jr. (1980). The role of visual experience in knowledge of spatial layout. Perception & Psychophysics, 28, 185-190.

18. Rieser, J. J., Guth, D. A., & Hill, E. W. (1982). Mental processes mediating independent travel: Implications for orientation and mobility. Journal of Visual Impairment & Blindness, 76, 213-218.

19. Smith, G. C. (1972). The stereotoner: A new reading aid for the blind. Proceedings of the 25th Annual Conference on Engineering and Medical Biology.

20. Stone, J. (1983). Parallel Processing in the Visual System. New York: Plenum.

21. Veraart, C., Orban, G.A., Wanet, M.-C.,& Richard, I. (1984). Design of sensory substitution systems for the blind. In P. L. Emiliani (Ed.), Rehabilitation of Visually Impaired. Dr. W. Junk Publ., The Hague.

22. Wanet, M.-C. & Veraart, C. (1984). Improvements in space coding by blind people by means of a sensory substitution system. Behavioral Brain Research, 12, 246.

23. Warren, D. H., Anooshian, L. J., & Bollinger, J. G. (1973). Early versus late blindness: The role of early vision in spatial behavior. American Foundation for the Blind Research Bulletin, 28, 191-218.

SONAR SENSORY AID AND BLIND CHILDREN'S SPATIAL COGNITION

Randolph D. Easton

Boston College

In the present report I would like to outline several findings from an empirical investigation which was conducted to assess the ability of blind school-age children to learn to use a sonar sensory aid to perceive and behave in small scale space. The particular aid we used is Leslie Kay's Trisensor (8) which is patterned after his earlier Binaural Sensory Aid (BSA). The basic principle on which these aids operate is that a small transmitter irradiates the field of view with very high frequency acoustic waves which encounter objects and surfaces in space. Reflected waves, which return to the observer as echoes, are detected by suitable transducers, and this information is transformed into an audible acoustic display which informs the user of the properties and structure of the environment. Like Kay's BSA, the Trisensor has binaural inputs from angled receivers which yield interaural differences in amplitude level which result in a sense of azimuth spatial location and movement. In addition it adds monaural information derived from a very narrow beam in front of the subject. This later design feature provides the user with high acuity information regarding objects directly ahead and was added in order to allow the Trisensor to function in a manner analogous to the dual modes of vision -- foveal and peripheral (14).

The use of sensory aids has sometimes met resistance from within the blindness community. It has been argued, for instance, that use of the aids might discourage skilled use of the remaining sensory modalities. A related concern with respect specifically to sonar sensory aid is that use of these devices might interfere with natural echo location skill (e.g., 13).

These questions have been debated for nearly three decades, but unfortunately debate alone will not answer the questions; they are empirical issues. Moreover, before these particular questions can be addressed empirically, the actual effectiveness with which the aids can be used by blind people needs to be determined. Surprisingly, little careful work has been done on the psychophysical features of sonar sensory aids (but see 3,12,17), though ample work exists on the physical/engineering features of the devices (8).

As mentioned, we initially chose to assess the ability of blind schoolage children to learn to use the Trisensor in <u>small scale space</u> (within reach). One could argue that training with a sensory aid in small scale space logically should precede training in large scale space. Developing infants are initially restricted to interacting in relatively small scale space, and only after the onset of mobility do they interact with a larger scale environment. The information processing demands of small scale space also seem less formidable than those in large scale space: An immobile observer maintains a fixed reference between the self and object as well as object-to-object relations in the small scale space. The empirical evidence regarding this issue is far from clear, however. Several studies have indicated that congenitally blind children more readily learn tasks in large scale space (reviewed in 16). Further, one study exists which demonstrates that the transfer from large to small scale space perception is easier for blind people than small to large scale space perception transfer (5). The efficiency of large scale space perception in these instances may be related to the sheer amount of afferent perceptual information generated during locomotion regarding the relation of self to the environment, information which David Lee has termed <u>exproprioception</u> (10).

Other studies in the literature, however, have not demonstrated that large scale space perception in congenitally blind children is easier than small scale space perception (e.g., 4,6). In addition, recent research conducted as part of a doctoral dissertation at Boston College suggests that both adventitiously and congenitally blind adults perform certain small scale space tasks with greater ease than large scale tasks (11). The upshot is that the issue of whether children should be <u>introduced</u> to sonar sensory aid training in large or small scale space is complicated, and in need of further empirical study.

Be this issue as it may, the study of blind children's ability to use sonar sensory aids in small scale space affords methodologically convenient opportunities to assess certain features of these sensory aids, and to assess the perceptual skills of the users. In our investigation we sought to design a study which

A.   SUBJECT CHARACTERISTICS

GROUP 1				GROUP 2		
	SEX	AGE	ETIOLOGY		SEX	AGE	ETIOLOGY
JOE	M	14	RET. BLAS.	DIANE	F	14	RLF
MIKA	M	11	CORTICAL	ANDREW	M	13	RLF
RENEE	F	10	OP. NRV.	T.J.	M	10	CORTICAL
KERRIE	F	11	RLF	JON	M	9	OPT. NRV.

B.   DESIGN OVERVIEW

GROUP 1	GROUP 2
- PRE TEST (HILL & REP/MOD/ROT)	- PRE TEST (HILL & REP/MOD/ROT)
- HAPTIC TRAINING (12 SES./6 WKS)	- TRISENSOR TRAINING (12 SES./6 WKS)
- INT TEST	- INT TEST
- TRISENSOR TRAINING (12 SES./6 WKS)	- HAPTIC TRAINING (12 SES./6 WKS)
- POST TEST	- POST TEST

Table 1: A. Subjects' age, sex, and cause of blindness. All were enrolled in public schools and had received direct service from Visuallyl Handicapped Education Specialists and Orientation and Mobility Specialists; B. Overview of Pre-Intermediate-Post test design.

would permit a) the quantitative assessment of children's ability to use the Trisensor, b) a comparison of Trisensor localization to haptic localization (since this is the principle means by which children obtain information in small scale space), and c) transfer of aid use to other perceptual-cognitive skills which do not involve use of the sensory aid.

Method

As can be seen in Table 1, our study made use of two independent groups of four congenitally blind children each (mean age = 11.5 yrs in each group). Three graduate student assistants traveled to the students' homes or schools for twice weekly, 45 min. sessions. All children were pretested without sensory aid on a battery of tests which included the Hill Performance Test of Selected Positional Concepts (7) as well as a series of perceptual/motor target localization tasks. The Hill spatial concept test required subjects to demonstrate their knowledge of spatial relations on four subtests by 1) touching body parts, 2)

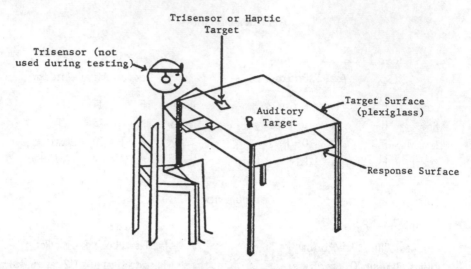

Figure 1. Testing and Training Apparatus. Top surface is used for presentation of targets; lower surface is used by subject to place a small dowel with the hand at a position which is directly beneath the perceived target position. Actual and perceived target location are readily determined by an X-Y coordinate system on each board. These values are used to compute angle and distance error.

positioning body parts, 3) positioning the body in relationship to objects, and 4) positioning objects in relation to each other. The perceptual/motor localization tests required subjects to locate natural sound sources using audition or vertical dowels using haptic exploration, and to replicate the perceived location of these targets (see Figure 1). In addition, on some of these tests subjects were required to model the targets by responding on a smaller surface 1/4 the size of the target surface, and on other trials they responded only after an imagined 90° rotation of the target surface.

After pretesting, the children began a training phase of the project: One group of subjects began haptic training while the other group began with Trisensor training. The training tasks were identical for each group except for the mode of input: Trisensor acoustic signals vs. hand/arm proprioception after free exploration. The shortest range setting of the Trisensor (2/3 m) was used in order to avoid the complicated acoustic display created by echoes returning from background clutter. All children were provided haptic feedback regarding the correctness of their responses. The first category of training involved four sessions (two 45 min. sessions per week) using Preliminary exer-

cises. These exercises involved locating with the Trisensor, or
through touch, an 18 inch tall, 1/2" dia. dowel (or two) which
was (were) placed on the top target surface. As in pretests,
subjects were required to place a small dowel directly beneath
the target dowel (see Figure 1). After completing preliminary
training the children were required to train on Intermediate
exercises. These exercises involved modeling the layout of one,
two, or three dowels on the target surface by placing a small
dowel on a response surface which was 1/4 the size of the target
surface (1 sq. ft.). In order to help teach this "scale down"
task, each trial was preceded by a trial where a subject was
presented a small response board with four or nine raised pegs.
The subjects' task was to indicate those pegs which were presented on the target surface. Again, four sessions (two weeks)
were spent on the intermediate exercises. Finally, the children
moved to Advanced exercises for an additional four sessions.
The advanced exercises entailed teaching subjects how to mentally
rotate the target surface 90° clockwise and imagine the layout of
targets in this position. One, two, or three targets were used
and the teacher asked the child to replicate an imagined rotated
array. Then, as a means of teaching, the target surface was
actually rotated so the child could experience the correct layout. The array of targets was then returned to its original
position and the child again attempted to replicate the array as
it would appear in rotated form. Feedback was provided regarding
the correct response and a new trial was begun.

    Within each category of training sessions, subjects always
began with the first exercise within the category and moved to
the next exercise only after criterion was met [two successive
trials in which the response dowel was placed within a four inch
square surrounding the target dowel (or two inch square for
modeling)]. Each day the subjects progressed as far as possible
into the series of exercises. The exercises were ordered in
terms of their apparent difficulty. Angular error and distance
error were recorded on every trial. At the beginning of each
training session a warm-up session was conducted which consisted
of replicating (haptically or with the Trisensor) a single dowel
on three trials and two dowels on a fourth trial.

    After the six-week training period all subjects again re-
ceived the battery of tests outlined above. At this point in
the project the two groups of subjects resumed training, but
those subjects who had received Trisensor training received
haptic training and vice versa. The same training regimen
of Preliminary, Intermediate, and Advanced exercises was again
administered over a six-week period. At the conclusion of the
second training period the testing battery was again administered.

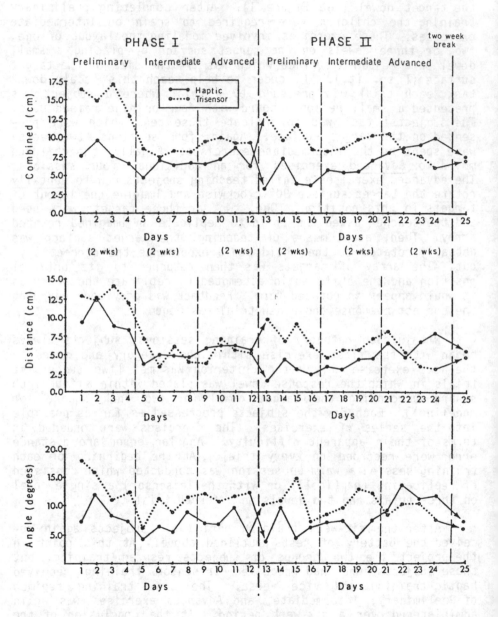

Figure 2. Absolute error in localization as a function of days (45 min) of training.

Results

     Training. Figure 2 presents the absolute error associated with single dowel trials as an index of haptic and Trisensor learning over sessions. Combined error is simply the direct distance between the target and response dowels, and can be broken into distance and angle components. Note that half-way through training the groups were switched to a different sensory input. The most noteworthy finding in these data is that while Trisensor localization was initially less accurate than haptic localization, after five or six hours of distributed practice the two input modes yielded comparable localization accuracy. This is an important finding in view of the fact that blind children rely extensively on haptic processing. In addition, the Trisensor has a potential range of some 5 m, which is well beyond reach (compared to the 2/3 m setting used in the present investigation).

     After the 12-week training was over and final testing was complete the children were each visited one last time (average two-week lapse since training ended) to assess their abilities to use the Trisensor. The data associated with day 25 in Figure 2 represent single dowel localization error using the Trisensor after two weeks (Group I) or eight weeks (Group II) without using the device. Clearly, the ability to use the aid had been retained over these time intervals.

     The Trisensor learning data in Figure 2 can be compared to somewhat analogous Trisensor training data presented in Figure 3. These data were previously obtained from six blindfolded-sighted college students (3). The students were trained with the Trisensor for 45 min. on each of five consecutive days. After a one-week interval they resumed training for four additional days.

     The data on the left side of the figure were obtained from standard localization targets which were always accompanied by haptic error feedback. The data on the right side of the figure were obtained from novel target positions used at the end of each daily training session. A comparison of the data from the children in Figure 2 and the adults in Figure 3 clearly points to the fact that our congenitally blind children learned to use the Trisensor as rapidly and accurately as sighted-but-blindfolded adults. This is particularly noteworthy since blindfolded sighted people presumably have at their disposal visual imagery or an internal visual metric onto which they can map target locations with a resultant increase in localization accuracy and precision (15). (The triangular data points connected with dotted lines in Figure

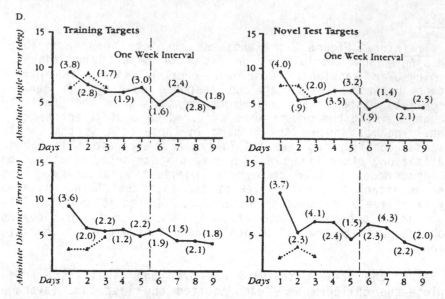

Figure 3. Localization data from six sighted-but-blindfolded adults: Absolute distance and angle error for training (feedback provided) and test (novel no-feedback) trials. The data are collapsed across 27 training trials and nine test trials that occurred each day. Standard deviations among the six subjects' means are presented parenthetically for each datum.

ABSOLUTE ERROR		# OF TARGETS	
		ONE	TWO
COMBINED	GRP 1	7.0	13.9
(CM)	GRP 2	7.5	8.3
		ONE	TWO
DISTANCE	GRP 1	5.0	7.8
(CM)	GRP 2	5.8	6.2
		ONE	TWO
ANGLE	GRP 1	6.3	10.1
(DEGREES)	GRP 2	7.5	11.7

Table 2. Trisensor localization accuracy for one versus two targets on day 25 experiment.

3 are from a 17 year-old congenitally blind woman. Her superior performance on the distance component of localization is likely attributable to the fact that she possessed perfect pitch!)

One small experiment conducted on the final assessment day of our project involved comparing localization accuracy of one vs. two targets. Table 2 presents the absolute error data associated with these conditions. (For the two target condition the error associated with each target is simply averaged.) ANOVA of the combined error index revealed that localization of the two targets was less accurate than localization of one target ($\underline{F}(1,6)$ = 3.3, $\underline{p} < .11$). (The acceptance of higher than usual $\underline{p}$ values will be discussed in a later section.) ANOVA of distance error revealed no significant effects, but ANOVA of angle error indicated poorer performance when two targets were present ($\underline{F}(1,6)$ = 6.5, $\underline{p} < .05$). Evidently, when two dowels were present the angular information provided by the Trisensor (monaural-center channel and/or binaural side channels) was more complicated and difficult to pick up or selectively attend.

An additional experiment on day 25 compared the side vs. center channel information provided by the Trisensor. Single dowels were localized with either side channel or center channel information only. (During the 12 hours of Trisensor training, of course, both channels of information had been simultaneously present.) As can be seen in Table 3, for the combined error index significantly more error was associated with the side channels than with the

ABSOLUTE ERROR		SIDE	CENTER
COMBINED	GRP 1	11.4	9.9
(CM)	GRP 2	12.7	7.8
		SIDE	CENTER
DISTANCE	GRP 1	7.2	7.9
(CM)	GRP 2	8.2	5.8
		SIDE	CENTER
ANGLE	GRP 1	12.9	8.6
(DEGREES)	GRP 2	15.7	8.5

Table 3. A comparison of side (binaural) and center (monaural) Trisensor information on day 25 experiment.

center channel ($F(1,6)$ = 5.7, p < .06). As can also be seen, the angle error associated with the side channel information caused the effect ($F(1,6)$ = 10.1, p < .02); distance perception accuracy with the side and center channels was comparable. Thus, side channel information specifying angular position provided by the Trisensor was apparently more difficult for the children to use.

It should also be noted that in this experiment, on half of the trials the target was placed before the Trisensor was activated, and on the other half of the trials the target was moved in from the periphery after the Trisensor was activated. In an earlier study performed with sighted-but-blindfolded adults we found that moving targets significantly reduced the relatively large error associated with the Trisensor side channels (3). In our study with the blind children, however, this manipulation did not have an effect (and hence the data are collapsed across this factor in Table 3). Unlike sighted adults, our congenitally blind children were unable to make use of the dynamic information created by moving targets to reduce angular error when using the Trisensor side channels.

The data from our training sessions have begun to reveal a number of important psychophysical characteristics of the Trisensor (compared to haptic input, one vs. two targets, side vs. center channels, pitch/distance vs. IAD/direction codes). Before considering these findings more generally, the results of aid training transfer to non-aid performance will be considered.

Transfer of training to non-aid performance. For purposes of the present report the effect of haptic and Trisensor training on the Hill Test of Selected Positional Concepts will not be discussed. The results have been reported in detail elsewhere (2) and will be alluded to in the discussion below.

The top panel of Table 4 contains data from the pretest which compares the ability of our subjects to replicate, model, and mentally rotate target arrays. These absolute error data are collapsed across the haptic vs. auditory and one vs. two target distinctions. As can be seen, prior to training the children performed replication and modeling of target arrays with comparable accuracy, while they experienced relatively more difficulty with the mental rotation task ($F(2,12)$ = 2.6, p < .12). (That modeling performance is comparable to replication in congenitally blind children is noteworthy, indicating that these children can "scale down" or transfer target arrays from a relatively larger scale space to a relatively smaller scale space.) In the bottom panel of Table 4, difference scores are presented based on the subject's performance of these same tasks after the entire 12-week training program was complete (both Trisensor and haptic train-

TEST ONE: ABSOLUTE COMBINED ERROR (CM)

REPLIC	MODEL	ROTATE
13.0	13.2	17.5

TEST ONE – TEST THREE: CHANGE IN ABSOLUTE COMBINED ERROR (CM)

REPLIC	MODEL	ROTATE
4.05	.73	-3.1

Table 4. Spatial Cognition tests performed without sonar sensory aid. Top panel: Localization accuracy for tests prior to training. Bottom panel: Change scores from pre to post test after all training.

CHANGE IN ABSOLUTE ERROR		TESTS 1-2		TESTS 2-3	
		HAP	AUD	HAP	AUD
COMBINED	GRP 1	.3	2.6	1.4	-.6
(CM)	GRP 2	2.2	4.7	4.1	.8
		HAP	AUD	HAP	AUD
DISTANCE	GRP 1	1.5	2.5	.7	-2.1
(CM)	GRP 2	1.3	5.3	4.2	1.0
		HAP	AUD	HAP	AUD
ANGLE	GRP 1	-3.6	.5	3.3	6.5
(DEGREES)	GRP 2	-.1	2.4	.8	-2.3

Table 5. Target replication accuracy change scores. Group I subjects received haptic training between tests 1 and 2, while Group II subjects received Trisensor training. The groups received the opposite type of training between tests 2 and 3.

ing). Since these difference scores are based on error values, positive numbers represent performance improvement. The only effect found was that replication ability had significantly improved ($\underline{t}$(7) = 3.8, $\underline{p}$ < .01), while modeling and mental rotation ability were not affected by training. Thus, the most generalized measures of perceptual/cognitive ability -- modeling and mental rotation -- were not affected by training, even though in later stages of training we made deliberate attempts to teach these skills.

The fact that the perceptual skill of target replication was affected by training is not a particularly surprising finding, since replication responding was a common component of all training exercises. When looking at this finding more closely, however, several noteworthy features become apparent. Data in Table 5 represent absolute error difference scores for phase I (tests 1-2) and phase II (tests 2-3) of the study. Recall that group I received haptic training during the first phase of the study and then transferred to Trisensor training. Group II began with Trisensor training and then transferred to haptic training. If the combined error data from group II are inspected, an interesting pattern emerges. After Trisensor training, replication of sounding auditory targets improved significantly ($t(3) = 2.9$, $p < .05$), whereas after haptic training, replication of haptic targets improved significantly ($t(3) = 1.65$, $p < .10$). It can also be seen that the effect for this group is principally located in the distance error data. While the haptic improvement is not surprising since the training and test tasks were comparable, the auditory improvement is an interesting and important effect. Evidently training with the Trisensor distance code (pitch) transferred positively to natural acoustic distance perception, the code being some complex variation of loudness (loudness alone, of course, would represent an ambiguous proximal cue to auditory distance).

Unfortunately, group I subjects do not show a similar pattern of results (even though their angle error improves significantly after Trisensor training). This pattern of differences between our Group I and II subjects was also found in other tests that we conducted but have not reported in the present paper. For example, our group II subjects improved significantly after Trisensor training on Hill's test of selected positional concepts (2).

Thus, while the rate of learning during Trisensor and haptic training was roughly comparable for these two groups of subjects (see Figure 2), they differed with respect to whether training transferred to non-sensory aid tests of spatial localization and concepts. Our group II subjects showed significant improvement on the Hill Test of spatial concepts following Trisensor training, showed a significant effect of Trisensor training on localization of natural sound sources, and improved significantly on haptic localization after haptic training. Group I did not show these effects. It seems unlikely that these effects are attributable to the particular sequence of Trisensor training followed by haptic training which group II received. In addition, teachers

were randomly assigned to children, with each teacher having at
least one child in each of the two groups. Thus it is difficult
to account for our group differences based on a teacher/group
confound. Our working hypothesis is that individual differences
play a prominent role in the successful use of sensory aids and
the assessment of their transfer to perceptual/motor tasks. A
reasonable interpretation is that the combination of motivational,
attentional, and perceptual factors contributed to the observed
effects for group II subjects. Motivation and attention span are
tremendously important variables in perception research (let
alone in work specifically with blind children), and in retrospect
it seems as though our group II children, for whatever reasons,
remained more attentive and motivated over the course of our
project.

SUMMARY AND DISCUSSION

     Our initial attempts to assess the ability of blind school-
age children have been of an exploratory, parametric nature. We
were fortunate to be able to locate eight totally blind children
in the Boston area who were free of other handicapping conditions
and whose schedules permitted participation in what proved to be
a rather lengthy and involved project. Still, our sample size is
small. Indeed, given the pilot study nature of the investigation
and the restricted sample with which we worked, several results
have been reported at non-standard levels of significance (i.e.,
p values $> .05$). The overall picture which emerges from this
project, however, seems reasonably unambiguous and interpretable.

     The finding of most importance in our project is that con-
genitally blind school-age children can learn to use the Trisensor
sonar aid to locate objects in near scale space (within reach).
They can learn to use the device for localization as accurately
as sighted-but-blindfolded college students. Furthermore, blind
children's localization accuracy with the Trisensor quickly
reaches a level comparable to their natural haptic localization
accuracy. This is an important finding given the very important
role played by haptics in the non-visually guided exploratory
activity of blind children. Additionally, it is important to
note in this context that the Trisensor can be adjusted so that
its range (within which objects are localizable) can be extended
well beyond reach, up to at least 5-6 m versus the 2/3 m setting
used in the current project. Thus, if blind children prove able
to use the aids to locate objects in large scale space they will
be able to extend their perception of the environment beyond
reach, perhaps providing sufficient advance information regarding
obstacles and perspective to facilitate the mobility process.
While the present results do not directly address the issue raised

in the introduction, whether sonar aid should be introduced in
small versus large scale space to be most effective, the findings
do point clearly to the need to assess next the effectiveness of
the Trisensor in relatively cluttered, larger spatial layouts.

Several specific results from our small scale project have
important implications for continued assessment of the aid in
more natural environments. First, we found that the children's
angular resolution of target position with the Trisensor was less
accurate when two targets were present than when one target was
present. This finding suggests that substantial training with
the aid may be necessary in more complicated, cluttered environments. We also found when that the children were provided only
binaural side channel information, angular resolution of target
position became less accurate, and moving the targets in from the
periphery failed to improve performance. In fact, performance
level for binaural-only perception of target direction was inferior to performance at the end of training when both center and
side channel information were present. In contrast to the angular
resolution results, perception of target distance was comparable
for the center vs. side channels, and was similar to the level of
error revealed at the end of training. Taken together these
results suggest that the interaural amplitude differences provided
by the Trisensor side channels represent a relatively complicated
code for direction which is somewhat more difficult to learn than
the pitch code for distance. For adults, movement of a target
apparently enhances the usability of the Trisensor IAD code, but
children continue to have difficulty using the code under moving
target conditions.

Several additional factors should be noted when considering
the relative effectiveness of the distance and direction codes of
the Trisensor. First, the IAD code for the Trisensor is very much
exaggerated compared to that used in Kay's earlier BSA, so that
objects appear too far off to the side. This design feature was
used to minimize wave interference created by the addition of the
center channels to the side channels (8). Thus without head movements one might expect users to have trouble with the cue set in
this fashion. Additionally, the side channels of the Trisensor
or BSA afford the user the opportunity to locate objects in the
periphery without head turning or scanning. Thus the issue of
the relative effectiveness of the IAD code in the Trisensor for
locating the direction of objects is complicated by several considerations and in need of further assessment (17, see also Warren
and Strelow, this volume for related comparisons of the two spatial codes).

The effects of haptic and Trisensor training on the children's more general spatial concepts and perceptual localization skill were not as clear-cut as our learning data. For one group of apparently well-motivated, attentive children, the effects of training did transfer to more general, nonsensory aid performance. While it is not surprising that haptic localization training resulted in improved haptic localization testing, these subjects also improved in their ability to locate the distance of natural sounding objects after Trisensor training. Since the codes for the spatial dimension of distance are different for the Trisensor and natural sounds, this finding represents a more general transfer of Trisensor learning. In addition, for this group of children, Trisensor training resulted in significant improvement on the Hill test of general positional concepts in blind children. Thus the effect of Trisensor training may extend beyond immediate learning to influence more abstract perceptual-motor processes which can be observed without sensory aid use. It is also important to note in this regard that our children only received 12 hours of distributed practice with the Trisensor. More extended training could result in a more valid test of the hypothesis of transfer of aid experience to perceptual-cognitive skills such as mental modeling and rotation.

The possibility that sensory aid use has beneficial effects beyond the immediate behavioral situation has many implications regarding the usefulness and suitability of these aids for visually impaired people, as well as for theoretical issues concerning sensory substitution in general (1). It may be that the Trisensor need not be regarded as a permanent visual prosthesis: Rather, a sonar sensory aid could be used in selected situations for specific tasks with a secondary consequence being the sharpening or "tuning" of other perceptual systems and of spatial conceptualization skill. Of course, for some individuals in particular situations the aid could be used more extensively and on a more permanent basis. Thus, in addition to continued assessment of these devices psychophysical characteristics (especially in large scale space), work should also be undertaken to assess blind people's preferred mode of interacting with the aids. Finally, from a theoretical point of view, research is needed to determine what the effect of extended processing of the sonar spatial layout information afforded by the Trisensor is on functional and morphological properties of the brain of a person or an animal born blind (see papers in this volume by Sonnier, Sonnier & Riesen, Strelow & Warren).

REFERENCES

1.   Bach-y-Rita, P. (1972). Brain Mechanisms in Sensory Substitution. New York: Academic Press.

2.   Easton, R. D. (1984). A quantitative evaluation of blind children's ability to use the Trisensor, a new generation sonar sensory aid. Paper delivered at the Louisville Workshop on Space Perception.

3.   Easton, R. D. & Jackson R. M. (1983). Pilot test of the Trisensor, a new generation sonar sensory aid. Journal of Visual Impairment & Blindness, 77, 446-448.

4.   Fletcher, J. F. (1982). Spatial representation in blind school children (Doctoral dissertation, University of Toronto 1981.) Dissertation Abstracts International, 42(10), 4362A.

5.   Gomulicki, B. (1961). The Development of Perception and Learning in Blind Children. Cambridge, England: The Psychological Laboratory.

6.   Herman, J. E., Herman, T. G., & Chatman, S. P. (1983). Constructing cognitive maps from partial information: A demonstration study with congenitally blind subjects. Journal of Visual Impairment & Blindness, 77, 195-198.

7.   Hill, E. W. & Hill, M.-M. (1980). Revision and validation of a test for assessing the spatial conceptual abilities of visually impaired children. Journal of Visual Impairment & Blindness, 74, 373-380.

8.   Kay, L. (1982). Spatial perception through an acoustic sonar. Christchurch, New Zealand, University of Canterbury.

9.   Kay, L. & Kay, N. (1983). An ultrasonic spatial sensor's role as a developmental aid for blind children. Transactions of the Opthamological Society of New Zealand, 35, 38-42.

10. Lee, D. N. (1978). The functions of vision. In H. L. Pick, Jr. & E. Saltzman (Eds.), Modes of Perceiving and Processing Information. New York: Lawrence Erlbaum.

11. MacWilliam, L. J. H. (1984). Relationships among five measures of survey level mental representation of space in the visually impaired. Doctoral dissertation, Boston College.

12. Rowell, D. (1970). <u>Auditory Display of Spatial Information</u>. Unpublished Doctoral Dissertation, University of Canterbury, Christchurch, New Zealand.

13. Supra, M., Cotzin, M. E., & Dallenbach, K. M. (1944). Facial vision: The perception of obstacles by the blind. <u>American Journal of Psychology</u>, 57, 133-183.

14. Trevarthen, C. B. (1968). Two mechanisms of vision in primates. <u>Psychologische Forschungen</u>, 31, 299-337.

15. Warren, D. H. (1970). Intermodality interactions in spatial localization. <u>Cognitive Psychology</u>, 1, 114-133.

16. Warren, D. H. (1977). <u>Blindness and Early Childhood Development</u>. New York: American Foundation for the Blind.

17. Warren, D. H. & Strelow, E. R. (1984). Learning spatial dimensions with a visual sensory aid: Molyneux revisited. <u>Perception</u>, 13, 331-350.

ACKNOWLEDGEMENTS

The research described in this report has been funded in part by a National Eye Institute grant (1 R01 EY04907-01) to principle investigators Randolph D. Easton and Richard M. Jackson. Other members of the research group include Research Associates Billie Louise Bentzen and Gary Snyder, and the children's graduate-student-teachers Sarah Stanton, Sandra Kruskel, and Tom Sullivan.

SPATIAL AWARENESS TRAINING OF BLIND CHILDREN USING THE TRISENSOR

Garry Hornby,* L. Kay,** M. Satherley,* N. Kay**

*New Zealand Psychological Service
**University of Canterbury

Improving the spatial awareness of blind children has obvious consequences for their later development of mobility skills and other areas of independent functioning. The use of ultrasonic spatial sensors for training spatial awareness in blind children has been a matter of considerable interest and research (1,5,10). Past investigators have been constrained to use binaural spatial sensors for such training, and there has been considerable debate as to their suitability for this purpose (3,6,9). Recently, a more highly developed ultrasonic spatial sensor has become available for experimentation. This device, called a trinaural sensor, or Trisensor has, in addition to the binaural channels, a high resolution central monaural channel (7, see also Kay, this volume).

The functioning of the Trisensor is in some respects analo-gous to that of foveal and peripheral visual systems, with the central channel modeling the high resolution capacity of the fovea and the side channels detecting objects or movement in the peripheral field (7). Evidence that the Trisensor does indeed function in this way has been provided by a pilot study conducted with blindfolded college students (4). This study also lent support to the claim that the effectiveness of the Trisensor has been increased by adding high resolution monaural information to the binaural feedback provided by previous devices.

In a pilot study, conducted with school-age blind children, data were collected which suggested that the Trisensor could be used to carry out various tasks involving spatial location, orientation, and transfer while seated at a table (8).

Subject	Sex	Age (years)	I.Q.	Onset of blindness	Diagnosis
Caren	F	7.9	81 - 91	Approx. 5 years	Glaucoma and Retina- blastoma
Trish	F	8.8	104 - 114	Birth	Optic nerve hypoplasia
Mary	F	10.3	73 - 83	Birth	Bilateral Retrolental Fibroplasia
James	M	10.11	104 - 114	Approx. 2 years	Congenital Glaucoma
Linda	F	11.6	65 - 75	Birth	RE- Retinal detachment LE - Micro- opthalmic & cataract
Sam	M	12.6	55 - 65	Birth	Congenital ocular deformity

Table 1. Relevant characteristics of the six subjects.

This paper presents the findings from a further, more intensive, study in which six school-age totally blind children, of
various ages and levels of intellectual functioning, undertook a
spatial awareness training programme using the Trisensor. The
programme consisted of 40 exercises involving spatial location,
discrimination, identification, and transfer tasks carried out
at a table and moving around the classroom. The aim of the study
was to determine whether blind children of various ages and
ability levels could learn to perform a variety of spatial tasks
using the Trisensor. Also of interest was whether the children's
ability to use the Trisensor at the table would transfer to tasks

in which it was necessary to move around the room and whether undergoing a series of exercises with the Trisensor would improve performance in spatial orientation tasks carried out without the Trisensor.

EMPIRICAL WORK

Method

   Subjects. Details of relevant subject characteristics are provided in Table 1. The children's ages at the start of the project ranged from 7 to 12 years, and their IQ (WISC verbal) ranged from 60 to 109. Four of the children were congenitally blind, while the other two lost their vision as pre-schoolers. All of the children were classified as being totally blind.

   Procedure. The project was conducted in a classroom, of size approximately 20 feet by 20 feet, which was set aside for the purpose. The children were withdrawn from their class pro- grammes for two 1/2 hour sessions per week for Trisensor train- ing. The project was carried out over a period of 9 months during which each child received approximately 35 hours of train- ing. The programme was conducted by two teachers who themselves had received training in the use of the Trisensor. The two teachers and the first author had previously spent two weeks with Professor Leslie Kay at the University of Canterbury gaining ex- perience with the Trisensor and developing the Trisensor Training Manual (2).

   The Trisensor Training Manual contains 40 exercises on spa- tial orientation, transfer, and discrimination (See Appendix 1). The first 20 exercises are conducted with the children seated at a desk using the table model of the Trisensor. The second 20 exercises are carried out with the children using the portable Trisensor. This model takes the form of a helmet which has all the electronics and battery installed within it.

   The first series of seven exercises is designed to teach object distance and direction codes. In Exercise 7 the children have to locate wooden rods placed on the table in various posi- tions and place a small rope circle over them. Exercises 8 to 11 are spatial transfer tasks, in which the children copy the pat- tern of rods placed on the table onto a small pegboard placed directly in front of them. The following two exercises concern the enumeration of up to eight rods placed on an arc in front of them.

Exercises 14 through 17 involve the discrimination and identification of different objects such as single and multiple rods and various textured surfaces. Exercises 18 through 20 are simple games designed to reinforce distance and direction codes. For example, Exercise 18 involves the children in building a block tower. Every time a block is put in place the tower is moved so that the child has to relocate it using the Trisensor before placing another block.

The second set of 20 exercises, which are conducted using the portable Trisensor, include some tasks which are simply replications of exercises carried out at the table and others which are mobility-type tasks. Exercises 21 to 27 are replications of Exercises 1 to 7 except that the children are standing up and using the portable Trisensor to detect large free-standing metal poles. In Exercise 27 the children have to locate the position of and walk directly toward a pole, placing the rope ring over it with one arm movement.

Exercise 28 involves discriminating between poles and wall boards in preparation for the introduction of several exercises involving wall boards. In Exercises 29 and 30 the children are taught to judge distances from wall boards, and in particular to recognise a "Halt" position, a safe distance from a solid surface. Exercises 31 through 34 involve the enumeration of up to 8 poles on an arc while standing still, or in a straight line while walking past them. The following two exercises require the children to walk through openings between two poles and then between two wall boards. Exercises 37 through 40 involve the discrimination and identification of different objects, including single and multiple poles and wall boards with different surface textures.

Experimental Design and Data Collection

A single-subject research design was used along with a pre- and post-test of spatial orientation. This methodology was employed because of the difficulties in establishing a control group due to the small number of totally blind subjects available for study (11).

Spatial orientation pre-post test. A simple test was designed by a mobility instructor to assess the children's spatial orientation prior to and following their involvement in the programme. The test required the children to walk between a table, a desk, and a chair which were set out in an isosceles triangle formation with equal sides of length 3 m and a hypotenuse side of approximately 4 m. It involved nine tasks in which the children were asked to walk from one piece of furniture to another given only instructions such as "Walk straight ahead and find the

desk. Then turn left and walk straight ahead to the chair."
Also included were four tasks in which children were seated at
the table and asked to represent the orientation of the chair,
table, and desk using magnetic tape. Each task was scored as
either correct or incorrect by both Trisensor teacher and mobility
instructor, giving a maximum score of 13. In the case of any disagreement between observers the response was scored as incorrect.

Single subject design. Data was collected on the children's
performance at all times during the programme. At least three
baseline measurements were taken for each of the exercises before
training was begun. The children were not given any guidance or
feedback on their results during baseline training.

A multiple-baseline design was used in the first seven exercises to determine if transfer of learning would occur on these
basic exercises involving distance and direction codes.

A series of 10 trials was used for each exercise during
each session in which it was administered. This enabled a score
out of a maximum of 10 to be computed which could then be displayed on a graph.

In the treatment phase, children were scored on each trial,
then given feedback on the accuracy of their response. If incorrect, they were then trained in the appropriate movements
required to obtain a correct response. Following this the next
trial was administered and the process repeated. Treatment
sessions for each exercise were administered until a criterion
level of performance was reached. For most exercises this was
100%, but for some exercises this level of accuracy was unrealistic and a lower criterion was established.

Results and Discussion

Single subject design. The data collected during each exercise are presented in Figures 1, 2 and 3. Complete data are
presented for one child, Mary. Data are also presented on the
average performance of all six children.

Figure 1 presents the children's performance on the first
seven exercises. For 6 out of the 7 exercises there was considerable learning during baseline, suggesting that the children
were improving in their use of the Trisensor simply by having
experience with it. Exercise 2, in which no improvement occurred
during baseline, involves learning the pitch-distance code. This
indicates that associating a high pitch with a distant object and
a low pitch with a near object is arbitrary and must be taught.
The direction code involved in Exercise 3 was learned during
baseline.

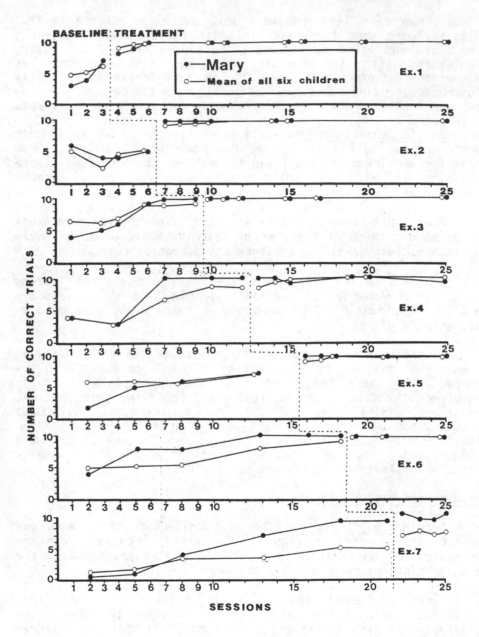

Figure 1. Results for one child and the average of all six children on the first seven table exercises involving the learning of distance and direction codes.

Once Exercise 2 was taught an immediate improvement was seen in Exercise 4 which involves both distance and direction codes. This, and the improvement during baseline in Exercises 5, 6, and 7, suggests that there was considerable transfer of learning among the various tasks. Once teaching was begun on each of the 7 exercises it took a maximum of 3 sessions before a satisfactory criterion of performance was reached. This criterion was set at 100% for the first six exercises and 75% for Exercise 7, which was a more difficult task.

Figure 2 presents the results of the children's performance on Exercises 8 through 17. Exercises 8 through 11 were learned relatively easily, showing that children could be taught to transfer spatial configurations of up to three rods, using the Trisensor, from a large board on the table to a small pegboard directly in front of them. The children achieved a high degree of accuracy when counting up to four rods in Exercise 12 but had more difficulty enumerating up to eight rods in Exercise 13. Findings from Exercises 14 through 17 indicate that the children quickly learned to discriminate and identify different objects and surface textures.

No data were collected on Exercises 18 through 20, which were simple games designed to reinforce distance and direction codes. However, the children did not enjoy taking part in the game as much as the other more formal exercises, a finding contrary to expectations.

Figure 3 presents the results of Exercises 21 through 40, which were carried out using the portable Trisensor. The high level of performance achieved, in baseline, on Exercises 21 through 27, which are replications of Exercises 1 through 7, indicates that the skills learned by the children on these table exercises transferred to their use of the portable Trisensor when standing.

The high level of performance attained in Exercises 29 and 30 suggests that the distance code learned at the table had transferred to the children's judgements of their distances from wall boards.

The children found enumerating poles that were set out on an arc, as in Exercises 31 and 32, more difficult than counting them as they walked past a line of poles, in Exercises 33 and 34.

Children needed little teaching to be able to walk through openings between two poles (Exercise 35) or between two wall boards (Exercise 36), following their previous experience with the Trisensor.

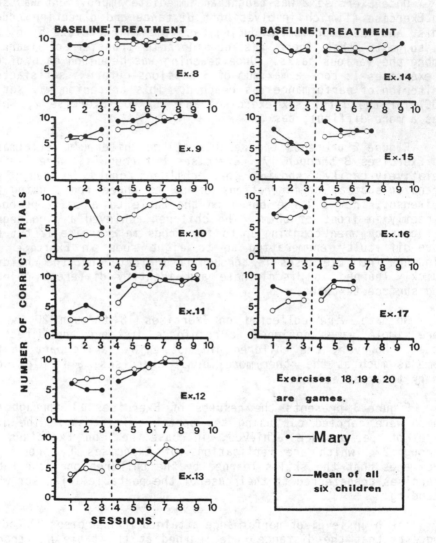

Figure 2. Results of the second series of table exercises involving spatial transfer, discrimination, and object enumeration.

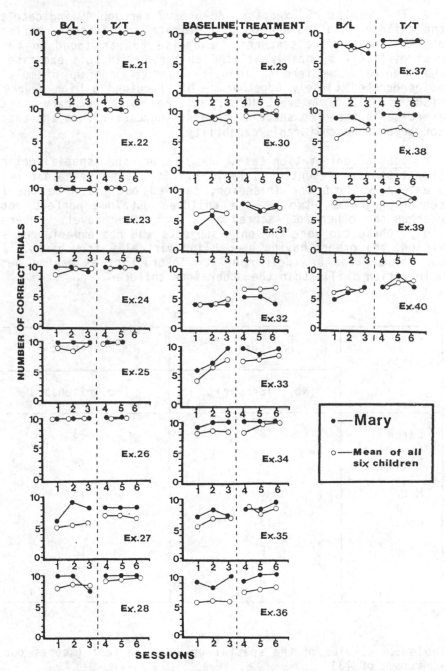

Figure 3. Results of the 20 exercises using the portable Trisensor to carry out spatial orientation, discrimination, and enumeration tasks.

The results of Exercises 28 and 37 through 40 indicate that the children had learned to discriminate and identify different objects and surface textures. Exercise 38 was found to be the most difficult by nearly all the children. In this exercise the children were required to identify objects made up of multiple poles bunched closely together. This required a high degree of discrimination. However, Helen attained 100% accuracy on this exercise in three consecutive trials, suggesting that the task is not beyond the children's capability.

Spatial orientation test. Results of the spatial orientation test are presented in Table 2. It can be seen that on the pre-test, without the Trisensor, carried out prior to the Trisensor programme, two of the children obtained perfect scores whereas the other four scored at a much lower level. Interestingly, these two were the only subjects who had experienced some vision, the others having been blind virtually from birth. They were also rated by their mobility instructors as having better orientation skills than the other four children.

Subject	Pre-test	Post-test
	(No Trisensor)	(No Trisensor)
Caren	13	13
Trisha	4	8
Mary	6	13
James	13	13
Linda	5	12
Sam	3	8

Table 2. Results of the spatial orientation test (scores out of a maximum of 13)

A post-administration of the spatial orientation test, without the Trisensor, was carried out in the month following completion of the Trisensor programme. The two children with perfect scores on the pre-test again obtained perfect scores. The others substantially improved their performance, in all four cases achieving at least twice as many items correct during the post-test than in the pre-test. This finding suggests that the spatial orientation of these four children had improved following undertaking the Trisensor programme. Since it was not possible to have a control group of blind children to whom the spatial orientation test was administered pre and post, but who did not undertake the Trisensor programme, the above results must be treated with caution. The findings from the spatial orientation test may be regarded as suggestive of positive changes, but a more rigorous experimental methodology needs to be employed before a definitive statement can be made.

CONCLUSION

The six blind children in this study successfully completed all 40 exercises in the training programme and thereby demonstrated their ability to use the Trisensor in a variety of spatial orientation, spatial discrimination, and spatial transfer tasks.

The data indicate that skills learned from the table exercises were transferred to later tasks carried out with the children moving around the room using the portable Trisensor.

Furthermore, results from the spatial orientation test suggest that the children may have improved in their spatial orientation (without the Trisensor) as a consequence of undertaking the programme. The implication of this finding is that the Trisensor may well have an important role to play in programmes designed to develop spatial awareness in blind children.

ACKNOWLEDGEMENTS

The authors wish to thank the following people for their assistance in conducting the project:

Steve Bellamy, Joan Speight, Lorraine Hutcheson, Adrian Pole, Tom Rogerson, and the staff of Homai College for the Blind; Mike Cusdin and Lyn Buttle of Canterbury University; Geoff Gibbs, Don McKenzie and Terry Small of the Royal New Zealand Foundation for the Blind; Don Brown of the Department of Education; and Carol Cunningham of Auckland Teachers College.

Funding for the project was provided by: the International Year of Disabled Persons - Telethon Trust; and the Royal New Zealand Foundation for the Blind.

REFERENCES

1. Aitken, S. & Bower, T. G. R. (1982). Use of the Sonicguide
    in infancy. Journal of Visual Impairment & Blindness, 76,
    91-100.

2. Bellamy, S., Hornby, G., & Satherley, M. (1984). Trisensor
    Training Manual: A Programme of Spatial Orientation, Trans-
    fer and Discrimination Training for Blind Children.   Auck-
    land: Auckland: Homai College for the Blind.

3. Bower, T. G. R. (1977).   Blind babies see with their ears.
    New Scientist, 73, 255-257.

4. Easton, R. D. & Jackson, R. M. (1983). Pilot test of the
    Trisensor, a new generation sonar sensory aid. Journal of
    Visual Impairment & Blindness, 77, 446-449.

5. Ferrell, K. A. (1980). Can infants use the Sonicguide? Two
    years' experience of project VIEW.   Journal of Visual
    Impairment & Blindness, 74, 209-220.

6. Kay, L. (1984). Learning to use the ultrasonic spatial sen-
    sor by the blind infant: Comments on Aitken and Bower.
    Journal of Experimental Child Psychology, 37, 207-211.

7. Kay, L. & Kay, N. (1983). An ultrasonic spatial sensor's
    role as a developmental aid for blind children. Trans-
    actions of the Opthalmological Society of New Zealand, 35,
    38-42.

8. Kay, L., Kay, N., & Hornby, G. (1984) The role of a high
    resolution spatial sensor in an educational setting. Journal
    of Visual Impairment & Blindness, 78, 260-262.

9. Kay, L. & Strelow, E. R. (1977). Blind babies need special-
    ly designed aids. New Scientist, 73, 709-712.

10. Strelow, E. R. (1983). Use of the Binaural Sensory Aid by
    young children.   Journal of Visual Impairment & Blindness,
    77, 429-438.

11. Van Hasselt, V. B. & Hersen, M. (1981). Applications of
    single-case designs to research with visually impaired
    individuals.   Journal of Visual Impairment & Blindness, 75,
    359-362.

APPENDIX 1

Trisensor Training Exercises
(For a more comprehensive description see 2).

1. Perceiving whether a vertical 60 cm wooden rod is or is not on the table in front of the child.

2. Perceiving whether the rod is far away or near to the child.

3. Perceiving whether the rod is on the left or right side of the child.

4. Perceiving whether the rod is far or near, and left or right. For example, "far away on the left."

5. Discriminating whether there are one or two rods on the table in front of the child.

6. Determining which of two rods on the table is nearer to the child, the one on the left or the one on the right.

7. Locating a rod on the table by placing a small rope circle over it. The rod is placed in various predetermined positions within the child's reach on the table.

8. Copying the position of a rod placed in one of four positions (far, near, left, right) on the table, on a small pegboard directly in front of the child.

9. Copying the positional pattern of two rods, placed in a large pegboard on the table, onto a small pegboard placed directly in front of the child.

10. Copying the positional pattern of three rods placed in triangular formations from the large to the small pegboard.

11. Copying the pattern of three rods placed in straight line formation from the large to the small pegboard.

12. Counting correctly from one to four rods placed on an arc of radius 75 cm in front of the child. Minimum separation of radius 30 cm.

13. Correctly counting from five to eight rods on an arc of radius 75 cm, with a minimum separation of 15 cm.

14. Discriminating between a single rod and stands with three or five rods bunched together.

15. Identifying a single rod, a three-rod stand, and a five-rod stand.

16. Discriminating among five surface textures attached to cylinders placed on the table in front of the child. The textures used were: Carpet; sandpaper; woodchip; corrugated cardboard; smooth plastic.

17. Identifying the above five surface textures.

18. Building a block tower by locating the blocks by means of the Trisensor and placing another block on top. The tower is moved to another location and the process is repeated.

19. Similar to Exercise 18. The child locates a block tower with the Trisensor, then attempts to place another block on top.

20. This game requires two players, both wearing Trisensors and seated at a circular table at approximately 75° to one another. The aim is to build a block tower as in the previous two exercises. But this time the two players compete in reaching for the block tower and attempt to place their block on top before the other player.

21. Perceiving whether a 2 m vertical metal pole is or is not on the floor, in front of the chld.

22. Perceiving whether the pole is far away or near to the child.

23. Perceiving whether the pole is on the left or right side of the child.

24. Perceiving whether the pole is far or near, and left or right. For example, "far away on the right."

25. Discriminating whether one or two poles are in front of the child on the floor, out of reach.

26. Determing which of the two poles is nearer to the child, the one on the left or the one on the right.

27. Locating the position of a pole on the floor, using the Trisensor. Walking directly toward the pole and placing a small rope ring over it with one arm movement.

28. Discriminating between a pole and a wall board.

29. Determining which of two wall boards placed vertically facing each other, 4 cm apart, is nearer to the child when the child is placed in various positions between the boards.

30. Determining a safe distance from a wall board when placed various distances from the board. In this way recognizing the safe-distance or "Halt" position.

31. Correctly counting from one to four poles placed on an arc of 2 m radius. Minimum separation of poles is 1 m.

32. Correctly counting from five to eight poles placed on an arc of 2 m radius. Minimum separation of poles of 50 cm.

33. Correctly counting from five to eight poles (minimum separation 50 cm) placed in a straight line, while walking past them.

34. Correctly counting from one to four poles (minimum separation 1 m) placed in a straight line, while walking past them.

35. Walking through a 75 cm opening between two poles without touching them.

36. Walking through a 75 cm opening between two wall boards without touching them.

37. Discriminating between a single pole and stands with three or five poles bunched together.

38. Identifying a single pole and three and five pole stands.

39. Discriminating among four surface textures, attached to wall boards, placed at right angles to each other, 2 m apart and 2 m from the child. The textures used were: A smooth wooden surface (gloss painted); a rough surface (brick veneer); a corrugated surface (wood panel); and a soft surface (carpet).

40. Identifying the above four surface textures.

SENSORY SUBSTITUTION IN BLIND CHILDREN AND NEONATES

Edward R. Strelow and David H. Warren

University of California, Riverside

In this paper we will examine the goals and strategies of developmental research using sensory aids. Considering how little is understood about the use of spatial sensors in adults, it may seem surprising that there has been any substantial amount of research with blind children and infants. However, as this paper and others in this volume make clear, developmental studies are a major part of current sensory aid research.

There are many reasons why one should be concerned with the remediation of the effects of blindness in children with sensory aids. The blind child's lifestyle has many unsatisfactory features, particularly due to limited independent mobility. It is also widely felt in rehabilitation circles that the behavioral deficits associated with problems such as blindness should be remedied early in life to prevent a cumulation of effects later in life. However, more generally the interest in developmental research with sensory aids reflects a strong orientation which has existed in psychological research for several years towards the understanding of developmental processes. Developmental sensory aid research has proceeded as much from a concern for understanding the nature of developmental processes as for the remediation of blindness (see Muir, Humphreys, Dodwell & Humphreys, this volume). In our own research, this interest with the underlying processes of development has led us to the use of animal research models in order to gain more precise experimental control over the early experience of neonates, and in order to investigate the impact of sensory substitution on neural development (see Sonnier and Sonnier & Riesen, this volume).

Effects of Blindness in Children

Children who are born nearly or totally blind show problems of general development, as well as more specific problems of spatial ability. The intellectual development of blind children is highly variable, ranging from above normal to grossly retarded (see 19 for a general review). While brain damage is frequently diagnosed or suspected in these latter cases; problems of serious developmental delay may occur even when there is no problem other than blindness (6). Space perception in particular shows a consistent pattern of disability into adulthood, irrespective of the extent of general disability, which is more severe the earlier the onset of blindness (19-21).

These difficulties with spatial activities severely limit the lifestyle of blind children especially as regards independent mobility. While there is limited data on this aspect of their development, Table 1, based on responses from parents of New Zealand children in a study by Strelow (15), illustrates the 'closeted' lifestyle of the school-age blind children in this study who even by the age of 10 were not managing even simple outdoor spatial activities around their own homes.

The Role of Electronic Spatial Sensors

Electronic devices, capable of remotely sensing objects in space and displaying this information to the blind, could potentially both assist independent mobility and reduce developmental delays due to problems of understanding space. Regular use might take place in a way analogous to the use of a hearing aid for the deaf. We are not yet in a position to achieve this goal, although the long-term prospects appear promising. Several types of sensors for the blind have been produced and several generations of particular technologies have appeared. As well, the considerable engineering and computer science interest in devising visual-type sensors (1) may, when applied to the problem of spatial sensing by the blind, lead to even greater advances. However, even if much improved technology were to become available, it is evident from the research which has taken place already, with adults and children, that the psychological issues raised by the use of these devices are far more difficult than occur in the use of hearing aids, and will require a great deal of examination.

The Perceptual Psychology of Artificial Sensors

Unlike a hearing aid, a spatial sensor poses major problems of learning and use. Whereas a hearing aid merely amplifies existing natural sounds, a spatial sensor creates novel, artificial stimuli. These represent environmental information in a manner with which the blind user is not initially familiar and the

	Debra (7)	Anton (8)	James (10)
Early Development			
Age of unsupported standing	14 (months)	18	11
Walk three steps	14	20	12
Walk across room	36	24	13
Lifestyle			
% time typically spent			
Indoors	80-100%	60-80%	40-60%
In yard or outbuildings	0-20%	20-40%	40-60%
Outside at yard	0-20%	0-20%	0-20%
% time child can be relied on to get to places:			
In the home	80-100%	80-100%	80-100%
In yard or outbuildings	0-20%	80-100%	80-100%
To places in the neighborhood	0-20%	0-20%	0-20%
Special routes known	-None	-to letter box	-to letter box -driveway to road -schoolgate to classroom

Table 1. Survey of school age children's mobility and perceptual-motor development based on parents' reports (15). Age of children ay time of study is in brackets.

concepts of space they present may be difficult to grasp because young blind users in particular have difficulty relating to spatial concepts (9,17,19-21).

In another paper in this volume (Warren & Strelow) we point out that there are many unknowns about how training should best take place with the binaural sensory aid.   These experiments trained blindfolded sighted adults to be sensitive to dimensions of the display signals and to learn what these signals correspond to in the external world.   This meant teaching the user to discriminate pitch, direction, and timbre, the stimuli respectively for distance, direction, and surface characteristics in this device, and secondly teaching what particular display stimuli indicate about properties of objects in the external world.   Because the subjects were blindfold-sighted college students, we avoided the problems created by the lack of perceptual-motor skill and spatial understanding which we would encounter with the blind, and particularly with blind children (9,19,21).   However, we obtained findings which indicate that some apparently reasonable practices of device training are probably not effective. The training of congenitally blind children, in all likelihood, poses even more difficult problems.

Problems of Training the Use of Spatial Sensors by the Blind

Many of the conceptual or physical skills required for sensing the environment by an electronic spatial sensor are poorly developed in blind children.   Sighted persons generally have no trouble maintaining an erect head position, or turning their heads to look at different locations.   However, a blind child may hold his or her head to one side or have a problem of body posture which interferes with both head turning and puposeful locomotion. If, for example, the sensor points down to the ground or to the side because of such a physical problem, no useful signals may be received as the person attempts to walk through the environment and the sensor will be useless.

Nor can an artificial means of display of space be easily comprehended unless the user already has a general understanding of the characteristics of spatial layout.   Such understanding can be assumed with sighted subjects and some blind adults, but younger children show deficiencies ranging from a lack of knowledge of the detail of the spatial environment to fundamental problems of body image (9).   Thus in dealing with younger subject populations we face the problem not just of teaching the sensor, but of dealing with a range of spatial problems over and above what would be encountered with blindfolded-sighted and even blind adults.   Just as poor head control can interfere with a subject's ability to obtain suitable signals from a sensor, lack of understanding of the environment can interfere with learning the relations between the display signals and the external objects that they specify.

Motivation of the blind child is also a major problem The college student will perform most tasks required by experimenters with reasonable grace. The adult blind may also have a strong motivation to learn the use of a sensor if, for example, there is a need to improve mobility in order to take a job. However, the blind infant or child is not likely to recognize the need for enhanced spatial sensing in his or her own life, nor be very amenable to the goal of collecting research data for its own sake.

Finally, nearly all age groups of the blind will have established perceptual-motor skills relevant to device use. If sensor use involves a change in these skills, there may be resistance to the new skills required for artificial sensing unless these skills relate closely to previous abilities. The blind adult may be used to particular techniques such as the use of echo cues and may resist the use of alternate cues. The blind child may instead be inattentive to spatial tasks in general. While the very young infant is without such effects of prior experience, he or she on the other hand lacks the basic perceptual-motor skills needed for tasks involving more than rudimentary device use.

Table 2 outlines several of the problems of training various subjects with spatial sensors. All groups face similar problems of learning the basic characteristics of the sensors and the correspondence between display signals and spatial objects. However, blind subjects face very much greater problems of motivation, spatial understanding, and perceptual-motor skill.

Research with Blind School-age Children

We will consider first the problems of children in the primary school age bracket, i.e., roughly 5-12 years of age. Several approaches to training have been tried by ourselves and others. Generally, it has not been difficult to show that school-age blind children can perform a variety of tasks with sensors; however, going beyond these preliminary efforts to the provision of practical training programs has proven difficult and at this time there is no clear rationale for one particular approach over another.

There are many questions about training that are currently unanswered: For example, how should training be started: Should one first teach sensitivity to the dimensions of the display, and its spatial correspondences, or instead concentrate on improving underlying skills such as head control? How should specific training tasks fit into an overall program to ensure that all important aspects of device use are covered? There is, for ex-

Aspects of skill in the use of Electronic Spatial Sensors	Subject Group			
	blindfold -sighted adult	blind adult	blind child	blind infant
differentiation of sensory dimensions of display	problem	problem	problem	problem
correspondence between display signals and spatial objects	problem	problem	problem	problem
perceptual-motor skills, head control, hand reaching	not a problem	sometimes a problem	problem	problem
understanding of spatial environment	not a problem	sometimes a problem	problem	problem
motivation to use sensor	not a problem	sometimes a problem	problem	problem
countervailing skills or tendencies	problem	problem	problem	may not be a problem

Table 2. Different aspects of the skill of using electronic spatial sensors pose different problems for different types of subjects.

ample, no guarantee that tasks suitable for developing sensitivity to the display will be useful for establishing spatial correspondences, or will assist motivation. It is difficult to put forward a program of training when there are so many psychological unknowns.

A Mobility Approach to Training

Before coming to Riverside I (E.S.) spent several years attempting to train blind children of varying ages, working in some cases over periods of up to two years with a binaural sensory aid adapted for work with children (4,15,16,18). The approach to training in this work involved a minimum of training on specific device skills and a maximum of involvement with real tasks in real space, and it was strongly influenced by the example of mobility training programs of the adult blind. It made few demands on psychological theory other than an assumption that something will be learned both about spatial layout and the sensing characteristics of the device from trial-and-error interaction with the environment.

A small amount of basic training was provided on a few skills such as teaching the children to keep their heads up, to scan to find objects, and to deal with the basic categories of information in the sensor, i.e., distance, direction, and surface characteristics. Training also included some simple exercises (e.g., games of finding poles) to teach general alertness, and specific skills, such as turning the head to orient to targets. The children were then allowed to learn more about the use of the sensors through interaction in real-world environments.

Settings were chosen for this interaction where the device might be effectively used. Training took place in comparatively safe settings such as parks near the home or in shopping centers. Not all such locations are equally appropriate to either training or use: For example, given a choice of having the child cross an open space or walk along beside a wall, one would choose the walk along the wall because it provides continuous signals from the device for the child to relate to his or her own movements, whereas walking across an open space is a dead-reckoning task for which the device provides no information except possible warning of unexpected obstacles.

The sensing device resembled the binaural sensory aid (10) which later became the Sonicguide. However, it also incorporated a novel, automatic-level-control to keep display signals audible, but not excessively loud, in spite of changes in background noise level (4,18). The range was set to about 4 m.

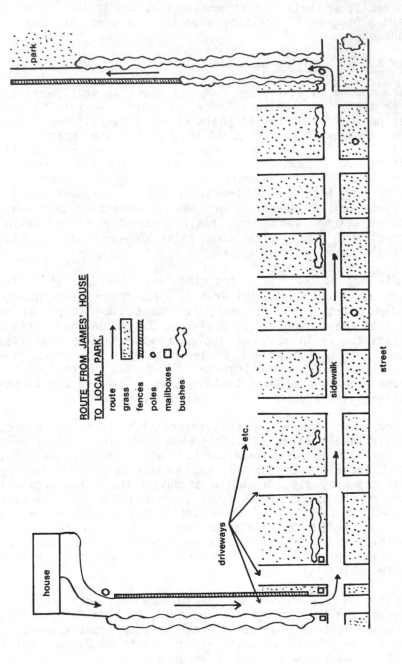

Figure 1.   Map view of a mobility travel route performed by a young blind child (from 15).

Four school-age children were trained. Two showed a good
ability to manage partly-supervised activities and some independent travel. An example is shown in Figure 1. Several of the
mobility tasks were accomplished at a commendable level of skill,
i.e., the children moved quickly and confidently in some difficult
travel situations. As well, all children showed testable levels
of skill in a number of component tasks such as shorelining and
object recognition, and the more successful children showed
performance fully worthy of the term skill (15).

It is possible that with continued practice on these routes
and the gradual introduction of other routes, the better children
would have advanced to very high levels of general spatial comprehension and device skill. However, whether or not this is likely
to happen, a major failure of this approach was that it worked
well with only two children. The other two children did not show
substantial benefit from this approach. Instead they manifested a
variety of problems which interfered with even simple device
activities: e.g., one child walked with a stride of only 4 inches,
and another was unable to keep his head upright and pointing
straight ahead. As well, there were problems of motivation to
use the sensor; fear of the environment was not obvious although
it may have also been an underlying factor. Nevertheless, under
some circumstances and with some children, this mobility-oriented
approach, providing minimal pretraining and then allowing supervised self-learning in natural settings, appears to be a reasonable approach to training, and introduces children to normal
mobility experiences.

Pretraining

One way to get a program usable by more children is to teach
the various subskills necessary for device use before moving onto
mobility tasks in large spaces. This approach has been tried
here in Los Angeles with the new short-range trisensors which
have enhanced resolution due to their additional central field
(11). The problem of the hard-to-move child is avoided by teaching aid skills using sit-down activities within arm's reach, with
the sensor set to about 1 m range. The procedures followed are
based partly on training procedures employed with adults (see 22;
also Warren & Strelow, this volume). After a series of such
activities was trained, the sensor was set to longer (4m) range
and a number of locomotor and mobility tasks were trained and
tested. Tasks followed in this approach are shown in Table 3.
One innovation in this program was the comparison of groups
receiving different training procedures specifically to determine
if the period of sit-down pretraining would improve later mobility
skills performed in larger space.

Pretraining	Locomotor Tasks	Travel Task
reach out and touch single targets to learn distance and direction correpondences	find and walk up to a single pole	walk a route inside a school building
discriminate and identify targets with different surfaces	walk around a single pole	walk a route outside the school building
recognize recorded signals of objects moving left, right, or forward	walk parallel to a row of objects	
	find several randomly scattered targets	

Table 3. Design of pretraining program of sensory aid instruction. The pretraining portion was conducted using short range settings. The loco-motor and travel tasks used long range settings.

Distance and Direction Pointing Errors

Direction

(random performance = 22 degrees; adult performance = 6 degrees)

Day 1	Day 2	Day 3	Day 4
15.2 (degrees)	14.9	14.7	14.9

Distance

(random performance = 12 cm; adult performance = 6 cm)

Day 1	Day 2	Day 3	Day 4
11.5 (cm)	12.0	12.0	10.6

Errors in Recognizing Surfaces

(covered with smooth wood, woodchips, sandpaper; maximum errors-18)

Day 1	Day 2	Day 3	Day 4
7.7	8.8	8.7	4.2

Errors in Recognizing Directions of Recorded Signals

(objects moving left, right or forward; maximum errors-21)

Day 1	Day 2	Day 3	Day 4
6.7	7.7	4.3	2.8

Table 4. Data from some pretraining activities (6 subjects).

The selection of results shown in Table 4 show that success was mixed. Some tasks, such as the recognition of surfaces and directions worked fairly well, i.e., we could demonstrate learning over days. Others, such as distance and direction learning, were less successful and failed to show an improvement over days. These procedures might work if longer training periods were employed (see Easton, this volume). However, on the basis of our adult work we suspect that the major problem is in our choice of tasks and the procedures for training. We doubt that fully successful training programs will be achieved without a much greater understanding of the processes of perceptual learning in these types of task.

We found little transfer from the pretraining device skills, learned in near space tasks, to the gross locomotor skills in larger spaces. That is, the pretrained group showed little advantage over the group that received device use for the first time on locomotor tasks. This lack of benefit may reflect the general lack of success of some of our training procedures; when better procedures are available, transfer may also be observed. We do not want to discredit totally the possibility that pretraining on near-space tasks is a useful precursor to device use in large spaces. Among other problems, we found that, in spite of our efforts to match subject groups on various characteristics, the pretrained group had an earlier average onset of blindness than the comparison group. Nevertheless, for the present, we regard the pretraining hypothesis as unproved.

Criterion Mastery Tasks

Before considering further the implications of the pretraining study, let us mention our most recent work. The failure to show learning on some tasks was particularly bothersome. If children are not able to develop device skills beyond their entry level of performance then it would not seem that their cognitive and perceptual skills are being aided by the sensor. We were struck by the possibility that some of the features of the training program devised by the group working with Kay in New Zealand (see Hornby et al., this volume) might give better results.

One characteristic of the New Zealand approach is that children progress through a sequence of tasks in which a criteria for learning is set on one task before the next is begun. Thus, unless the task is excessively easy or difficult, this approach guarantees that learning can be demonstrated. Of course the success of the entire program still hinges on the choice of training items. As in our previous work, there was some arbitrary choice of training items; all appear reasonable, or have "face validity." The list of tasks that we chose has some resemblance to that of

the New Zealand group. One notable difference was that there
were no short-range tasks; instead, all tasks were carried out in
larger spaces with a setting of about 4 m of sensing range. This
change is in part a response to the problems that we noted previously about the transfer from short-range to long-range tasks.
However, we should add that the mobility requirements of these
tasks were not as demanding as those of the first "mobility"
approach to training so we did not anticipate that locomotor control would be as much of a problem as in the first study. Travel
of "routes" was not a part of the study; only simple locomotor
tasks were employed such as walking alongside a row of objects.

    The tasks are shown in Table 5. Table 6 shows that all
tasks could be trained to a criterion of 8 correct trials out of
10 with all subjects within an average of 1.2 to 2.2 sessions. No
subject required more than 8 training sessions of 1/2 hour each.

Purpose		Description
1. Basic awareness of signal	-	large target present or absent in front of child; child says yes/no
2. Hold head level	-	small target present or absent at head height; child says yes/no
3. Left-right discrimination	-	object on left or right 45° to side; child says left/right
4. Near-far discrimination	-	object at 1.5 or 3 m; child says near/far
5. Smooth/rough surface	-	object at 1.5 m, either a smooth pole or a wire mesh; child says smooth/rough
6. Locomotor control: target approach	-	child faces pole at 4 m, walks up and touches pole
7. Locomotor control: orient and approach	-	child faces away from pole, turns 180° to face pole, walks up and touches pole
8. Stopping distance	-	child walks up to wall, stops at arm's reach +/- 10 cm
9. Locomotor control Walk between objects	-	child walks 7.5 m between two rows of poles, 2 m apart

Table 5. Criterion mastery tasks.

Sessions to Criterion   1 - 3 sessions per task

$\overline{X}$

1. Basic awareness of signal   -   1.6

2. Hold head level   -   1.8

3. Left-right discrimination -   1.2

4. Near-far discrimination   -   1.4

5. Smooth/rough surface   -   1.8

6. Locomotor control   -   1.8

7. Locomotor control
      orient and approach   -   2.2

8. Stopping distance   -   2.2

9. Locomotor control
      walk between objects   -   1.8

Table 6.   Criterion mastery tasks (5 subjects)

The training procedure outlined here provides a systematic introduction to children of the use of the binaural/trisensor type of sensory aid. It still leaves open the many questions noted earlier about the most appropriate form of training to achieve the best performance, but it nevertheless provides a means of bringing a child to the level of self-guided spatial activity in a variety of controlled spatial settings. In the next section, we will discuss how this approach to training might be further applied.

ISSUES: USE AND USEFULNESS

There have been several attempts now to train children with spatial sensors. However, the goal of general use of spatial prostheses on a daily basis, as with hearing aids, still eludes us with children. The mobility-clinical approach shows some success and may be appropriate to a limited number of children who might have particularly patient and dedicated teachers, or parents capable of understanding some of the capabilities and limitations of the technology, and of sustaining the interest of these children. Its major benefit is that it does introduce children to useful mobility skills. However, this approach will not be easily applied to a large number of children. Various attempts to pretraining can be shown to work in the limited sense that children can actually use the devices to learn the tasks. However it remains to be shown that such training is useful either in preparing the child for real world activities, such as mobility, or that it will provide general benefit to perceptual-motor or cognitive skills. We cannot guarantee general success in using electronic spatial sensors without a better understanding of the complexity of the skill with which we are dealing. The next section will address one of the issues we consider most important.

Sensory Substitution and Spatial Cognition

One current problem we are examining is the usefulness of spatial sensors for spatial comprehension in lifesized spaces (as opposed to table-top settings). Thus we have begun, with some of the children trained as in the last study, to determine the impact of a sensor on their ability to comprehend the layout of real-life spaces. The understanding of layout has been largely neglected to the present time in studies of spatial behavior of the sighted and the blind (see Haber, this volume; and 17). In effect we are asking: What does a person understand about the arrangement of objects in the environment as he or she walks through this environment? Presumably even the blind child has some conceptualization of the spaces through which he or she travels, although it is not a very good understanding of the environment. We believe that it will be instructive to determine both how good this understanding is in a particular spatial setting and how it is affected by the experience of using a sensor.

We believe that the issues of spatial cognition are important to the use of sensory aids because we suspect that if the ability to conceptualize space is inadequate, incoming spatial stimuli from either natural non-visual senses or a sensory aid do not enter as information, but instead are ignored or simply confuse the user. A major part of the problem of device use by children and adults may be the lack of basic cognitive skills and dispositions that are necessary to process the information that the sensory systems provide. However, we presume that these basic skills can be built up by appropriate training and that electronic spatial sensors are important tools by which this can occur.

STUDIES OF NEONATES

To the present time, more developmental studies have been conducted with blind infants than with school-age children. Most of this work has used very short exposures to the sensors, and little has been tried in the way of systematic training. In some cases little was likely to be achieved for the simple reason that the headphone arrangement that provided the auditory display did not work effectively (2,3,12). As might be expected then, much of this work has been inconsequential. Nevertheless the more successful studies have shown that infants are capable of a number of simple reactions to the sensors, and this has maintained interest in the possibility of early intervention with blind infants by electronic means (for reviews, see 16, 19, and Muir et al., this volume).

Partly in response to the unsatisfactory nature of much of the work with infants, we have developed an alternative strategy for studying neonates, using animal subjects. There are several advantages to the use of animal subjects: Firstly, it is possible to control the experience of animal subjects in a precise fashion; secondly, long exposures can be tried; and thirdly, the neural development of the animals can be examined.

The work with animals has allowed us to relate the use of spatial prostheses to the substantial and still-growing research literature of the last 20 to 30 years that has shown that the early years are a period of great plasticity of behavioral and neural development. The developing organism is particularly sensitive to qualitative and quantitative aspects of experience and can potentially be set along a variety of paths of more or less appropriate development. The psychological and biological literature based on animal studies is very suggestive about the importance of early stimulation on basic behavioral and neural development. This work, reviewed in the paper of Sonnier and Riesen (this volume), shows that there is a complex dependency of behavioral and neural development on the opportunities for stimulation provided by the environment.

ANIMAL STUDIES

Rationale

Our basic approach has been to examine the perceptual skills of animals reared blind from birth with Kay-type sensors worn on the head. We have to the present time examined two animals reared with sensors from the 7th day of life. We are currently undertaking a study of more animals, with the collaboration of Sonnier and Riesen, in which we will also examine neural development. The first study was performed with a binaural device, the second with a trisensor (TSA).

To the present time, our chief concern has been whether an animal would be able to interpret the sensor's information through its own interaction with the environment rather than through a specific, experimentally structured training program. This approach is followed partly because, as in the work with blind adults and older children, we do not know what an optimal training strategy may be. Partly, though, our rationale is based on the belief that the conditions for self-learning will be met in such a study far better than in work with human children or adults. The points in favor of self-learning are several: Firstly, the Kay sonar devices contain a large amount of information (distance, direction, and a reasonable degree of object resolution and recognition) which could potentially aid the perceptual skills of the animal. Secondly, we are providing this exposure to the sensor before alternate habits either of blindness or of the use of vision are established. Thirdly, the exposure is continuous, unlike the very restricted exposure given to human subjects, thus providing much more spatial information over time. Finally, the animal's learning is based on self-initiated motor activity, a feature of natural learning which appears to be important even though the precise reason is a matter of controversy (5,8,14,22). All of these assumptions are, of course, amenable to investigation with this animal paradigm.

Methods

In our work with the first animal, the experimental procedures were still being worked out. The procedure required that the animal be born in the dark, where it was then left with the mother for 7 days in order to ensure survival before being placed in the experiment with eyes sutured and covered, and with a sensory aid in place. Large amounts of time were required to monitor the equipment and the animal: Over 1000 hours of work were put in by undergradute assistants alone over the duration of this 34-day study.

The study proved difficult but essentially feasible. We were able to give this animal almost continuous exposure from its 7th day. Most significantly, we obtained a number of indices of behavioral use of the sensor by the animal which encouraged us to consider a second animal raised with the sensor for 90 days using improved procedures. We will present this later study in detail.

The Second Animal Study

The animal in the second study wore a capsule weighing 35 gm, containing the earphones and part of the electronics, which was fixed to its head with elastic straps. The remainder of the electronics were in a pivoting control box mounted at the top of the cage and connected to the capsule by a flexible cable. The cable was attached to the back of a jacket worn by the animal and thus did not impede head movements or tangle as the animal moved around in the cage.

The rearing environment was a plexiglas cage, 1.3 m square and 1.5 m high, with a metal grill floor. The cage was a semi-enriched spatial environment containing various objects, which along with the walls and the floor, created signals for the sensor. These objects included a 'surrogate mother' containing a feeding bottle and heating coils, a small wooden box for climbing, a 20 cm diameter rubber ball and a 6 cm diameter plastic ball with a bell inside which jingled when moved.

A 106 by 76 cm mobility box, with the surrogate in the center and six 2.5 cm diameter vertical poles randomly located in the open space, provided a novel setting to assess exploration and the avoidance of obstacles.

Volume levels of the sensor were set at about 53-68 db and were controlled by an automatic level control (ALC) which provided up to 15 db of gain with changes in background noise levels. Thus the TSA signals remained consistently above background noise but never totally dominated hearing. The sound levels also varied with target size and position. A 2.5-cm diameter target produced a maximum sound level of 53 dBA at .3 m from the sensor, with the ALC switched off. Sensing range was about 2/3 m with a range code of 10 kHz/m. This code allowed the detection of objects as close as 2 cm.

The subject was a female stumptailed macaque (Macaca arctoides), born in a light-proof room and left with her mother for 7 days in the dark. The eyes were then bandaged, and the sensor was fastened to the head over the eyes and snout so that it provided a second cover for the bandage to guard against visual exposure. Visual experience throughout the experiment was limited to short periods when the device and bandage were removed in dim light to inspect the animal or repair the device. The animal remained in this cage for a period of 90 days except for short periods of testing outside the cage, or for veterinary care or maintenance of the sensor. The device was operable for 84% of the animal's waking and sleeping experience. During device-off periods the head bandage remained in place.

Data Collection

Observations were made of the animal's free behavior for 90 days in the animal's home cage and in the mobility box. Starting at 15 days of age, systematic observations were made of percep-

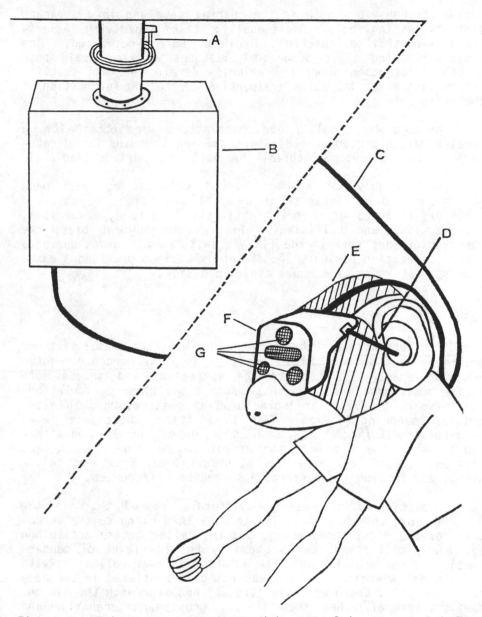

Figure 2. Trisensor arrangement with control box suspended from top of cage and sensor capsule on animal's head. A. Electrical commutator; B. Control box; C. Connecting cable; D. Earphone tube; E. Cloth helmet; F. Sensor capsule; G. Ultrasonic transducers: Center circular transducer is transmitter, left and right circular transducers receive left and right channels, large oval transducer receives center channel to give trisensor amplitude peak.

tual-motor behaviors both in the rearing cage and in a separate mobility testing box. Additionally, tasks involving experimentally-controlled reaching behavior were performed. The rationale behind these behavioral measures was to obtain both general information about the animal's development and specific information about its actual responsiveness to the information of the sensor.

The cage and mobility box observations were obtained by a focal sampling procedure (13) which sampled behavior in 20 categories during 30 second intervals for half-hour periods (Table 7).

Each category was scored 1 if it occurred at least once during each 30-sec interval or 0 if it did not. The observed behaviors included gross motor activities, posture, mannerisms, vocalizations, and collisions. To prevent judgment bias, the observer did not know if the TSA was switched off or on during a given observation period. The aid-off situation provided a baseline against which to compare aid-on behavior.

RESULTS

Checklist data. In the rearing cage, with the sensor switched on, the animal showed higher levels of adaptive perceptual-motor behavior, spent less time on the surrogate, and showed more active behaviors, such as gross motor activities, manipulation, and "visual" behaviors including head up posture, hand in view, and head scanning (cf Table 7). In addition, there were fewer behaviors indicating stress, such as mannerisms and loud vocalizations. With the aid off, the animal became more passive and distressed. Several categories of observations (posture, collisions, and feeling the surrogate) showed no differences.

Inspection of the day-by-day totals showed that in the mobility box, the animal did little more than cling to the surrogate for the first three weeks, but thereafter became active and not unduly distressed (as is shown by the low level of mannerisms). In the mobility box, the animal had fewer collisions with the aid on, whereas this item was not differentiated in the home cage. As well, there was more "visual" behavior with the aid on. However, several other items (e.g., gross motor behavior and manipulation) showed higher levels with the aid off.

The pattern of activity in the rearing cage suggests a specific influence of the artificial sensory information on perceptual behavior rather than a general arousal effect. For example, neither of the "distress" behaviors increased with the aid on, as would occur if arousal were the explanation. As well,

Behavior	(Total Possible)	Cage Behavior			Mobility Box		
		Aid On	Aid Off	P*	Aid On	Aid Off	P*
Rests on surrogate	(60)	14	24	.01	20	18	ns
Gross motor (locomotes, climbs objects)	(180)	35	22	.01	26	30	.01
Manipulation (walls, balls)	(180)	26	9	.01	22	31	.01
'Visual behaviors' (head up, hand in view, scanning)	(180)	50	29	.01	27	17	.01
Mannerisms (jerking, digit suck, self groom)	(180)	21	37	.01	15	16	ns
Vocalization (shriek, EEE sound, grunt and misc.)	(180)	10	17	.01	10	14	.05
Erect posture	(60)	5	3	.05	1	2	ns
Bizarre posture	(60)	8	8	ns	5	2	.01
Collisions	(60)	1	1	ns	5	10	.01
Feels surrogate	(60)	42	44	ns	39	48	.01

*P for a test of proportions between Aid On and Aid Off conditions.
Cage Behavior: Mean of 10 periods (Aid On)   Mobility Box Behavior: Mean of 7 periods (Aid On)
              Mean of 8 periods (Aid Off)   Mean of 8 periods (Aid Off)

Table 7. Summary of observations of checklist behavior--second pilot study with neonate macaque.

in the mobility box, gross motor activities were lower with the sensor switched on and yet visual behaviors were higher. On the other hand, familiarity with the home cage seems to explain the uniformly low collision rate here as compared to the mobility box. Nevertheless, in the mobility box the animal had fewer collisions with the aid on than off, suggesting that it gained some ability to detect and avoid obstacles with the sensor.

Reaching task. In order to investigate the animal's alertness to aid and natural sounds and the device's potential interference with normal hearing, 18 controlled reaching trials were performed twice a week in a chair outside of the cage with the sensor either switched off or on. These reaching data (Table 8) provide clear indication of the animal's ability to interpret device signals. With the aid on, there was a significant amount of reaching to static and looming targets, showing that the animal responded to aid signals as designating objects. The large targets used did not necessitate accurate reaching; however, because the animal needed to respond within a 10-second time limit, the reaching responses to the aid signals indicate a considerable alertness to the auditory display.

With the aid off, the reaching tasks showed the expected low level of spontaneous response to looming and static presentation of silent objects. Further, there was no difference between the aid-on and aid-off reaching to normal soundmaking objects, indicating that the TSA signals did not interfere with reaching to normal sound.

Task	Aid On	Aid Off	P*
Silent Objects			
a) Looming presentation	19/48	5/48	.01
b) Static presentation	28/48	6/48	.01
Normal sound-making objects (Rattles, etc.)	19/48	18/48	ns

*P from a test of proportions between Aid On and Aid Off conditions.

Table 8. Assessment of reaching behavior of macaque in restraining chair. (Sum of eight sessions for each task and condition, six trials per session.)

Overall, the results support the conclusion that the animal was alert to the sensor's signals, that it could interpret these as indicating objects in space, and that aspects of its free behavior were guided by the sensor's information. The results of these two studies demonstrate the potential for animals to learn the use of sensory substitution devices by feedback from their own activities (e.g., 8).

GENERAL CONCLUSIONS

We have presented data from two very different populations, neonate animals and blind human children. In spite of differences in the two groups, there are several underlying points of continuity. The question of how to train the novel display of the artificial sensor is a major concern with both groups. Learning does not automatically take place within the limited exposure to the aids given most blind adults and children. Developing soundly-based training programs which ensure the most effective use of a sensor and which allow the blind user to gain useful skills is a major problem in the human work.

Sensory disorders such as blindness may be alleviated by the use of sensory prostheses such as the TSA from early infancy. To the present time, blind human infants have not been presented with sensory substitutes for more than a few hours a day, and the results have not been clearly beneficial for general spatial development (16). The perceptual-motor development of blind infants could potentially be improved by the earlier and more continuous application of a sensory aid in appropriate environments. However, because the developmental sequence which could occur with artificial information is not known, intensive use of such aids with human infants should be approached with great care. For example, we do not know the effects of continuous exposure of an auditory display on the development of hearing, although the present data with the animal does not suggest obvious interference with normal listening skills.

If the results of the current studies with animals show clear benefits, by comparison with control groups, from early use of sensors, then this would provide incentive for a similar approach with human infants. However, much will also depend on what is discovered about neural cortical development under these conditions of rearing. At the moment we do not know whether or not there will plastic brain changes arising from these rearing conditions and if so, whether or not they will be advantageous to the animals (see Sonnier and Sonnier & Riesen, this volume for detailed discussion of neural and behavioral plasticity).

Much of our interest in the animal study is in examining the interaction of neural and behavioral interactions in development. At the moment we simply do not know the limits of CNS plasticity. Because sensory substitution devices provide a novel but lawful restructuring of spatial experience, the possibility exists that they may produce significant reorganization of neural structures. Alternatively they may have very little impact. This question is, we believe, illustrative of the significance of substitution devices as research tools, irrespective of their potential as aids to the blind (see also Sonnier, Sonnier & Riesen and Warren & Strelow, this volume).

ACKNOWLEDGEMENTS

This work was supported by the Parsons, Wallace, and Riverside Foundations, by BRSG2-507-RR07010-16 awarded by the Biomedical Research Support Grant Program, Division of Research Resources, National Institutes of Health, and by a University of California Intramural Research Grant to D. H. Warren.

REFERENCES

1.   Ballard, D. H. & Brown, C. M. (1982). Computer Vision. New
      Jersey: Prentice-Hall.

2.   Bower, T. G. R. (1977). Blind babies see with their ears.
      New Scientist, 73, 255-257.

3.   Bower, T. G. R. (1977). Babies are more important than
      machines. New Scientist, 73, 712-714.

4.   Boys, J. T., Strelow, E. R., & Clark, G. R. S. (1979). A
      prosthetic aid for a developing blind child. Ultrasonics,
      17, 37-42.

5.   Day, R. H. & Singer, G. (1967). Sensory adaptation and
      behavioral compensation with spatially transformed vision
      and hearing. Psychological Bulletin, 67, 307-322.

6.   Fraiberg, S. (1971). Intervention in infancy: A program for
      blind infants. Journal of the American Academy of Child
      Psychiatry, 10, 40-62.

7.   Gibson, E. J. (1969). Principles of Perceptual Learning and
      Development. New York: Appleton-Century-Crofts.

8.   Held, R. & Hein, A. (1963). Movement-produced stimulation in
      the development of visually-guided behavior. Journal of Com-
      parative and Physiological Psychology, 56, 872-876.

9.   Hill, E. & Blasch, B. B. (1980). Concept development. In
      R. L. Welsh & B.B. Blasch (Eds.), Foundations of Orientation
      and Mobility. New York: American Foundation for the Blind.

10.   Kay, L. (1974). A sonar aid to enhance spatial perception
      of the blind: Engineering and evaluation. The Radio and
      Electronic Engineer, 44, 605-626.

11.   Kay, L. (1982). Spatial perception through an acoustic sen-
      sor. Report, University of Canterbury.

12.   Kay, L. & Strelow, E. R. (1977). Blind babies need special-
      ly designed aids. New Scientist, 73, 709-712.

13.   Rhine, R. J. & Flanigon, M. (1978). An empirical comparison
      of one-zero, focal-animal, and instantaneous methods of
      sampling spontaneous primate social behavior. Primates, 19,
      353-361.

14. Riesen, A. H. & Aarons, L. (1959). Visual movement and intensity discrimination in cats after early deprivation of pattern vision. Journal of Comparative and Physiological Psychology, 52, 142-149.

15. Strelow, E. R. (1980). The use of the binaural sensory aid by pre-school and school-age children -- final report. New Zealand Scientific Research Committee.

16. Strelow, E. R. (1983). The use of the binaural sensory aid by pre-school children. Journal of Visual Impairment & Blindness, 77, 429-438.

17. Strelow, E. R. (1985). What is needed for a theory of mobility: Direct perception and cognitive maps -- Some lessons from the blind. Psychological Review, 92, 226-248.

18. Strelow, E. R. & Boys, J. T. (1979). Canterbury child's aid: A binaural spatial sensor for research with blind children. Journal of Visual Impairment & Blindness, 73, 179-184.

19. Warren, D. H. (1984). Blindness and Early Childhood Development. New York: American Foundation for the Blind, 2nd edition.

20. Warren, D. H., Anooshian, L. J., & Bollinger, J. G. (1973). Early versus late blindness: The role of early vision in spatial behavior. Research Bulletin of the American Foundation for the Blind, 26, 151-170.

21. Warren, D. H. & Kocon, J. A. (1974). Factors in the successful mobility of the blind. Research Bulletin of the American Foundation for the Blind, 28, 191-218.

22. Warren, D. H. & Strelow, E. R. (1984). Learning spatial dimensions with a sensory aid: Molyneux revisited. Perception, 13, 331-350.

23. Welch, R. B. (1978). Perceptual Modification: Adaptation to Altered Sensory Environments. New York: Academic Press.

USE OF SONAR SENSORS WITH HUMAN INFANTS

D. W. Muir,* G. K. Humphrey,** P. C. Dodwell,*
and D. E. Humphrey**

 *Queen's University
**University of Lethbridge

When we first became interested in studying the possibilities of using Kay's sonar aid as a prosthesis for blind infants and children, some six years ago, we subscribed to a widely held belief that those who had never had visual experience lacked to an extraordinary degree the ability to represent space and spatial relations to themselves (26,50,51). Such individuals, it appears, lack adequate concepts of space and geometry. Given the lively new scientific interest in perception in infancy that began during the 1960's (13), and the important new discoveries that soon followed in visual physiology about the plasticity of the mammalian visual system during certain "critical" periods (31,39), it seemed altogether plausible that the deficiency under discussion was due to lack of appropriate stimulation during some critical period of development of the brain. We believed the stated doctrine that the severest deficits only occurred in those who had lacked visual experience in their earliest years. A spatial sensor that could supply relevant information, albeit through a different sense, seemed like an exciting possibility for remedying - if not fully redressing - some of the deficit. Given the nature of visual critical periods, and the general knowledge about plasticity in young organisms, it seemed clear that to obtain maximum benefit the stimulation should be started at a very early age. Thus began our cooperative research with Leslie Kay on the use of his infant sonar aid.

Our hope and expectation was that, by introducing the aid to blind infants in the first year of life, dramatic changes from the previously reported deficits in spatial understanding would be obtained. Once this had been established, we intended to investigate the amount of sensor use needed to achieve maximal benefit. As we shall show, it is still too early to state whether any long-range changes occur as a result of wearing the aid at a young age, but we are reasonably sure of two things. First, getting an infant or young child to wear and use the aid on a consistent basis is far more problematical than we had supposed, and second, in order to make best use of the aid at any one time, it is necessary to take account of the infant's general cognitive, emotional, and social state. Aid use and training do not occur in a psychological vacuum.

Bower (5) has also considered the usefulness and potential effectiveness of sonar aid use by blind infants. His theoretical position, a fairly extreme form of the Gibsons' Differentiation Theory (19) holds that a "primitive unity of the senses" exists at birth. The claim is that newborns will respond to certain amodal or abstract properties of stimuli such as intensity, rhythm, and direction in space, but they fail to distinguish between sounds, sights, and touches as sources of stimulation. What emerges in development, according to Bower, is the ability to differentiate sensory input in various ways, including the formation of specialized functions within each modality. This process is supposed to begin sometime between 3 and 9 months of age and, once completed, is irreversible.

Bower argues that provided the experience occurs very early in life, a congenitally blind baby will automatically substitute information from a prosthetic device which delivers the appropriate abstract, relational information via another modality. To support this differentiation theory, Bower (5) presented evidence that a blind 4-month-old could "see with his ears" when he first wore the Sonicguide designed by Kay (28). This device is an ultrasonic spatial sensor which produces an audible stereophonic image of objects located at different positions in space. The infant was reported to have made immediate use of the Sonicguide's distance (pitch) and directional (interaural amplitude difference) cues, reaching out for silent objects moved into the aid's receptive field, responding with affect toward the mother when she entered the field, defending himself from looming objects, and reaching for objects toward which he was lowered. Recently, Aitken and Bower (1) reported that such dramatic "perceptual" use of the aid upon initial exposure to the device was restricted to infants who were less than 13 months of age. Because a few older infants failed to use the aid, Aitken and Bower concluded that the congenitally blind who do not receive early aid experience --

in contrast to those who do -- will never develop the geometric
spatial representation system which normally is accessed through
vision.

While Bower's theory is more extreme than our hypothesis, he
shared a common hope for the early introduction of prosthetic
devices, although we never made any specific predictions as to
what the critical period in human development might be. The
notion of amodality of stimulation in early infancy is also quite
foreign to our way of thinking. We will evaluate the evidence
for and against Bower's position, beginning with a brief overview
of the developmental course of the sighted infant's spatial
responses to visual and auditory stimuli. This involves first
auditory and visual orientation toward objects and people, then
reaching and grasping near objects, and finally moving out in
search of distant objects. This will be followed by a summary of
several recent reports on the use of some form of sonar aid by 23
congenitally blind infants and pre-school children. Finally,
practical difficulties, methodological problems, and ethical
issues encountered in this work are discussed, emphasizing the
need for improved research designs and new spatial sensors.

DEVELOPMENT OF AUDITORY AND VISUAL LOCALIZATION RESPONSES IN SIGHTED INFANTS

Localization Responses of Sighted Infants

The argument that infants respond equivalently to the spatial properties of auditory and visual input has, at best, limited support. A comparison of localization responses to sights and
sounds by infants of different ages illustrates the complexity of
these developmental functions. Both auditory and visual targets
will elicit a slow (3 - 5 second latency) but reliable head turn
(toward the source on about 80% of trials) in neonates (30,38).
In fact, in a conflict paradigm when visual and auditory targets
are presented simultaneously on opposite sides, newborns will
turn toward the sound as often as toward the sight, suggesting
that there is little dominance of one modality over the other at
birth, at least for the elicitation of a head turn (36). However,
there is one striking difference between the two modalities at
birth: Their fields are not coincident. The "effective" visual
field (i.e., the area in space within which a target reliably
elicits an orienting response) is narrow, approximately 20 - 30
degrees on either side of the midline (23,48). By contrast, the
"effective" auditory field is at least 180 degrees wide. For
example, sound sources 90 degrees from the midline elicit more
reliable responses than those at 45 degrees (16).

The lack of comparability of auditory and visual responses becomes even more evident for infants between 1 1/2 and 4 months of age. During this period, infants turn less, or stop turning, toward off-centered sounds, even though they are tested under the same conditions as when they were newborns (35). At the beginning of this period, their effective visual field expands (2) and visual stimuli appear to "capture" their attention (19). When auditory and visual stimuli are presented on opposite sides to 2 1/2month-olds, they always turn toward the visual stimulus and seem to ignore the fact that the sound is in a different direction (15).

It is noteworthy that at the time infants stop turning to sounds, visual attention to certain stimuli such as schematic faces appears to peak (14). This relationship between the two response functions is shown in Figure 1.

By 3 - 4 months of age, infants demand novel visual experiences, rapidly becoming bored with repeated presentations of stationary abstract visual displays and objects. This response had led to the development of the visual habituation research paradigm (for a review see 13) which has been used extensively by investigators to study the nature of early perceptual processing. Investigators compare both the rates of decline in fixation time during habituation and the degree of recovery of looking, follow-

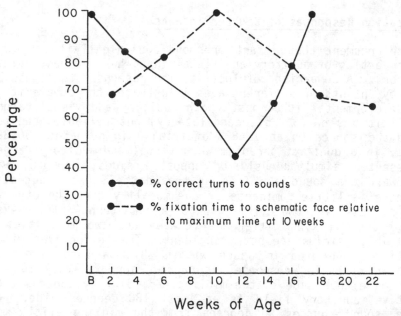

Figure 1. Comparison of auditory localization and visual attention as a function of age weeks (14,35).

ing a drop in fixation, to changes in various aspects of a visual display. It is interesting to note that although 3- to 4-month-olds show interest in some configural changes of certain abstract visual patterns, we have found that they appear to be more interested in elementary, but important, spatial transformations of the patterns. These are dilations (expansion), rotations, or lateral shifts through translation (27).

We are not suggesting that infants fail to respond to a sound's location between 1 1/2 and 3 months of age; however, their responses become more diversified, perhaps reflecting the development of intermodal attentional processes and increased sensitivity to social exchanges. For example, Bundy (9) reported that 8-week-olds detected shifts in the interaural arrival time of identical sounds presented to the two ears by exhibiting renewed interest in an auditory-visual display following a shift. Demany, McKenzie, and Vurpillot (11) have reported that 1/2 to 3-month-olds showed visual habituation to an unchanging visual stimulus associated with a repetitive sound sequence; their visual interest, to the same visual target, increased after the associated sound sequence changed in rhythm. In localization testing, infants of this age increase their smiling and vocalization to sound presentations, compared with their neonatal performance (33).

By 3 months of age, infants are using the direction of their gaze to modulate social exchanges. They engage in "face-to-face conversations" with their mothers, orienting toward and away from them to initiate and temporarily interrupt the dialogue. If this conversation is changed by the mother's suddenly freezing or acting depressed, almost all infants will begin to avert their gaze and many will become upset (10,20).

Rather suddenly, at approximately 4 1/2 to 5 months of age, infants again turn toward sounds as reliably as they did during the newborn period, but now they are faster (mean latency less than 1 sec) and more accurate in locating the sound within a hemifield (34). Indeed, when presented with sounds 30 and 60 degrees from the midline along the horizontal plane, these 4 1/2-month-old infants rotate their heads an average of 30 and 48 degrees, respectively, comparable to the performance of adults tested under similar conditions. The most important difference between adult and infant performance is that infants fail to locate sounds in the other planes with equal facility. Although a 4 1/2-month-old turns toward sounds along the vertical median plane at better than chance levels, he responds slowly and rarely locates the exact position of the sound within the hemifield (17). Infants begin to locate sounds off the horizontal plane more reliably and accurately between 9 - 12 months of age (40,52).

A further point worth noting is that while a 4 1/2-month-old plays the "turn to sound alone" game willingly for many trials, by 6 months of age, such behavior can only be maintained by visual reinforcement procedures (32). Thus, the construction of auditory space appears to develop slowly during the first year of life and is characterized by peaks and troughs in the performance of localization responses. By comparison, the effective visual field of infants expands steadily during the first few months of life as they establish pattern preferences and use visual localization responses to search for novel experience and to modulate social interactions.

Reaching and Locomotion of Sighted Infants

Although conflicting evidence exists, newborns and very young infants appear to exhibit a poorly controlled reaching response in the direction of visual stimuli (12,24). By 5 - 6 months of age, just after they begin to turn again to sounds, infants will reach out, grasp, and manipulate nearby objects (53). Recently, von Hofston (25) described a U-shaped function for the developmental course of reaching which parallels that for auditory localization. He reports that the frequency of arm extensions directed toward the object of fixations (prereaching) declines at about 7 weeks of age and then increases in frequency at 16 - 19 weeks of age. In the more mature form, the beginning of the directed reach is accompanied by hand shaping.

A single published report by Wishart, Bower, and Dunkeld (54) claims that infants will reach for sounding objects presented in the dark, in a manner equivalent to visual targets, beginning at around 5 months of age. Unfortunately, no control trials or comparative details of the response characteristics of visually and auditorily elicited reaching were described in this report. A preliminary analysis of results of a study in our laboratory on responses to both glowing visible-but-silent and invisible-sounding objects presented in the dark suggests that on occasion 4- to 5-month-olds will reach out and grasp for an invisible sound, but this response is less frequent and might be characterized as groping, compared with the more accurate, visually elicited responses. Although reaches for invisible sounds could indicate that sounds are taking on substance for infants of this age, in subsequent months the visually elicited reach becomes refined, less obligatory, and more selective while, according to Wishart, et al. (54), the reach to invisible sounds disappears at 6 - 7 months and begins to recover by 11 - 12 months of age. It is at this latter age that infants begin to search for visible sounding objects which are made to disappear from sight, a form of searching that is based on sound cues alone (4,49).

Newborns, if properly supported, make "automatic walking" response which become increasingly difficult to elicit with age. However, volitional locomotion does not appear until the latter part of the first year of life, thus furnishing yet another example of a response of an apparently reflexive nature that disappears (is suppressed?) at one stage of development, to re-appear in a more mature form at a later stage. An interesting shift in the infant's spatial memory for a distant object's location occurs when infants become mobile. Most studies report egocentric coding, where objects are localized relative to en-vironmental landmarks, beginning around 9 - 12 months of age, particularly if the landmarks are salient or familiar (see 3 for a review). Thus we see that even in the sighted infant, there are many psychological, physiological, and social factors that have to be considered if we want to understand the course of development.

AUDITORY LOCALIZATION AND LOCOMOTOR DEVELOPMENT OF BLIND INFANTS

Congenitally blind infants develop postural skills such as sitting, rolling over, and standing at about the same age as sighted babies, but are delayed in crawling and walking (18). Fraiberg suggests that these locomotor delays result from the absence of visual lures which attract the sighted infant and thus elicit the more complex "voluntary" response. She argues that for the blind child sound provides the only distance in-formation identifying objects beyond reach. Sound does not come to represent solid objects until an infant enters Stage 4 in the development of Piagetian object permanence. This occurs at approximately 9 - 10 months of age when sighted babies recover objects that disappear under a screen, and shortly thereafter both sighted and blind infants begin to search for hidden objects which continue to sound. As evidence, Fraiberg stresses that no blind infant in her sample ever used any form of forward pro-gression before learning to reach for sounds. Unfortunately, detailed normative data on the development of auditory locali-zation and reaching for sounds by the blind are not available. Fraiberg did chart reaching to sound but only in the midline position, thus we do not know the developmental course of direc-tional reaching.

On the basis of evidence from four case studies, large in-dividual differences are to be expected among blind babies, both in localizing and reaching for sounds. Schwartz (1984) reports that a 28-week-old blind baby failed to turn or reach for sounds presented from different directions after 12 weeks of training, while a younger blind infant, 20 weeks old, began to raise his hand on the side of the sound after a brief sound-play period and rapidly acquired the ability to reach and grasp sounding objects after a few weeks of training. In our experience with two young, blind infants, one did not localize or reach for sounding objects at birth, three, or six months of age, but with training quickly acquired the responses. The other infant did not turn his head to sound during the neonatal period, but did at a 6-month assessment, and with no training on our part localized and reached for sounding objects in the first formal assessment given at 7 months of age (22). We will discuss these results later.

If Bower is correct in his prediction of instantaneous and appropriate inter-sensory substitutions with the Sonicguide's signals by the very young infant, we would expect to see immediate coordinated sensory-motor activity when the aid is first turned on, provided the infant is less than 13 months of age. If Fraiberg is correct, however, this might occur only after an extended period of training in localization and reaching for sound sources. In any case, we initiated our own research hoping that early sonar aid experience would allow our blind infants to discover and maintain contact with silent objects out of reach, enabling them to develop a spatial frame of reference for the distant world and to provide them with a lure to explore it.

Sonar Aid Responses of Blind Infants Under 13 Months of Age

Reports exist on ten congenitally blind infants less than 13 months of age who were given sonar aid experience.[1] Although the test protocols for each infant differ and the data in some cases consist of informal observations, a general picture of the young blind infant's response to the aid's signal does emerge. Results described below are summarized in Table 1. As noted earlier, Aitken and Bower's (1) 5- to 13-month-old congenitally blind infants were reported to make immediate use of the Sonicguide's signals. They reached for objects brought into the midline of the aid's receptive field after 10 - 25 trials, and four babies swiped at or reached for objects presented laterally. These were "clinical observations," so details such as the total number of trials given, the exact position of the objects in the aid's field and the actual form (e.g., 1 or 2-handed, hand shape), speed, and accuracy of these responses were not reported. The lack of details and the absence of control trials with the aid turned off makes the results difficult to evaluate (see 45). All 5 infants also were reported to make a defensive response by interposing their hands between their face and an approaching object. It is possible, however, given the increase in intensity and distortion in the signal which occurs when an object approaches too close to the receivers, that the response may have been either an attempt to reach for the object or to remove the aid. Aitken and Bower observed few tracking responses and no

instances of placing responses (reaching for the edge) when the
infants were lowered toward a surface. Furthermore, the results
of three of Aitken and Bower's infants studied on a long term
basis are less encouraging. Two infants continued to use the aid
to reach for silent objects, but their use was intermittent. The
third infant refused to wear the aid after the initial session.
Another infant given the aid at 14 months, but not assessed initially, failed to show any use after 4 months of experience.

     Other investigators working with blind infants between 6 and
10 months of age have failed to observe the responses that Bower
reported on the initial session, but have found that infants can
use the sonar aid adaptively with some practice. Schwartz (42)
reported that a 6-month-old initially tried to remove the aid;
this was overcome by turning it on before the aid was placed on
his head. After it was in place, he would quiet and listen for
an extended period. Following a few weeks of experience, he
began to raise his arm when an object entered the aid's field and
after several more weeks reached for objects signaled by the aid.
Ferrell (15) also reported no immediate response when the Sonicguide was first introduced to a 6-month-old blind infant, but
after 2 months of exposure to the aid the baby began to use the
aid for reaching. Strelow (45) failed to observe any initial
responses by a 10-month-old blind infant and obtained only three
reaching reponses after 70 trials over a number of training sessions. However, after a break in the program for several months,
and once reliably reaching for naturally sounding objects was
observed, this baby began to reach consistently and accurately
for objects signaled by the aid.

     We (22) have placed the aid on two congenitally blind in-
fants beginning when they were 6 and 8 months old. Our first
infant, Kathy, fussed when the aid was first placed on her head,
but appeared attentive as soon as it was turned on, quieting and
stopping her rocking. She failed to track, reach for, or show
defensive responses toward silent objects moved into the aid's
receptive field. This was not surprising given that she did not
turn toward or reach for naturally sounding objects. The aid was
removed and she was trained to make these responses over the next
10 weeks. At the beginning of training, bilateral arm raises
increased dramatically but, by the end of training, the responses
were primarily with the arm ipsilateral to the sound. The results of tests of her reaching accuracy, conducted during this
training period, are shown in Figure 2. Despite the high frequency of arm movements during a trial, Kathy's initial ability
to contact the sounding object was low, increasing from 12 1/2%
on lateral trials after the first two weeks of training to exceed
50% for combined lateral and midline trials after 10 weeks of

Younger Infants	Age (mo.)	Response during initial session	Age (mo.)	Response with experience/training
1-a (SC)	5	Reach-Defensive		
2-a (AN)	6	" "	19	Exploration during mobility
3-a (SN)	8	" "	15-20	Intermittent mobility
4-a (BG)	13	" "	None	
5-a (SI)	13	" "		
6-b (Andrew)	6	Quiet/Alert	7	Reach
7-c (Julie)	6	Quiet/Alert	8	Reach
8-d (Alfred)	10	Grasp speakers	13	Reach and place
9-e (Kathy)	6	Quiet/Alert	9	Reach, touch speaker and in mobility
10-f (Ted)	8	Quiet/Alert	8 (+1 week)	Reach
11-a (NN)	14	?	14	None
12-a (LR)	18	None-Fuss		
13-a (JT)	18	None-Visual Response	15-20	
14-a (MP)	20	None-Fuss		
15-c (May)	14	Quiet	25	Reach; 29 avoid obstacles

Table 1. Summary of aid use by congenitally blind infants before and after 13 months of age from 7 reports (a. Aitken and Bower, 1982; b. Schwartz, 1978; c. Ferrell, 1980; d. Strelow, 1983; e. Harris, et. al., 1984; f. Muir, Dodwell, Humphrey, & Humphrey, 1984; g. Humphrey & Humphrey, 1984; h. Strelow, Kay, & Kay, 1978). The age at which infants clearly demonstrated a response when a silent target was presented within the aid's field of view is underlined, and responses on the initial test session are compared with those on later sessions.

Table 1. (cont.)

Older Infants	Age (mo.)	Response during initial session	Age (mo.)	Response with experience/training
16-c (June)	14 1/2	Quiet	20	Reach; 24 avoid obstacles
17-c (April)	26 1/2	Quiet-Reach	28.5	Reach; 32 avoid obstacles
18-d (Daniel)	30	None	30+	After 1 year- intermittent use in mobility
19-d (Martha)	26	Cry	<u>26</u>	3rd session-reach in mobility
20-d (Marg)	21	Reach		Later in mobility
21-f (Bell)	21	Quiet-Smile	22-4	Play with sound; 36 mo. avoid obstacles
22-g (Lee)	19	Reach	19+	Continues to reach
23-g (Eddy)	31	Avoided and explored objects	31+	Runs and reaches
24-h	30	Reach after 30 trials on 3 days	34	Some obstacle avoidance and following

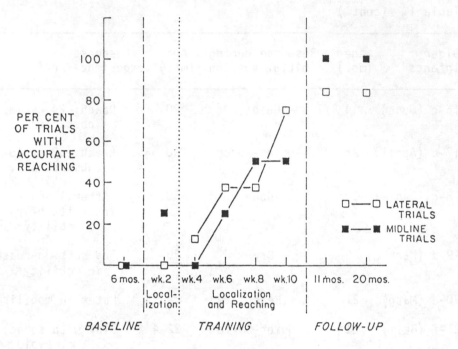

Figure 2. Successful reaches for sounds prior to, during, and after training (22).

training. Thus her ability to locate a sound's position was still immature and slow (average latency to contact of 10.2 sec), compared with sighted infants reaching for visible targets.

The aid was reintroduced to Kathy, after she was habituated to a headband, when she was 9 months old. When the aid was turned on, she reached for the carpet and then touched one of the aid speakers. When a silent object was presented she reached toward it without making contact on 4 of 8 trials and not at all on trials with the aid turned off. Furthermore, she tracked silent objects moved in the aid's field on 7 of 11 aid-on trials and never during aid-off trials. Over the next few months the parents placed the aid on Kathy for about one hour a day and carried out specific exercises during feeding and play time. Kathy learned to anticipate the approach of a spoon containing food (our attempt to instruct her on the distance code for the 1 m range). Reaching with the aid turned on and turned off was assessed by videotaping the number of contacts she made when silent objects were presented to her left, and right, and in the midline. As can be seen in Figure 3, more reaches were elicited when the aid was operating, e.g., 40% correct at 19 months, but

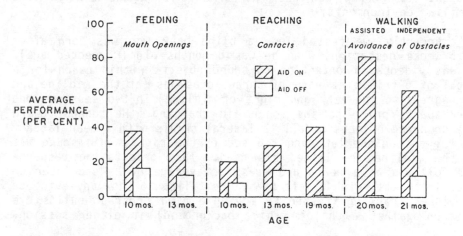

Figure 3. Summary of results of tests with the sonar aid switched on and off during meals (anticipatory mouth openings to an approaching spoon), when objects were presented within the Aid's field of view (accurate reading), and during walks (avoiding obstacles) as a function of age (22).

she was much more accurate in obtaining sounding objects (100% in the midline and 82% on lateral trials) at 11 and 20 months of age. This discrepancy in performance may be due to the mismatch between the natural localization cues and the single, mismatched, interaural amplitude cue used by the aid. That is, the aid presents only one directional cue (Interaural Amplitude Difference) versus at least three for normal hearing (time, phase and intensity differences) (See 44). Also, the set IAD may not match the level required for normal hearing by a given subject (see 41). Poor motivation for using the aid's signal while working in near space also may have lowered her performance; in many cases she simply engaged her normal sweep and grope strategy, grasping the object upon contact.

The most consistent, continued use of the aid occurred when Kathy was walking. At 19 months of age, with the aid's range set at 1 m, Kathy was encouraged on walks during training to find hidden objects. During assessments, she avoided objects in her path or reached for them prior to contact. As shown in Figure 3, her performance was clearly better with the aid on than off.

In general, throughout the program, we found that although Kathy could use the aid adaptively when she wore it for practice, she appeared to habituate to its signal. Furthermore, she rarely asked to wear the aid and was content to navigate around her home without it, giving her best performance with the aid in less familiar environments.

Recently, we tested Ted, a blind baby who was born after 29.5 weeks gestation, when he was 8 months old (corrected age). He was videotaped orienting to sound objects within reach for a total of 6 trials at each of three locations (at the midline and 90 degrees to the left and right of midline) in two sessions one week apart, prior to any sonar aid training. He turned toward the sounding objects on all 12 lateral trials with a mean latency of 1.1 sec on the left and 2.5 sec on the right; when sound was at the midline, he lifted his head. This orientation response was followed by a reach and grasp an average of 24 sec later on 7 of 18 trials, with a left bias. He failed to show any evidence of visual tracking (tested by moving a high contrast bull's eye pattern against a uniform white background) at either session.

When the aid was first placed on his head, Ted reached for the headband and then quieted, appearing to listen to the aid's signals with his head held up as objects were brought into the aid's field, but he showed no tracking or reaching during the entire 40 min session. No placing responses were observed when he was slowly lowered to a surface either three times with the aid turned on or three times with it off. He did, however, smile in response to his mother's looming face and voice with the aid on. At the second visit, Ted's responses were more dramatic. On the first trial with the aid switched on, he reached for the aid after 35 sec; he appeared to make accidental contact on the second trial after 11 sec, and reached with increasing speed on the next three. He reached with both hands for silent objects brought toward him alone the midline on the last 5 of 6 trials, with a mean latency to contact of 9.3 sec. No responses were recorded when the aid was switched off. In a third session, Ted refused to reach for silent objects with the aid and sounding objects with or without the aid, presumably due to his unusual fussiness that day.

It appears that young infants find the signals from the aid to be novel and interesting, as they typically quiet and attend to the aid's sounds when it is first introduced. There is some evidence that the young infant will, quite readily, reach for aid-signaled objects, but, at least in most cases reviewed, such reaching only occurs if the infant is already reaching reliably for naturally sounding objects. Unfortunately, Aitken and Bower (1) make no mention of the response of their infants to naturally sounding objects, so we do not know if their experience fits this pattern. When the infants do reach for aid-signaled objects, either immediately or with training, they appear to reach most reliably on midline presentation and do not show a great deal of appreciation for the aid's directional cue. Most reaches are two-handed reached toward the midline in the infants we have tested. Furthermore, the reaches are inaccurate in comparison to the blind infant's reach for naturally sounding objects, especially on lateral presentations. Thus, although young blind infants can use the aid to reach for objects and sometimes do this with little or no training, they do not appear to use all of the information that is potentially available. Training in aid use appears to help, as our work with Kathy suggests, but the "level" of aid use achievable by a blind infant does not, in our experience, seem to be very high.

Sonar Aid Responses of Infants Over 13 Months of Age

Aitken and Bower based their argument for a "critical period" for aid experience primarily on the results of three infants between 18 and 20 months of age who failed to respond on initial test sessions. However, the evidence is not convincing given that two of their infants were distressed by the procedures and screamed, while the third had residual vision. It is interesting to note that Fraiberg (18) has reported that the infants in her study showed stranger anxiety or avoidance at a median age of 12.5 months. Ted's parents spontaneously reported the same phenomenon when he was 12 months old. Also, Lee, who reached for aid-signalled objects at 19 months only did so for his mother, not for the experimenter. Perhaps the older babies in Aitken and Bower's study were not rejecting the aid as much as the "strangers" testing them.

Other investigators have found that most older infants do respond adaptively to the aid's signals, some almost immediately and others after training. Ferrell (15) reported that with the aid switched on, two 14-month-olds began reaching accurately for the presentation of silent toys after 5 to 10 months of experience, and a few months later, while walking, used the aid's signal to avoid obstacles. A 26.5 month old child, tested by Ferrell, responded as soon as the aid was turned on by scanning and reaching for her mother. After a two-month break, she pursued her father and avoided objects while walking, and by 32 months of age was using the aid to reach accurately for silent objects presented in the aid's field of view. Strelow (45) reported that a partially crippled, developmentally delayed 21-month-old blind child, who had begun reaching for natural sounds one month earlier, reached for a silent toy signaled by the aid after four presentations during the first session. In subsequent sessions, she improved her performance and responded significantly more often when the aid was operating than when it was switched off. Later on in the training program, during formal assessments, she used the aid signal to discriminate reliably between objects within and outside her reach, and eventually she attempted to move toward persons silently entering the aid's field. Other 2 1/2-year-olds in this study showed much less ability, or interest, in using the aid although they eventually would reach on occasion for objects signaled by the aid. In both cases incompatible mannerisms and motor activities appeared to be hindering aid use. Finally, Strelow, Kay, and Kay (47) reported that a developmentally delayed 30-month old child reached for silent objects after six sessions of five trials over three days. After four months more work, this child showed some obstacle avoidance and ability to follow people. As well, his listening skills were improved.

In our own studies, we placed Kay's Binaural Sensory Aid on Belle, who was born 3 1/2 months premature, when she was 21 months of age (corrected for prematurity). Both her speech and motor development were delayed, but she could stand well and was just starting to walk forward. She exhibited many self-stimulating movements, tactile defensiveness (withdrawing from any contact), and kept her hands at shoulder height. On the first session, when the aid was turned on, Belle quieted, smiled, and then moved her head in a scanning motion when objects were placed in the aid's field. She also smiled when food on a spoon was brought to her mouth. However, there was no tracking or reaching for silent objects in the aid's view. For several months, on a regular basis, the parents played games while she wore the aid, and reported that she readily accepted it, calling it a "hat." She was observed to move her arms and fingers excitedly when the aid was turned on and enjoyed playing with the sound by moving her head. During feeding, she began to open her mouth to the sound of an approaching spoon; however, she never seemed to explore actively using the aid, but this is not surprising given her tactile defensiveness. Although the parents reported that she would sometimes avoid obstacles while walking with the aid on, but not when it was off, we were not able to verify this until at age four she was recorded as she approached and stopped before a bush, tree, or a person. Sometimes she would name the object and then reach for it.

More dramatic results were obtained by Humphrey and Humphrey (26), who placed the Sonicguide on two blind infants at 19 and 31 months of age. Both children demonstrated an ability to reach for and grasp sounding objects during formal assessments (7/17 trials for the younger and 8/8 trials for the older child). In the first session the younger child, Lee, reached for a silent object entering the aid's field for four successive trials out of seven, beginning on the second presentation. He never responded with the aid switched off. Subsequently, he wore the aid to play aid games with his parents for about 20 minutes per day and was videotaped during biweekly assessments. He continued to reach for objects signaled by the aid, was observed tracking objects, and began to reach more rapidly for preferred than non-preferred objects (e.g., a wallet) and to smile when his brother silently entered the aid's field, suggesting some degree of object discrimination.

The older child, Eddy, who was walking proficiently, was standing when the aid was first turned on and immediately moved toward objects and smiled while exploring them, first by scanning with the aid and then with his hands. He would not sit passively and refused to keep the aid in place when it was not operating. He continued to wear the aid for 1/2 to 2 hours per day. Follow-up assessments on Eddy's reaching four months after the aid was introduced showed that he reached for aid-signaled objects on 30 of 35 trials. Both midline and 30° left and right test trials were given. He was most successful on midline trials, making no errors. Interestingly, on successful lateral trials he would often scan with his head until the signal amplitude was balanced in the two ears and then reach out in the direction his head was pointed to contact the object.

Although Eddy would tolerate reaching assessments for a while, he preferred to use the aid while mobile to locate objects, explore surfaces, and avoid obstacles. His smiling confidence while using the aid to explore novel environments contrasted sharply with his drooping posture, slow hesitant steps, collisions, and eventual immobility when the aid was removed. Two further observations are noteworthy. After only two weeks of aid use, he freely ran down a hallway with the aid on, while previously he refused to run forward at all. Furthermore, in outdoor exploration, he avoided poles and walls, chose to explore some trees, fences, and especially cars, and commented on unusual obstacles in his path on the sidewalk, such as garbage cans, without touching them. His performance suggests that he can recognize depths and textures and guide his path accordingly.

SUMMARY AND DISCUSSION

The research reviewed on sensory development in sighted infants suggests that certain aspects of early development are characterized by peaks and troughs. The relation between the development of visual attention and changes in the auditory localization response is one particular example in which a "peak" in one response system is contemporaneous with a "trough" in another. At this point, as early as two months of age, vision seems to become dominant in controlling infant attention, but both earlier and later there appears to be more "sharing" between these two systems. Such complex relations are not adequately

described by a simple differentiation view of intersensory development in which a process begins and ends at a particular time.

From our review of 23 case studies it is clear that both
congenitally blind infants and older pre-school children can make
some use of the information supplied by a sonar aid, provided they
will cooperate and attend to the changes in the aid's signals.
Typically, blind infants less than one year of age first quiet
when the aid is turned on and then, provided they have attained
the stage of reaching for naturally sounding objects, almost
immediately (or very rapidly with training) begin to reach for an
approaching object. Although it may not be absolutely necessary
that a child is reliably reaching for sounding objects before the
sonar aid is used effectively, the research reviewed suggests
that infants are more likely to use the aid if they are reaching
(22,34,43,45). The most consistent use is in reaching for objects
presented at midline. There is no strong evidence to suggest
that infants use the interaural amplitude difference cue to
perceive off-center targets or that they have a fine appreciation
of the distance code. This should not be taken as suggesting
that the aids could not be of benefit, however, as reaching for
objects at midline has been seen as a crucial milestone for the
blind infant (e.g., 18).

There is little support for Bower's "critical period" hypothesis that very young infants use the aid in a different and
more sophisticated manner than older children. Many children
past the supposed critical age (13 months) have shown immediate,
or rapid, appreciation of the information signaled by the aid.
The quality of their responses is at least at the level of the
younger infants. We would argue that the forms of assessment
used by Aitken and Bower (1) are most appropriate and interesting
to young infants, but do not engage the interest of older infants
and young children. So their finding of a "critical period" for
introducing the aid may not be as closely tied to sensory differentiation as they suggest, but may be more a function of
motivation, which is closely tied to the available skills of the
child. Indeed if there is any trend, it is for older children,
especially those that are mobile, to make more effective use of
the spatial information signaled by the aid (26,45).

The importance of both novelty and need in maintaining aid
use is equally clear. The principle of the infant's continual
search for novel visual experience, beginning as early as 2 - 3
months of age, appears to be true later on for the auditory
input produced by the aid. Thus we see rapid habituation during
training sessions, even with tasks which include social or food
rewards. Moreover, as soon as the infant solves a particular
problem without benefit of the aid, its use in that context often

declines. Examples of such declines are the refusal of infants
to use the aid for reaching when they have developed a "sweep or
grope" strategy for locating nearby objects (1,22), and refusal
to use the aid as an obstacle detector in walking once the spatial
layout of a particular environment has been mastered (8,27).
Perhaps this is why responsiveness to the sonar aid appears to
emerge so gradually. The trainer's inventiveness declines with
time until a new motor milestone inspires the presentation of
novel tasks.

A number of methodological issues need to be considered when
sonar aids are placed on young infants. We still have no clear
indication of the best age at which to introduce the aid. Although
it may serve as a focus for social stimulation in infants who are
premobile and less than 13 months of age, more spontaneous use
appears in the older, mobile child. Parents should always be
made aware of those limitations of the aid's use at various
developmental stages that are a function of the child's natural
activities. If this is not done, the parents will surely experience a sense of failure when rapid and dramatic advances in
aid use fail to occur. Our experience suggests that it may be
important to require children to have achieved some minimum level
of aid-related skills prior to the introduction of the aid. For
example, premobile infants can use the aid's signal for reaching
but only seem to do so once they are already reaching for sounding
objects. Furthermore, the presence of behaviors which interfere
with attention to the aid's signals (e.g., rocking or facing the
floor) should be minimal if we are to expect the infants to make
effective use of the aid (e.g., 45).

Another issue involves who should do the training, and for
how long. In most studies, the aid is given to the parents along
with suggestions about how to carry out various short daily
exercises with the aid in operation. This places an extraordinary
demand on the parents to develop novel situations for using the
aid, given the infant's tendency to habituate. Once novelty has
diminished for the parents, they seem to consider this task a
chore and may convey their frustrations to the infant, particularly when the infant becomes uncooperative. Possibly, parents
may not be as successful as a specially trained sonar aid instructor who only works with the infant on, say, a biweekly
basis. Once the infant begins to assert his/her independence
from the parents, the aid may simply become a focal point for
confrontation, with its signals ignored by both parties.

We initially expected the aid to become a partial substitute
for vision and assumed that our subjects would eventually demand
full time use. Instead, we found that each skill took time to
train, sometimes with limited success, and rarely was there any

demand by the infant to be given the aid. Possibly with a lighter, smaller, less cumbersome unit (our aid's headband was 1 1/4" high and 3/4" thick at the front, where the transmitter and receivers were packaged, and weighed 1/4 lb., while the encased battery pack weighed 1 5/16 lbs.), which could be powered for long periods of time without battery change, extended use will become more frequent. Also, an FM transmitter-receiver to be used by parents and professionals for monitoring the aid's signal (22) during testing and training would help reduce the number of wires surrounding the child and interfering with his or her mobility.

Perhaps the greatest need at this point is for properly designed experimental assessments and follow-up programs which will determine the degree to which the aid is used by children of different ages and any residual benefit that early use may have on later spatial understanding. Although Bower suggested that aid experience during the early months of life might keep a blind child on track, meeting developmental milestones on time, other forms of infant stimulation, such as simple training to attend to sounding objects as well as enriching tactile experience and novel environments may be more effective (18,43). Also, Tronick and Brazelton (2) have suggested that with support, resourceful parents can be helped to interpret the limited ability of blind infants to communicate, and with continued effort can help their infants to reduce "blindisms" and achieve motor milestones on time. Again, however, we must recognize the fact that there are large individual differences. The only convincing way to determine the actual effects of early aid use would be to conduct a study in which aids are assigned to one group and a different training program to another, on a random basis; given the limited availability of infants, it is unlikely that such a study will be carried out. Alternatively, the very least we should be expected to do in our research is to provide clear evidence of aid use during our evaluation program by comparison of behavior with the aid turned on and with it switched off (22,45). One major problem that we have experienced with such a procedure is that some of the infants we have worked with refuse to keep the aid in place unless it is operating. A method which we hope will show promise in demonstrating that early aid experience is beneficial is to compare the performance of children who have such experience with those who do not as they are trained on a new spatial task whose solution is materially assisted by correct use of aid signals. If early aid use has made a memorable impact, the experienced child might be expected to perform in a superior manner.

CONCLUSIONS

We conclude that our own hopes and expectations when we embarked on this research were naive and very optimistic. There is little doubt that some young children, like adults, can benefit greatly from the use of a sonar-type device as a substitute for vision. So far there is not a great deal of evidence to show that major changes in mental abilities can be engineered by early introduction of the aid. However, the final word on this awaits more extensive, and in particular more long-term, developmental research.

It is very evident that to understand how the aid can be used effectively with young children, and to assess its impact on their mental development, requires an intimate knowledge of the course of normal cognitive growth. The sonar aid is no panacea for the problems of the blind child, which is not to say that great improvements in the way it is introduced and used may not still be possible. We hope they will be.

ACKNOWLEDGEMENT

This research was supported by grants from the National Sciences and Engineering Research Council of Canada to P. C. Dodwell and D. W. Muir (A-0044), and to G. K. Humphrey (A-8289), and from the Ministry of Health and Welfare to P. C. Dodwell and D. W. Muir, and a Postdoctoral Fellowship from the Alberta Heritage Foundation for Medical Research to D. E. Humphrey. Special thanks to Kathy, Ted, Belle, Eddy, and Lee and their respective parents for making this research possible and to Sarah Dawe and Audrey Bailey for typing this manuscript.

1. Two models of the sonar aid have been used in the research reported in this paper, both being variations on Kay's (28) basic design. The commercially available Sonicguide was used by Aitken and Bower (1); Ferrell (15); and Humphrey and Humphrey (26); a research model of the Binaural Sensory Aid provided by L. Kay's group was used by Schwartz (42); Harris et al. (22); Muir, Humphrey, Humphrey, & Dodwell (37); and Strelow (45). See Strelow and Boys (46) report for a review of the aid's properties.

REFERENCES

1.   Aitken, S. & Bower, T. G. R. (1982). Intersensory substi-
     tution in the blind. Journal of Experimental Child Psychol-
     ogy, 33, 309-323.

2.   Als, H., Tronick, E., & Brazelton, T. B. (1980). Affective
     reciprocity and the development of autonomy: The study of a
     blind infant. Journal of the American Academy of Child
     Psychiatry, 19, 22-40.

3.   Bertenthal, B. I. & Campos, J. J. (1983). Self-produced
     locomotion: An organizer of emotional, cognitive and social
     development in infancy. In R. Emde & R. Harmon (Eds.),
     Continuities and Discontinuities in Development. New York:
     Plenum Press.

4.   Bigelow, A. E. (1983). Development of the use of sound in
     search behavior of infants. Developmental Psychology, 19,
     317-321.

5.   Bower, T. G. R. (1977). Blind babies see with their ears.
     New Scientist, 73, 255-257.

6.   Bower, T. G. R. (1979). The origins of meaning in percep-
     tual development. In A. D. Pick (Ed.), Perception and its
     Development: A Tribute to E. J. Gibson. Hillsdale, NJ:
     Erlbaum.

7.   Boys, J. T., Strelow, E. R., & Clark, G. R. S. (1979). A
     prosthetic aid for a developing blind child. Ultrasonics,
     17, 37-42.

8.   Bullinger, A. (1984). Blindness and sensory aids for babies.
     Unpublished manuscript.

9.   Bundy, R. F. (1980). Discrimination of sound localization
     cues in young infants. Child Development, 51, 292-294.

10. Cohen, J. F. & Tronick, E. Z. (1983). Three-month-old in-
     fants' reaction to simulated maternal depression. Child
     Development, 54, 185-193.

11. Demany, L., McKenzie, B., & Vurpillot, E. (1977). Rhythm
     perception in early infancy. Nature, 266, 718-719.

12. DiFranco, D., Muir, D. W., & Dodwell, P. C. (1978). Reach-
     ing in very young infants. Perception, 7, 385-392.

13. Dodwell, P. C., Humphrey, G. K., & Muir, D. W. (In Press). Shape and pattern perception. In L. B. Cohen & P. Salapatek (Eds.), Handbook of Infant Perception. New York: Academic Press.

14. Fantz, R. L. (1961). The origin of form perception. Scientific American, 204, 66-72.

15. Ferrell, K. A. (1980). Can infants use the Sonicguide? Two years experience of project VIEW! Journal of Visual Impairment & Blindness, 74, 209-220.

16. Field, J., DiFranco, D., Dodwell, P. C.,& Muir, D.W. (1979). Auditory-visual coordination of 2 1/2 month old infants. Infant Behavior and Development, 2, 113-122.

17. Forbes, B. (1981). Orientation differences in sound localization abilities of 4 to 5 month old infants. Unpublished master's thesis. Queen's University.

18. Fraiberg, S. (1977). Insights from the Blind: Comparative Studies of Blind and Sighted Infants. New York: Basic Books.

19. Gibson, J. J. & Gibson, E. J. (1955). Perceptual learning -- Differentiation or Enrichment? Psychological Review, 62, 32-41.

20. Gurella, J. & Muir, D. (1985). Experimental manipulations of mother-infant interactions. Isolating the effective components. Paper presented at the 17th Banff International Conference on Behavioral Sciences, Banff, Alberta.

21. Haith, M. M. (1978). Visual competence in early infancy. In R. Held, H. Leibowitz, & H. L. Teuber (Eds.), Handbook of Sensory Physiology, 8. Berlin: Springer-Verlag.

22. Harris, L., Humphrey, G. K., Muir, D. W., & Dodwell, P. C. (1985). The use of the Canterbury Child's Aid in infancy and early childhood: A case study. Journal of Visual Impairment & Blindness, 79, 4-11.

23. Harris, P. & MacFarlane, A. (1974). The growth of the effective visual field from birth to seven weeks. Journal of Experimental Child Psychology, 18, 340-348.

24. Hofsten, C. von. (1982). Eye-hand coordination in newborns. Developmental Psychology, 18, 450-461.

25. Hofsten, C. von.   (1984).   Developmental   changes   in   the
    organization of prereaching movements. Developmental Psycho-
    logy, 20 378-388.

26. Humphrey, G. K. & Humphrey, D. E.   (In Press). The use of
    binaural sensory aids by blind infants and children: Theo-
    retical and applied issues. In F. Morrison, C. Lord, & D.
    Keating (Eds.), Applied Developmental Psychology, Vol. 2.
    Toronto: Academic Press.

27. Humphrey, G. K.,   Humphrey, D. E.,   Muir, D. W., & Dodwell,
    P. C. (in press). Pattern perception in infants: Effects of
    structure and transformations, Journal of Experimental Child
    Psychology.

28. Kay, L. (1967).   Ultrasonic spectacles for the blind.   In
    R. Dufton (Ed.), Proceedings of the International Conference
    on Sensory Devices for the Blind. London: St. Dunstan's.

29. Landau, B., Spelke, E. & Gleitman, H. (1984). Spatial know-
    ledge in a young blind child. Cognition, 16, 225-260.

30. Maurer, D. & Lewis, T. I. (1979). A physiological explana-
    tion of infants' early visual development. Canadian Journal
    of Psychology, 33, 232-252.

31. Mitchell, D. E. (1978). Effect of early visual experience on
    the development of certain perceptual abilities in animals
    and man. In R. D. Walk & H. L. Pick, Jr. (Eds.), Perception
    and Experience. New York: Plenum Press.

32. Moore, J. M., Thompson, G., & Thompson, M. (1975). Auditory
    localization of infants as a function of reinforcement con-
    ditions. Journal of Speech and Hearing Disorders, 40, 29-34.

33. Muir, D. (1982). The development of human auditory locali-
    zation in infancy.   In R. W. Gatehouse (Ed.), Localization
    of Sound: Theory and Applications.   Groton, CT: Amphora
    Press.

34. Muir, D. (In Press).   The development of infants' auditory
    spatial sensitivity.   In S. E. Trehub & B. A. Schneider
    (Eds.), Auditory Development in Infancy.   New York: Plenum
    Press.

35. Muir, D., Abraham, W., Forbes, B., & Harris, L. (1979). The
    ontogenesis of an auditory localization response from birth
    to four months of age.   Canadian Journal of Psychology, 33,
    320-333.

36. Muir, D. & Clifton, R. (1985). Infants' orientation to the location of sound sources. In G. Gottlieb & N. Krasnegor (Eds.), The Measurement of Audition and Vision During the First Year of Life: A Methodological Overview. Norwood, NJ: Ablex.

37. Muir, D. W., Humphrey, G. K., Dodwell, P. C. & Humphrey, D. E. (1985). The perception of vector patterns by 4-month-old infants (Unpublished manuscript).

38. Muir, D. W. & Field, J. (1979). Newborn infants orient to sounds. Child Development, 50, 431-436.

39. Muir, D. W. & Mitchell, D. F. (1973). Visual rsolution and experience: Acuity deficits in cats following early selective visual deprivation. Science, 180, 420-422.

40. Northern, J. L. & Downs, M. P. (1978). Hearing in Children. Baltimore: Waverly Press.

41. Rowell, D. (1970). Auditory Display of Spatial Information. Ph.D. dissertation, University of Canterbury.

42. Schwartz, M. A. (1978). Specific auditory enrichment program for congenitally blind infants. Unpublished manuscript.

43. Schwartz, M. A. (1984). The role of sound for space and object perception in the congenitally blind infant. In L. P. Lipsitt & C. Rovee-Collier (Eds.), Advances in Infancy Research, Vol. 3, Norwood, NJ: Ablex.

44. Searle, C. L., Braida, L. D., Davis, M. F. & Colburn, H. S. (1976). Model for auditory localization. Journal of the Acoustical Society of America, 60, 1164-1175.

45. Strelow, E. R. (1983). Use of the Binaural Sensory Aid by young children. Journal of Visual Impairment & Blindness, 77, 429-438.

46. Strelow, E. R. & Boys, J. T. (1979). The Canterbury Child's Aid: A binaural spatial sensor for research with blind children. Journal of Visual Impairment & Blindness, 73, 179-184.

47. Strelow, E. R., Kay, N., & Kay, L. (1978). Binaural sensory aid: Case studies of its use by two children. Journal of Visual Impairment & Blindness, 72, 1-9.

48. Tronick, E. (1972). Stimulus control and the growth of the infants' effective visual field. Perception & Psychophysics, 11, 373-376.

49. Uzgiris, I. C. & Benson, J. (1980). Infants' use of sound in the search for objects. Paper presented at the International Conference on Infant Studies, New Haven.

50. Warren, D. H. (1984). Blindness and Early Childhood Development (Second edition). New York: American Foundation for the Blind.

51. Warren, D. H. Anooshian, L. J. & Bollinger, J. G. (1973). Early vs. late blindness: The role of early vision in spatial behavior. American Foundation for the Blind Research Bulletin, 26, 151-170.

52. Watrous, B. S., McConnell, F., Sitton, A. B., & Fleet, W. F. (1975). Auditory response of infants. Journal of Speech and Hearing Disorders, 40, 357-366.

53. White, B. L., Castle, P., & Held, R. (1964). Observations on the development of visually-directed reaching. Child Development, 35, 349-364.

54. Wishart, J. G., Bower, T. G. R., & Dunkeld, J. (1978). Reaching in the dark. Perception, 7, 507-512.

DEVELOPMENTAL BRAIN RESEARCH, DEPRIVATION, AND SENSORY AIDS

B. J. Sonnier and A. H. Riesen

University of California, Riverside

A major goal of brain research is to develop a better understanding of the correspondence between changes in central nervous
system (CNS) processes and changes in behavior. Studies of the
CNS are approached with the assumption that morphological and
physiological features consistently observed under normal developmental conditions are essential to the functional and behavioral interactions that enable members of a species to compete
and reproduce successfully in their environment. Since the very
nature of brain research makes it difficult, if not impossible,
to use human subjects, animal models are used to examine genetic
and experimentally induced disorders in an attempt to gain
insight into CNS processes underlying developmental patterns,
mechanisms of plasticity, and relationships between brain and
behavioral organization. Assessments of changes in brain and
behavioral development occurring under abnormal conditions are
also used to evaluate the capacity of an organism to compensate
for developmental differences and to survive trauma to the CNS or
abnormal sensory input, such as occurs with the loss of vision or
with the use of a sensory substitution device.

Although species differences occur, members of the mammalian
line share enough common principles of evolution and development
to allow us to make some inferences about human development from
animal studies. For example, while critical or sensitive periods
of maximum plasticity are observed more often in immature mammals, all mammals, including humans, appear to retain a degree of
of brain and behavioral plasticity throughout their lifetime.
Relationships between the formation of brain and behavioral response patterns and the basic processes underlying changes in the

functional organization of these patterns during mammalian development are not yet understood. We are only beginning to appreciate the nature and importance of developmental processes, and to see that human sensory and nervous capabilities are designed to acquire, integrate, and act on specific information necessary to survival. We may not yet comprehend the full nature or extent of these stimulus relationships, but we do know that the organization of brain and behavioral response patterns in mammals can influence and be influenced by the way in which information is processed.

Sensory Substitution

Perceptions are based on combinations of both current and past information obtained through the sensory systems, with behavioral capacity determined by the kinds of relations among stimuli that can be perceived (41,66,132). When sensory modalities or the stimuli that are available to them are altered, alternative response strategies are developed, but these strategies are usually less efficient or appropriate than those developed under normal conditions. Why is this so? Recent theories of perception (e.g., 25) question the uniqueness and exclusiveness of the importance of information from any given sensory channel to perceptual development, and they argue that the acquisition of perceptual skills is the result of an education of attention to relevant information from any source.

By this reasoning, the importance of the visual system to the development of spatial-motor skills may not be a result of inherent genetic processes which favor the visual system, but instead may be a result of the fact that more salient spatial information is carried by electromagnetic wavelengths of light, which the visual system has evolved an ability to process efficiently, in comparison to that carried by other stimuli, such as by sound or touch. Thus theoretically, any aspect of neural, behavioral, or perceptual development which is normally influenced by information obtained visually, such as the acquisition of spatial-motor skills, could be influenced by a different sensory modality if sufficiently salient information could be provided to that modality by an alternate means, such as the use of a sensory substitution device.

It is apparent that some environmental factors can cause independent acceleration or depression of growth in certain neurons in specific brain areas (27,108,125) as well as enhance, prevent, or retard the development of specific social, spatial, or learning skills (33). We need to determine exactly what is necessary for optimal biological and behavioral development and how these factors relate to each other.

The role of the information content of specific versus general sensory stimulation in the induction, facilitation, and/or maintenance of ontogeny of developmental processes is not adequately understood. Sensory substitution techniques (2,3,4) could be used to examine the effect of certain types of stimulus information on developmental processes and to test the exclusivity of specific sensory channels for the learning of spatial-motor skills. For example, one could present salient information about the spatial environment to blind subjects through auditory or tactile channels in controlled experimental situations. Such data could be useful to those interested in the acceleration or alteration of certain forms of sensory or motor skills to compensate for deficits, e.g., those developing training programs to assist blind subjects in the use of nonvisual sensory cues to enhance their spatial-motor skills. This approach would also provide a test of Gibson's (25) theory.

A subject should ideally be able to use the information obtained from a sensory substitution device rapidly, efficiently, and effectively. In order for this to happen, certain conditions will have to be met. The patterns of stimulation produced by a sensory substitution device should lawfully represent the spatial locations of objects in the immediate environment, and the input patterns should vary in accordance with the user's self-initiated activities. The impact of the form or information content of device-generated stimuli can be assessed relative to several aspects of both brain and behavioral development.

Sensory substitution techniques can be used to examine specific plastic properties of sensory systems and to determine the role of polysensory neurons in providing alternative modes for the development of response strategies. Sensory prostheses can be used to develop experimental animal models for evaluating the type and extent of behavioral abnormalities and neurological deficits that are associated with, or have the potential to become associated with, any form of specific deprivation, such as early blindness. One might also be able to assess the effectiveness of early intervention training to compensate for sensory loss and species-typical preparedness or constraints and their effects on adaptive capacity.

With creative imagination, the application of sensory substitution techniques may prove to be just as useful in solving basic research problems as we hope they may be in solving applied ones.

DEVELOPMENTAL BRAIN RESEARCH

Justification

Brain research has demonstrated that analyses of even the smallest cell assemblies often provide useful information about the developmental consequences of genetic change or environmental manipulation (10,27,28). In fact, quantitative and qualitative differential changes in the spatial configuration of neurons during development may eventually prove to be the most significant contributing factor to changes in functional integration (1,18,79,80,81,82). Although each class of neurons normally makes rather specific types of connections, their general connectivity patterns vary with the area in which they are located and exhibit many plastic properties, especially in the immature organism. Functional integration of sensory data involves all types or classes of neurons, and neuronal interplays of excitation and inhibition form the basis of complex cortical processing. One of the major goals of developmental brain research is to acquire a better understanding of those factors which have the potential to influence CNS organizational properties during maturation.

Comments

Although we find it necessary to break complex developmental processes down into their component parts in order to study them, we must not forget that the separation is only conceptual. Development is an ontogenous, unified process with orderly, recognizable patterns resulting from or accompanied by the formation of new constituents, their growth or integration into larger units, and their arrangement in space (23). Evolutionary processes ensure the survival of life forms in changing environments through the retention or alteration of old systems and the development of new ones; an example of this evolution is the neocortex. The neocortex appears to increase the range of variability of response capacity in mammals, thus allowing for more rapid and efficient behavioral adaptation during environmental change.

Surprisingly little is known about the development, evolution, or function of the brain, especially the neocortex. This is regrettable, as one of the truly unique characteristics of primates is their tendency toward a high degree of cerebral development with the rest of the body relatively unspecialized. Increases in cerebration result in increased potential for association or integration of stimulus input and for voluntary control of behavioral responses.

FACTORS INFLUENCING DEVELOPMENT

Genetics

Genetic material and plastic properties of the CNS interacting with the environment provide the basis upon which experience
may build or shape the mode or capacity for responding in an
organism (34). Hereditary and environmental influences on behavior
cannot be separated, because the reception, integration, and
interpretation of all sensory data is subject to both influences
simultaneously. All behaviors are complex events, and the tabula
rasa concept of newborn organisms is not tenable. It is altogether
possible that some behaviors may be expressed through genetically
generated and functionally related body parts in much the same
way as the knee-jerk reflex or a physical characteristic like the
shape of the ear is expressed.

Although it is generally accepted that abnormal conditions,
whether deficiencies or excesses, can have long-lasting effects
on brain structure and function, and influence the biology and
behavior of the organism as a whole, genetic restraints on the
potential for change in developmental processes have not been
determined. Some invariant aspects of neuronal components may
exist to provide a stable framework within which the variable
aspects can assure adaptive flexibility.

Plasticity

Human and other primates have acquired a remarkable capacity
for adaptation to changes in environmental conditions, and have
developed many variations in the complexity of their social interactions (40). Experimental control of the human environment
is virtually impossible, but studies of the effects of environmental manipulations on other animals allow us to speculate about
how certain changes might affect the human species. We know that
some forms of deprivation in animals often result in abnormal behavior patterns that show a degree of similarity to those present
in certain types of human behavioral disorders, such as mental
retardation and emotional disturbance. Neuroanatomical and
physiological alterations of the CNS have also been observed in
some deprivation experiments, but their precise relationship to
behavioral ontogeny, such as the development of pathological
behavior patterns, is not known.

The CNS appears to retain a degree of plasticity throughout
the lifetime of an organism, and environmental factors determine,
shape, direct,or modulate ongoing neural development and behavior,
which in turn affect each other (34,36,63,64,107,108,109,112).
Development of the CNS is a very complex process, especially in

primates, and abnormalities with persisting consequences can occur at any stage of the process, either pre- or postnatally. While most cortical neurons are present at birth, establishment of definitive connectivity continues, extending over several years in the human species, and progression of myelinization correlates with that of maturation and stabilization of functional ability.   Cortical connective complexity in human and other primates, in conjunction with the duration of myelinization processes, offers some explanation for the extended duration of psychomotor development, such as that found in children.

Differentiation and growth, beginning shortly after mitosis, exhibit a caudo-rostral medio-lateral maturation gradient (57, 65, 73), and vital functions are established prior to others (141). Mammalian neocortical differentiation is characterized by extensive cell migration to the final formation of six rather distinctive layers. Retention or prolongation of certain steps may result in maturational delays or pathological changes in CNS development. All adaptive changes, such as those often reported found in experimental situations, should be evaluated relative to their actual survival value over time in a normal environment as opposed to their value in an artificial environment.

Sensory

Sensory afferents ultimately converge on the neocortex, which is considered the major locus of sensory integration and behavioral coordination in primates (31,65,134). The organization of the CNS is relatively independent of sensory receptor organization in the mammalian line; for example, the organization of visual cortex does not particularly reflect retinal organization. The sequence of sensory modality maturation may be common to all mammals, proceeding in the order of tactile, vestibular, auditory, and visual modalities (32). Decreases in overlap between the connectivity of somatosensory and motor areas occur with increases in complexity of cortical organization such as that found in primates (68). Neural components of the different systems are similar; e.g., all systems contain pyramidal neurons, but there are many differences in connectivity, and some neurons in the different areas have rather specific stimulus requirements.

The form of neuronal structure may not be directly determined by type of sensory input, but pathological conditions in the CNS and/or abnormal features in sensory receptor development, or in the sensory information impending on them, can result in suboptimal development of certain skills. One example is reduced acquisition of spatial-motor skills in the blind. Behaviors that do not appear until much later can also be affected; this has been reported for audition, gustation, olfaction, and vision (89), as well as for general energy levels and intellectual functioning (142).

Neurons

Experimental manipulations may affect the locus, size, or number of a type of neuron, but they do not appear to affect basic characteristics of the general cell types, such as shape and polarity of the soma; however, restrictions on cellular plasticity are not known. Capacity for variation usually enhances adaptive capability, so the different classes of neurons probably contribute to increased potential for variability in control of responses in some way. Neuronal size may be related to functional requirements, and the eventual survival and form or pattern of neurons and their processes could be dependent on the connectivity of the cortex as an integrated "unit" or "whole" rather than on any one influencing factor.

Axons

As cells migrate and begin to reach their destinations in the cortex, they are still developing, and there is a sudden rise in axon growth at this time which correlates with increased appearance of other response components, such as dendrites and synapses (14,16,22,71,72). This occurs region by region, and the sequence is fairly invariant. Synaptic contacts appear to be nonrandom, specific, and sequential in development, but specific selectivity may be lost with maturation. Finally, for some contacts to mature, they appear to require functional validation, e.g., use in the formation, maintenance, or completion of an actual response, whether it is appropriate or not, to mature (57).

Axon growth is probably controlled by a combination of factors, and under normal conditions, any or all of the following may influence axon growth: a) target cell type and locus; b) competition for contact sites; c) substrate elements; d) positioning of neuron of origin of axon relative to other neurons; e) connectivity hierarchies; and f) neuron of origin or destination interactions with other cells (37,48,58,128). Axon decussation patterns appear to be determined quite early in development, but ongoing interactions with other axons are still important. For instance, the degree of connectivity normally controlled by each of the eyes can be altered, and subsequent cortical reorganization can occur postnatally (45,59,101). Cortical crossing at the midline to innervate appropriate laminae has been observed following lesions of visual cortex (92) and somatosensory cortex (69,70). The growth and reshaping of axons to establish normal visual callosal connections indicate that some interhemispheric connections are transitory and may serve as substrate for developmental plasticity in the CNS (50,51,52).

There is evidence for greater brain and behavioral plasticity in neonatally-lesioned animals compared to adult-lesioned ones. Adult striate-lesioned rabbits were compared to infant-lesioned ones on a battery of behavioral tests, and while infant-lesioned rabbits were not different from normals on any task studied, there were differences in the adult-lesioned group (129). The infant-operated rabbits showed shorter latencies from lateral cortex than did either adult-operated or normal ones, indicating the establishment of a novel thalamocortical organization following the neonatal lesions. Cortical innervation of the denervated left red nucleus (RN) after complete removal of the left hemisphere (hemispherectomy) has been demonstrated in cats using injections of tritiated leucine and proline to the primary motor cortex of the intact right hemisphere. Terminal field areas were much more symmetrical in the RN of neonatally-lesioned kittens, and bilateral innervation of the thalamus, present in the neonatally-lesioned group, did not occur in the adult-lesioned group (126, 139). More behavioral recovery was also observed in the neonatally-lesioned cats, and only trained observers could discriminate the kitten-lesioned cats from control cats with both hemispheres intact.

Dendrites

Although there are temporal and spatial regularities in dendritic development between mammals, dendritic development becomes more complex as one approaches the human species, (94,95), and dendritic differentiation is affected by many environmental factors. Dendrites appear to have evolved as increases in the surface contact area of neurons, and they enhance cellular potential for integrative organizational complexity (12,91,117, 118,119,123,124).

Each type of neuron has a characteristic pattern of branching, and since dendrites participate extensively in synaptic interactions, they tend to respond to altered input in different ways. The number and orientation patterns of dendrites are sensitive to environmental influences, and they are important factors in the development of connectivity relationships, because dendrites provide the major proportion of membrane surface area for integration of synaptic input (91,102,103,104). Under normal conditions, most dendrites run parallel to the axons with which they form synaptic relationships. This growth pattern increases the probability of axonal contact and produces a tendency to distribute by laminae (12,140).

General

Neocortical organization can be affected by many environmental manipulations; however, evolutionary increases in the size and surface area of the neocortex appear to have extended the range of an organism's control over the environment. This is thought to be based on larger neuronal populations, greater diversity of neuronal connections, and increases in the complexity of their interactions (121). Neocortical complexity is most advanced in man, who has developed an amazing, and sometimes frightening, ability to modify and control his environment. The possibility of being able to control modifications of developmental organizational processes in order to enhance compensation in the advent of a sensory deficit presents a significant scientific and technological challenge.

DEPRIVATION AND THE DEVELOPING BRAIN

Abnormal Input

Various influences on neocortical quantitative parameters, such as laminar thickness, axon length, and dendritic number or orientation patterns, have been observed in experimental conditions using deprivation and/or enrichment techniques. Studies of the developmental consequences of altered rearing environments provide further insight into factors other than genetic mechanisms that have the potential to influence connectivity patterns in the CNS, and consequently behavior. Knowledge about these factors may eventually become useful in the treatment of neural disorders, particularly in the development of techniques to alter abnormal innervation patterns. The consideration of this possibility is important, as the persistence of abnormal innervation patterns can prevent the formation of more functionally appropriate connections, and the probability of this is thought to increase subsequent to functional validation or use of an inappropriate connection (8,67).

We know that relatively long-lasting or permanent changes can occur in the brain as the result of experience and/or breeding. Two examples of this are well known. One, the brains of domesticated animals are smaller than those of the feral born even for some time following their return to the wild (44). Two, decreases in dendritic spine densities and changes in spine morphology have been related to mental retardation (49,83,84,100), but it is difficult to determine exactly which aspects of the changes are directly relevant to the disorder. We cannot say there is an actual loss of spines resulting from or causing the retardation, as the changes could be due to afferent reduction, intracortical connectivity alterations, lack of maturation of neuronal support systems, or failure of a class of neurons to complete a developmental stage.

Experimental investigations have shown that many aspects of neuronal development, such as dendritic orientation or branch number, axonal growth processes, spine density or morphology, and synaptogenesis, are affected by manipulations of the environment or changes in sensory and/or motor information available to the organism (7,26,34,35,36,111,114,115,130,135,136).   Visual and motor experience appear to be of utmost importance to developing mammals, especially primates.

Visual deprivation

Some synapses in the visual cortex appear to develop without stimulation, but their number may be reduced by certain manipulations of stimulus input. After 45 days of binocular occlusion, kittens exhibited a 30 percent reduction in synapses related to binocular input, and there was a rise in synapse formation after stimulus exposure (15). There is a reduction of or lack of increase in synapse formation in visual cortex with dark rearing, but synapse development may reach normal after some exposure to the light stimulus (113,137,138).

Visual deprivation experiments with kittens indicate that an entire population of neurons can be affected when only a subset receives stimulation (19,131). Constant exposure to light has been shown to increase synaptic contact with spines on pyramidal neurons in laminae IV and V in rats (93). Laminae II and IV decrease in thickness with visual deprivation, suggesting that lack of light may have a selective effect on pyramidal neurons (38). Auditory response cells in the cat were observed to increase from 11 percent to 42 percent in all layers of the superior colliculus after binocular deprivation (105), but visually responsive units did not decrease nor were visual responses depressed by nonvisual activity, thus indicating an increase in multisensory neurons.

The preceding results are only a small sample of available evidence, but they are enough to stress the importance of a specific extrinsic stimulus, in this case light, to the visual system and to point out the possibility of alternative modes of processing in the absence of light.

Nonvisual deprivation

Prior research has mainly focused on the effects of visual deprivation or the manipulation of visual stimuli, but other sensory modalities are now being investigated. In studies of stumptail monkeys (Macaca arctoides) that received varying degrees of somatosensory stimulation and motor activity, spineless stellate cell branching in lamina IV decreased in primary somatosensory and motor areas only in the two most deprived conditions, but all of the experimental animals showed decreased branching in the secondary motor area (111,125). Socially deprived but motorically enriched animals, who were consistently high in the active use of ladders, a trapeze, and other objects, showed a degree of dendritic branching in primary somatosensory cortex that was greater than in all other groups, including mother-reared controls. Abnormal behavior patterns were observed in all experimental groups by three months of age, and many of the observations were similar to those described for autistic, retarded, and emotionally disturbed children, or for children maternally deprived by long periods of hospitalization or placement in an orphanage (46,47). Attempts to alleviate effects of social isolation rearing by placing some of the animals that had been reared in the most deprived condition back into the social colony at three months of age were not very successful. Any unusual excitement in the colony, such as mating or fighting, tended to result in the emergence of the isolation behaviors.

Single factor explanations of deprivation effects are not adequate, and too many studies confound sensory deprivation with social deprivation. Whatever the form that deprivation effects take, they tend to last for a long time in primates. Isolation of an infant involves more than a lack of social interaction with parent figures and other conspecifics. The infant is also deprived of the passive movement normally obtained through parental handling, and motor activity is limited to self-induced movement or to those forms of activity related to its care and maintenance. This may account for some of the abnormal behaviors observed in primate deprivation experiments (110,111,125,130) and in infants that are blind or placed in an orphanage at birth (98,99). The enriched isolated environment of the stumptail monkeys in our study provided adequate support for dendritic development in primary motor and sensory areas, but evidently this was not sufficient for the development and integration of normal behavior patterns.

Excessive cortical branching, as was the case in the socially deprived monkeys with increased opportunity for motor activity, may be as deleterious to some behavioral functions as subnormal branch counts appear to be. Perhaps there is a very limited range within which dendritic development of certain cells can vary, between or within the different brain areas, without affecting the emergence, integration, and onotogeny of normal socially interactive behaviors. Acceleration or retardation of specific

behavioral skills can occur in the presence or absence of a
variety of abnormal CNS patterns: Structure-function relations
of this type require further clarification.

Mechanisms of Alterations

Reorganization, recovery, or compensation subsequent to CNS
damage usually occurs more readily in young, immature organisms,
but some aspects of contact specificity appear to be lost during
maturation, resulting in a delay of appearance of effects (13,74,
75,78). This makes it difficult to assess the true impact of CNS
damage or sensory loss in an immature organism.

Mechanisms underlying alterations in the brain following
subjection to pathological conditions are not well understood,
but are considered to take any one of, or combination of, the
following terms: a) sprouting of available afferents or the
utilization of a projection system that is within about 250 um of
the damaged system (60,74,76,120); b) rerouting of immature
afferents (30,77); c) demasking or disinhibition of redundant or
otherwise previously noneffective afferents (29,86,87,88); d)
retardation or acceleration of afferent and/or synapse development
(60,75). One of the major problems associated with evaluation of
deficits is, of course, related to our present inability to
predict or prevent the development of detrimental or pathological
integration subsequent to sensory loss or system trauma, especially in the immature organism. The probability of functional or
behavioral deficits is thought to increase as an organism matures,
with increases in probability of permanent deficits positively
correlated with increases in amount of damage to existing systems
or with increases in degree of pathological system integration
present.

Development of stereotyped responses, such as jerking and
spastic movement, has been observed in the absence of integrated
cortical rhythms (62), so a certain degree of synchronous wave
activity between the different areas of the brain may be necessary for normal functioning.

During brain growth, there are obvious increases in the maturation of neurons at intermittant time periods, sometimes
referred to as "spurts," and overlap or redundancy of cells types
appears to be characteristic of the neocortex (53,54,55). Every
component of lamina IV capable of forming asymetric junctions is
a potential recipient of thalamic input, and it is possible that
any cell type in any lamina could receive thalamic input, given
the right innervation or stimulus conditions (9,96). Are synchronous growth patterns between the various components of the
CNS, i.e., synchrony of neuroanatomical development, necessary

for the developmental ontogeny of normal brain and behavioral response patterns? How are the development of these response patterns related to each other? What are the conditions necessary for nonpathological redirection or reorganization of thalamic input to occur? The answers to questions like these may be of considerable importance to the successful development and application of sensory substitution techniques.

SUMMARY AND SPECULATIONS

1. The evolutionary history and phylogenetic characteristics of a species are important considerations in the formation of developmental hypotheses, because these factors combine with environmental experience to influence the range and quality of response capability in any subject. The demands of many test situations exceed the range of response capacity of their subjects, and bring us no closer to understanding how functionally adaptive adjustments to deviations from normal developmental patterns occur. Temporal factors, maturation rate or level, response capacity, adjustment potential, motivation, and environmental history should be given very careful consideration in the selection of subjects and design of test situations, especially in relatively new research areas like sensory substitution.

Lower primates acquire many social and spatial skills similar to those evident in the human species, and sensory substitution experiments with animals, such as these primates, may be the only practical way to acquire an understanding of the potential benefits and limitations inherent to each of the different types of devices currently available or in the planning stage. Sensory substitution experiments using animals are the only way we can examine the impact of device use on neurological and physiological aspects of developmental processes, and these experiments must be done prior to device use in blind human infants.

2. Both quality and quantity of environmental interactions, with emphasis on those involving parental figures and conspecifics, are extremely important to the normal ontogeny of brain development and of formation of behavioral response patterns. Current sensory substitution device designs preclude their practical use in animal experiments involving rearing with conspecifics; however, with devices used in isolation rearing environments it is possible to control and manipulate the type and amount of sensory information available to an animal at any given time. Justification for experiments using what is basically a pathological rearing environment lies in the degree of stimulus control, which is necessary to determine relationships between changes in CNS development and in acquisition of spatial-motor behaviors.

Caution must be exercised in interpreting the results of sensory substitution device use in isolation environments, because effective device use by human subjects may be related to how they perceive device-use impact on their interactions with peers, especially those peers whom they categorize as "significant others" and those who are without sensory deficits. Those subjects who have had positive, supportive relationships with parental figures and other conspecifics may find it easier to cope with their deficit. Whether or not this would enable them to learn to use a sensory substitution device more readily and effectively than those subjects with negative relationships is an open question.

3.   Active, self-initiated interactions with the environment are necessary to provide the reafferent information essential to the development of good spatial-motor skills (42). Many visually impaired persons simply do not negotiate their spatial environments enough to acquire or maintain spatial-motor skills, and this is thought to be one of the major factors underlying the motor retardation observed in some blind children. Another important factor could be neglect of or over-protection of the visually impaired child by parental figures.

Research with sensory substitution devices allows control of the sensory information available, which can help to determine the types and amounts of reafferent information necessary for development of spatial-motor skills. However, motivation to use sensory substitution devices effectively in the real spatial environment will depend on many other factors such as whether the devices are efficient, compact, affordable, and cosmetically acceptable. Cosmetic acceptability may prove to be the greatest limitation of the success of sensory substitution devices outside of test or laboratory situations.

4.   The idea of finite critical periods may need further assessment, but there are periods of apparent maximum sensitivity to environmental stimuli during CNS development (15,16,90). If the critical period concept applies to the development of sensory response capabilities related to integration of stimuli necessary for acquisition of spatial-motor skills, then sensory substitution devices should be introduced at the more sensitive periods for maximum compensation or substitution for the loss of normal sensory input.

One would expect the more sensitive periods to be at a time of maximum organization of CNS processes, such as is the case in an immature organism, or at a time of maximum reorganization of CNS processes, which apparently occurs following CNS trauma. Sensory substitution research should direct some of its efforts toward identification of sensitive periods, and define the role of these periods in organization and reorganization of sensory response systems and related behaviors. Perhaps there is a time when an area, such as visual cortex, has a more heterogeneous response capability relative to integration of those stimuli, other than light, that can be used to coordinate spatial-motor activity in the absence of vision.

5. Degree of recovery from trauma and/or compensation for a deficit are related to the age of an organism, stage of maturation, extent of damage, and availability of existing inputs (29). While we cannot reliably assess individual potential for reorganization of CNS or behavioral processes, both basic and clinical research evaluations of subjects who have demonstrated recovery or compensation subsequent to a variety of insults to the CNS indicate that adaptation or reorganization begins at the time of the insult, or very soon after. This implies that therapeutic techniques, including sensory substitution, should be introduced at an early age, or as soon after trauma, such as visual loss, as is possible in order for the intervention to attain maximum success. True recovery for the loss of a sensory modality, such as vision, may not be possible in the real neurophysiological sense, but compensation for the deficit by another sensory modality would serve to enhance psychological and behavioral adaptation to the loss.

6. Functional validation or use is a key factor in whether the development of connectivity patterns is normal or abnormal (57), and connectivity patterns and other morphogenetic changes are probable, and to be expected, in the event of sensory loss. Therefore, the goal is to discover, facilitate, and manipulate those CNS alterations that will allow spatial-motor functioning, even though the final forms or patterns of the alterations are ultimately abnormal.

Intuitively, another valid reason for early introduction of therapeutic or compensatory intervention measures, such as sensory substitution devices, is to prevent the formation or integration of inappropriate connections that can develop the potential to interfere with or prevent compensation or behavioral recovery. One of the most interesting challenges in sensory substitution research relative to visual deficits is to define those stimulus information characteristics that are necessary for the formation of CNS organizational patterns appropriate to development or maintenance of spatial-motor skills, and at the same time, identify and control or eliminate the impact of those factors that interfere with or prevent compensation for the deficit.

7. Stimulation, dominance, and competition of afferents and efferents and the ultimate destination of efferents play an important role in the development of response characteristics of neurons (17,20,21,63,106,127). Broader tuning curves than those normally observed in mice were reported for mice reared in an acoustic environment that repetitively entrained activity in a large proportion of primary auditory afferents for 11 to 16 days, starting on the eighth day. This suggests that the normal frequency tuning of the neurons was prevented or delayed by synchronizing the pattern of activity imposed on the auditory pathway, and that activity in the auditory system, as in the visual pathway, is critically involved in ontogenetic fine tuning (116).

There is little doubt that timing and type of sensory stimulation play an important role in shaping, or even determining, the final form or pattern of neuronal response characteristics. Appropriate times for sensory intervention and characteristics of stimulus information that are necessary for the development of neuronal response patterns that are involved in the acquisition, implementation, and maintenance of spatial-motor behaviors should be determined experimentally. Computer and animal modeling techniques should be developed to eliminate those aspects of timing and sensory substitution device generated stimuli that have the potential to interfere with or prevent spatial-motor interactions.

8. Selective cell changes or losses can occur in a population of neurons, and an entire population can be affected by lack of stimulation to a subset of one of its neurons (24,122). Alternatively, sensory substitution device generated stimuli could affect an entire population of neurons by stimulating a subset of its neurons, and prevent some of the cell losses that occur subsequent to a sensory deficit. Time schedules for naturally occurring neuronal death have been reported for neurons involved in motor functioning (39), and it might prove to be of interest to examine the effects of sensory loss and enhancement on the timing and amount of cell death in this population of neurons.

Sensory substitution device effects on CNS processing capabilities need to be examined experimentally. If "spatial" cortex contains auditory and tactile response units, or any other kinds of response units, that have the potential to respond to sensory stimuli other than visual, then there must be a way to develop device generated stimuli that will facilitate or maintain neuronal processes in spatial-motor integration areas, stimuli that will enhance the acquisition of spatial-motor skills in immature blind subjects or prevent spatial-motor behavior losses in those that become blind at maturity.

9. Orientation, growth, and responsiveness of cell processes are directly related to geometric or spatial aspects of
environmental stimuli, at least in the visual system (5,6,11,97).
Sensory substitution techniques might provide an effective way of
testing for this in other systems, i.e., tactile and auditory.

Systematic studies of correlations between the various types
of device generated stimuli, response behavior, and changes in
neurons and their processing capabilities are needed in the
sensory substitution research area. Combinations of sensory
substitution techniques, animal models, and computer technology
that are currently available should be used to develop practical,
creative, and feasible approaches to understanding sensory physiology, and perhaps, for learning to control and manipulate environmental effects on other brain and behavioral processes.

10. If there is more than one afferent system available
to cortical neurons at any given time, then these systems need
to be identified. Demasking or disinhibition of redundant afferents would make it easier for a system to attempt to correct
for trauma or failure by providing an efficient means for acquiring an alternative response system (29,57,61,73,87).

If redundant afferents exist in the sensory system, definition of their properties is important to sensory substitution
research goals. Sensory substitution intervention techniques
would be more effective if we knew how to supplement or enhance
the natural compensatory sensory stimulus-response alternatives
available to an organism when a modality, such as vision, becomes
nonfunctional.

11. Smooth stellate neurons deserve further study, since
they appear rather early in development and are thought to be
involved in inhibitory functions, which are very important to
most behavioral organization (43,56,57,133). Changes in these
neurons may play an important role in determining the success or
failure of the reorganization of response capacity and/or of the
activation of natural alternative afferent systems subsequent to
sensory loss, such as occurs with a visual deficit, or following
introduction of sensory substitution techniques, such as use of
a tactile or auditory device.

We do not know the prerequisite conditions for optimal functioning of smooth stellates, but hypothesize that too little or
too much inhibition of sensory input by these interneurons will
prove to be detrimental to the effective use of sensory substitution devices in developing spatial-motor skills.

12. Different patterns of morphogenesis appear to reflect differences in functional activity at the cortical level (85). If cortical functional activity changes with the use of a sensory substitution device, as it probably will, then corresponding or correlated changes should become apparent in neuronal and behavioral adaptation patterns.

Observations of behavioral changes that occur in conjunction with changes in CNS functional activity patterns should prove useful in identifying those characteristics of device input that prove to be detrimental to the individual device user, so that such characteristics can be altered or eliminated. Beneficial characteristics could also be identified and enhanced. Sensory substitution devices may have to be tailored to individual user needs much in the same way as some other prostheses, or in the way that medications are prescribed.

COMMENTS

At the present time, we can only speculate about the nature of the physiological basis of effective sensory substitution, because there simply is not enough data to do otherwise. However, currently we can make and test some rudimentary hypotheses, most of which involve plastic properties of the CNS. In essence, when we ask questions about the basis of sensory substitution, we are also asking questions about the nature of processes underlying CNS plasticity and compensation.

Since primary cortical areas may contain components that are much more responsive to well-defined aspects of specific environmental stimuli, such as sound, light, or touch, association or secondary cortical areas may be the major locus of adaptation relative to the changes in morphology and integrational capability thought necessary for recovery from sensory loss. Plastic properties of secondary motor, auditory, somatosensory, and possible visual areas may determine the degree of effectiveness of sensory substitution device use. Plastic changes between brain areas may also be involved; for example, with use of a sonar cue device, there may be increases in and/or changes in connectivity patterns between auditory and motor cortical areas. Subcortical changes in areas like the medial geniculate nucleus of the thalamus and the colliculi are also likely to be involved.

If there is a modality overlap, and neurons exist that share access to multimodal input, then these neurons are likely to be more numerous in association areas than in primary input areas. Then, we can expect to find dendritic branch pattern changes, dendritic spine differences on pyramidal and spiny stellate neurons, and connectivity alterations associated with compensation for a sensory deficit to be much more dramatic in the cortical association or secondary areas. One of the problems is to identify and provide those stimulus information characteristics which will enhance the plastic changes that are related to and necessary for compensation for sensory loss; this can only be accomplished through systematic experimental analyses using animal models.

Another problem is to define those differences in recovery processes, or in the degree and mode of expression of plasticity, that exist between immature and adult organisms, and which may require different sensory intervention techniques. We can expect these differences in processes to be reflected in the way and in the effectiveness with which immature and adult organisms adapt to a sensory deficit, with and without sensory intervention or use of a sensory substitution device. For instance, other sensory processing modes or connections, such as those with polysensory neurons, may be easier to access in immature organisms, and there may be sensitive periods after which sensory alternatives if not appropriately functionally validated, may become inaccessible. In essence, this means that more connective alternatives may be available to the immature organism; however, it may also be possible that the probability of forming aberrant connections is higher. In adults, some sensory processing alternatives may no longer exist, and some may have become associated with a specific modality, such as vision. Thus, there may be fewer compensatory alternatives, and those that are present may be more difficult to access through another modality, such as audition; however, the risk of generating aberrant connectively through sensory intervention may be lower in adult organisms than in immature ones.

The eventual outcome of any therapeutic technique, including use of a sensory substitution device, is related to the plastic properties of the CNS. The basic principles underlying CNS plasticity observed in developmental processes, recovery from trauma, and in response to altered environments, are the same principles that underly sensory substitution or compensation, so to understand the physiology of sensory substitution, we must first know more about plastic processes.

There is much to be learned about plastic processes, and this knowledge has potential value in alleviating suboptimal behavioral functioning in the handicapped, and for improving the quality of human life in general. We should begin to think beyond the immediate and urgent problem of developing specific skills in the handicapped, such as spatial-motor skills in the blind, and look upon sensory substitution techniques as tools or methods

with which to identify and manipulate the plastic properties of
the CNS and to develop a better understanding of the ways in
which brain and behavior organizational patterns affect each
other and shape the ontological course of all organisms throughout
their lifetime.

ACKNOWLEDGEMENTS

This work was supported by NIH grants 1 RO1 EY05224-01 and
5 RO1 HDIO408, and by the Center for Social and Behavioral Science
Research, University of California, Riverside.

REFERENCES

1.   Altman, J. (1967). Postnatal growth and differentiation of
     the mammalian brain, with implications for a morphological
     theory of memory. In The Neurosciences: A Study Program,
     G. Quarton, T. Melnechuk, & F. Schmitt (Eds.). New York:
     Rockefeller University Press, 723-743.

2.   Bach-y-Rita, P. (1972). Brain Mechanisms in Sensory Substi-
     tution. New York: Academic Press.

3.   Bach-y-Rita, P. (Ed.) (1980). Recovery of Function: Theo-
     retical Considerations for Brain Injury Rehabilitation.
     Baltimore: University Park Press.

4.   Bach-y-Rita, P. (1983). Tactile vision substitution: Past
     and future. International Journal of Neuroscience, 19, 13-
     19.

5.   Blakemore, C. & Cooper, G. (1970). Development of the brain
     depends on the visual environment. Nature (London), 227,
     477-478.

6.   Blakemore, C. & Mitchell, D. (1973). Environmental modifi-
     cation of the visual cortex and the neural basis of learning
     and memory. Nature (London), 241, 467-468.

7.   Borges, S. & Berry, M. (1976). Preferential orientation of
     stellate cell dendrites in the visual cortex of the dark
     reared rat. Brain Research, 112, 141-147.

8.   Changeux, J. & Danchin, A. (1976). Selective stabilization
     of developing synapses as a mechanism for the specification
     of neuronal networks. Nature, 264, 705-711.

9.   Christensen, B. & Ebner, F. (1978). The synaptic architec-
     ture of neurons in opossom somatic sensory-motor cortex: A
     combined anatomical and physiological study. Journal of
     Cytology, 7, 39-60.

10. Coleman, P. & Riesen, A. H. (1968). Environmental effects
     on cortical dendritic fields. I. Rearing in the dark.
     Journal of Anatomy, 102, 363-374.

11. Coleman, P., Flood, D., Whitehead, M., & Emerson, R. (1981).
     Spatial sampling by dendritic trees in visual cortex. Brain
     Research, 214, 1-21.

12. Colonnier, M. (1964). The tangential organization of the visual cortex. Journal of Anatomy (London), 98, 327-344.

13. Cotman, C., Matthews, D., Taylor, D., & Lynch, G. (1973). Synaptic rearrangement of the dentate gyrus: Histochemical evidence of adjustments after lesions in immature and adult rats. Proceedings of the National Academy of Sciences (USA), 70, 3473-3477.

14. Cragg, B. (1972). The development of synapses in cat visual cortex. Investigative Opthamology, 11, 377-385.

15. Cragg, B. (1975). The development of synapses in kitten visual cortex during visual deprivation. Experimental Neurology, 46, 445-451.

16. Cragg, B. (1975). The development of synapses in the visual system of the cat. Journal of Comparative Neurology, 160, 147-166.

17. Cragg, B., Anker, R., & Wan, Y. (1976). The effect of age on the reversibility of cellular atrophy in the LGN of the cat following monocular deprivation: A test of two hypotheses of cell growth. Journal of Comparative Neurology, 168, 345-354.

18. Crelin, E. (1976). Development of the nervous system. A logical approach to neuroanatomy. Clinical Symposia, 28, No. 1, CIBA.

19. Cynader, M. & Mitchell, D. (1980). Prolonged sensitivity to monocular deprivation in dark reared cats. Journal of Neurophysiology, 43, 1026-1040.

20. Duffy, F., Burchfiel, J., & Snodgrass, S. (1976). Ammonium acetate reversal of experimental amblyopia. Neuroscience Abstracts, 2, 1109.

21. Duffy, F., Snodgrass, S., Burchfield, J., & Conway, J. (1976). Bicuculline reversal of deprivation amblyopia in the cat. Nature (London), 260, 256-257.

22. Eayrs, J. & Goodhead, B. (1959). Postnatal development of the cerebral cortex in the rat. Journal of Anatomy (London), 93, 385-402.

23. Ebert, J. & Sussex, I. (1970). Interacting Systems in Development. New York: Holt, Rinehart & Winston.

24. Garey, L. & Blakemore, C. (1977). Monocular deprivation: Morphological effects on different classes of neurons in the lateral geniculate nucleus. Science, 195, 414-416.

25. Gibson, J. J. (1979). The Ecological Approach to Visual Perception. Boston: Houghton-Mifflin.

26. Globus, A. & Scheibel, A. (1966). Loss of dendritic spines as an index of pre-synaptic terminal patterns. Nature (London), 212, 463-465.

27. Globus, A. & Scheibel, A. (1967). The effect of visual deprivation on cortical neurons: A Golgi study. Experimental Neurology, 19, 331-345.

28. Globus, A. & Scheibel, A. (1967). Pattern and field in cortical structure: The rabbit. Journal of Comparative Neurology, 131, 155-172.

29. Goldman, P. (1974). An alternative to developmental plasticity: Heterology of CNS structure in infants and adults. In: D. Stein, J. Rosen, & N. Butters (Eds.), Plasticity and Recovery of Function in the Central Nervous System. New York: Academic Press.

30. Goodman, D., Bogdasarian, R., & Horel, J. (1973). Axonal sprouting of ipsilateral optic tract following opposite eye removal. Brain, Behavior and Evolution, 8, 27-50.

31. Gordon, M. (1972). Animal Physiology: Principles and Adaptations (Second Edition). New York: Macmillan.

32. Gottlieb, G. (1971). Ontogenesis of sensory function in birds and mammals. In: E. Tobach, L. Aronson, & E. Shaw (Eds.), The Biopsychology of Development. New York: Academic Press.

33. Gottlieb, G. (1978). Epilogue. In: G. Gottlieb (Ed.), Studies on the Development of Behavior and the Nervous System. Early Influences. New York: Academic Press.

34. Greenough, W. (1975). Experimental modification of the developing brain. American Scientist, 63, 37-46.

35. Greenough, W. (1976). Enduring brain effects of differential experience and training. In: M. Rosenzweig & E. Bennett (Eds.), Neural Mechanisms of Learning and Memory. Cambridge: MIT Press.

36. Greenough, W. (1977). Experimental modification of the developing brain. In: I. Janis (Ed.), Current Trends in Psychology. Readings from American Scientist. Los Altos, CA: Kaufmann.

37. Gutmann, E. (1976). Neurotrophic relations. Annual Review of Physiology, 38, 177-215.

38. Gyllensten, L, Malmfors, T., & Norrlin, M. (1965). Effect of visual deprivation on the optic centers of growing and adult mice. Journal of Comparative Neurology, 124, 149-160.

39. Hamberger, V. & Oppenheim, R. (1982). Naturally occurring neuronal death in vertebrates. Neuroscience Commentaries, 1, 39-55.

40. Handler, P. (1970). Biology and the Future of Man. New York: Oxford University Press.

41. Hebb, D. (1949). The Organization of Behavior. New York: Wiley.

42. Held, R. & Hein, A. (1963). Movement-produced stimulation in the development of visually-guided behavior. Journal of Comparative and Physiological Psychology, 56, 872-876.

43. Hendry, S. & Jones, E. (1981). Sizes and distributions of intrinsic neurons incorporating tritiated GABA in monkey sensory-motor cortex. Journal of Neuroscience, 1, 390-408.

44. Herre, W. (1966). Einige Bemerkungen zur Modifikabilitar, Vererbung und Evolution von Merkmalen des Vorderhirns bei Saugetieren. In: R. Hassler, & H. Stephan, (Eds.), Evolution of the Forebrain. New York: Plenum Press.

45. Hubel, D., Wiesel, T., & LeVay, S. (1977). Plasticity of ocular dominance columns in monkey striate cortex. Philosophical Transactions of the Royal Society, London, Series B, 278, 377-409.

46. Hunt, J. M. (1979). Psychological development: Early experience. Annual Review of Psychology, 30, 103-143.

47. Hunt, J. M., Mohandessi, K., Ghodssi, M., & Akiyama, M. (1976). The psychological development of orphanage-reared infants: Intervention with outcomes. Journal of Genetic Psychology Monographs, 94, 117-226.

48. Hunt, R. & Jacobson, M.   (1974). Neuronal specificity re-
    visited. In: A. Moscona & A. Monroy (Eds.), Current Topics
    in Developmental Biology, Vol. 8. New York: Academic Press.

49. Huttenlocher, P.   (1974). Dendritic development in neocortex
    of children with mental defect and infantile spasms.
    Neurology, 24, 203.

50. Innocenti, G.   (1981). Growth and reshaping of axons in the
    establishment of visual callosal connections. Science, 212,
    824-827.

51. Innocenti, G.   (1981). The development of interhemispheric
    connections. Topics in Neuroscience, June, 142-144.

52. Innocenti, G.   (1981). Transitory structures as substrate
    for developmental plasticity of the brain. In: M. W. Hoff,
    G. Van & Mohn (Eds.),Functional Recovery from Brain Damage.
    Developments in Neuroscience, Vol. 13. New York: Elsevier,
    305-333.

53. Jacobson, M. (1970). Development, specification and diver-
    sification of neuronal connections. In: F. Schmitt (Ed.),
    The Neurosciences: Second Study Program. New York: Rocke-
    feller University Press.

54. Jacobson, M. (1974). A plentitude of neurons. In: G. Gott-
    lieb (Ed.), Studies on the Development of Behavior and the
    Nervous System: Aspects of Neurogenesis, Vol. 2. New York:
    Academic Press.

55. Jacobson, M. (1974). Through the jungle of the brain: Neu-
    ronal specificity and typology re-explored.   Annals of the
    New York Academy of Science, 228, 63-67.

56. Jacobson, M. (1975). Development and evolution of type II
    neurons: Conjectures a century after Golgi.   In: M. Santini,
    (Ed.), Golgi Centennial Symposium: Perspectives in Neuro-
    biology. New York: Raven Press.

57. Jacobson, M. (1978). Developmental Neurobiology (Second
    Edition). New York: Plenum Press.

58. Jacobson, M. & Hunt, R. (1973). Origins of neuronal speci-
    ficity. Scientific American, 228, 26-35.

59. Kalil, R. (1972). Formation of new retino-geniculate con-
    nections in kittens after removal of one eye. Anatomical
    Record, 339-340.

60. Kalil, R. & Schneider, G. (1975). Abnormal synaptic connections of the optic tract in the thalamus after midbrain lesions in newborn hamsters. Brain Research, 100, 690-698.

61. Kasamatsu, T. & Adey, W. (1974). Recovery in visual cortical neurons following total visual deafferentation. Brain Research, 74, 105-117.

62. Komisaruk, B. (1977). The role of rhythmical brain activity in sensori-motor integration. In: J. Sprague, & A. Epstein (Eds.),Progress in Psychobiology and Physiological Psychological Psychology, Vol. 7. New York: Academic Press.

63. Kratz, K. & Spear, P. (1976). Effects of visual deprivation and alternations in binocular competition on responses of striate cortex neurons in the cat. Journal of Comparative Neurology, 170, 141-152.

64. Kratz, K., Spear, P., & Smith, D. (1976). Postcritical-period reversal of effects of monocular deprivation on striate cortex cells in the cat. Journal of Neurophysiology, 39, 501-511.

65. Langman, J. (1973). Medical Embryology. (Second Edition), Baltimore: Williams & Wilkins.

66. Lashley, K. (1949). Persistent problems in the evolution of the mind. Quarterly Review of Biology, 24, 28-42.

67. LaVere, T. (1980). Recovery of function after brain damage: A theory of the behavioral deficit. Physiological Psychology, 8, 297-308.

68. Lende, R. (1969). A comparative approach to the neocortex: Localization in monotremes, marsupials and insectivores. Annals of New York Acadamy of Sciences, 167, 262-276.

69. Leong, S. (1976). A qualitative electron microscope investigation of the anomalous corticofugal projections following neonatal lesions in the albino rat. Brain Research, 107, 1-8.

70. Leong, C. (1976). An experimental study of the corticofugal system following cerebral lesions in the albino rat. Experimental Brain Research, 26, 235-247.

71. Lidsky, T., Adinolfi, A., & Buchwald, N. (1975). Develop-
     ment of corticocaudate connections in kittens. Anatomical
     Record, 181, 410.

72. Lidsky, T., Buchwald, N., Hull, C., & Levine, M. (1976). A
     neurophysiological analysis of the development of cortico-
     caudate connections in the cat. Experimental Neurology, 50,
     283-292.

73. Lund, R. (1978). Development and Plasticity of the Brain.
     An Introduction. New York: Oxford.

74. Lund, R. & Lund, J. (1971). Synaptic adjustment after de-
     afferentation of the superior colliculus of the rat.
     Science, 171, 804-807.

75. Lund, R. & Lund, J. (1971). Modification of synaptic pat-
     terns in the superior colliculus of the rat during develop-
     ment and following deafferentation. Vision Research, II
     (Sup. 3), 281-298.

76. Lund, R. & Lund J. (1972). Development of synaptic pat-
     terns in the superior colliculus of the rat. Brain Research,
     42, 1-20.

77. Lund, R. & Lund, J. (1973). Reorganization of the retino-
     tectal pathway in rats after neonatal retinal lesions. Ex-
     perimental Neurology, 40, 377-390.

78. Lund, R. & Lund, J. (1976). Plasticity in the developing
     visual system: The effects of retinal lesions made in
     young rats. Journal of Comparative Neurology, 169, 133-154.

79. Marin-Padilla, M. (1970). Prenatal and early postnatal
     ontogenesis of the human motor cortex: A Golgi study. I. The
     sequential development of the cortical layers. Brain Re-
     search, 23, 167-183.

80. Marin-Padilla, M. (1970). Prenatal and early postnatal on-
     togenesis of the human motor cortex: A Golgi study. II. The
     basket-pyramidal system. Brain Research, 23, 185-191.

81. Marin-Padilla, M. (1971). Early postnatal ontogenesis of
     the cerebral cortex (neocortex) of the cat(Felis domestica):
     a Golgi Study. Z. Anat. Entwickl.-Gesch., 134, 117-147.

82. Marin-Padilla, M. (1972). Prenatal ontogenetic history of
     the principal neurons of the cat (Felis domestica): A Golgi
     study. II. Developmental differences and their significance.
     Z. Anat. Entwickl.-Gesch., 136, 125-142.

83. Marin-Padilla, M. (1972). Structural abnormalities of the cerebral cortex in human chromosomal aberrations. Brain Research, 44, 625-629.

84. Marin-Padilla, M. (1974). Structural organization of the cerebral cortex (motor area) in human chromosomal aberrations. A Golgi study. I. D. (13-15) trisomy. Patau syndrome. Brain Research, 66, 375-391.

85. Marty, R. & Scherrer, J. (1964). Creteres de maturation des systemes afferents corticaux. Progress in Brain Research, 4, 223-236.

86. Merrill, E. & Wall, P. (1972). Factors forming the edge of a receptive field: The presence of relatively ineffective afferent terminals. Journal of Physiology (London), 226, 825-846.

87. Merrill, E. & Wall, P. (1978). Plasticity of connections in the adult nervous system. In: C. Cotman (Ed.), Neuronal Plasticity, New York: Rayen.

88. Millar, J., Basbaum, A., & Wall, P. (1976). Restructuring of the somatotopic map and appearance of abnormal neuronal activity in the gracile nucleus after partial deafferentation. Experimental Neurology, 50, 658-672.

89. Mistretta, C. & Bradley, R. (1978). Effects of early sensory experience on brain and behavioral development. In: G. Gottlieb (Ed.), Studies on the Development of Behavior and the Nervous System. Early Influences. New York: Academic Press.

90. Mitchell, D., Griffin, F., Wilkinson, F., Anderson, P., & Smith, M. (1976). Visual resolution in young kittens. Vision Research, 16, 363-366.

91. Mungai, J. (1967). Dendritic patterns in the somatic sensory cortex of the cat. Journal of Anatomy (London), 101, 403-418.

92. Mustari, M. & Lund, R. (1976). An aberrant crossed visual corticotectal pathway in albino rats. Brain Research, 112, 37-42.

93. Parnavelas, J., Globus, A. & Kaups, P. (1973). Continuous illumination from birth affects spine density of neurons in the visual cortex of the rat. Experimental Neurology, 40, 742-747.

94. Percheron, G. (1979). Quantitative analysis of dendritic branching. I. Simple formulae for the quantitative analysis of dendritic branching. Neurosciences Letters, 14, 289-293.

95. Percheron, G. (1979). Quantitative analysis of dendritic branching. II. Fundamental dendritic numbers as a tool for the study of neuronal groups. Neurosciences Letters, 14, 295-302.

96. Peters, A. & Feldman, M. (1977). The projection of the lateral geniculate nucleus to area 17 of the rat cerebral cortex. IV. Terminations upon spiny dendrites. Journal of Neurocytology, 6, 669-689.

97. Pettigrew, J. & Freeman, R. (1973). Visual experience without lines: Effect on developing cortical neurons. Science, 182, 599-601.

98. Prescott, J. (1971). Early somatosensory deprivation as an ontogenetic process in the abnormal development of the brain and behavior. In: E. Goldsmith & J. Mooe-Jankowski (Eds.), Medical Primatology. New York: Karger.

99. Prescott, J. (1979). Somatosensory deprivation and its relationship to the blind. In: Z. Jastrzembska (Ed.), The Effects of Blindness and Other Impairments on Early Development. New York: American Foundation for the Blind.

100. Purpura, D. (1974). Dendritic spines "dysgenesis" and mental retardation. Science, 186, 1126-1128.

101. Rakic, P. (1976). Prenatal genesis of connections subserving ocular dominance in the rhesus monkey. Nature (London), 261, 467-471.

102. Rall, W. (1962). Electrophysiology of a dendritic neuron model. Journal of Biophysics, 2, 144-167.

103. Rall, W. (1962). Theory of physiological properties of dendrites. Annals of the New York Academy of Sciences, 96, 1071-1092.

104. Rall, W. (1974). Dendritic spines, synaptic potentency and neuronal plasticity. In: C. Woody, K. Brown, T. Crow, & J. Krispel (Eds.), Cellular Mechanisms Subserving Changes in Neuronal Activity, Los Angeles: BIS. UCLA.

105. Rauschecker, J. P. & Harris, L. R. (1983). Auditory compensation of the effects of visual deprivation in the cat's superior colliculus. Experimental Brain Research, 50, 60-83.

106. Riesen, A. H. (1962). Sensory deprivation. Progress in Physiological Psychology, 1, 117-147.

107. Riesen, A. H. (1978). Ontogenese von gehirn und verhalten. Die Psychologie Des 20. Jahrhunderts, 16, 763-782.

108. Riesen, A. H. (1982). Effects of environments on development in sensory systems. In: W. Neff (Ed.), Contributions to Sensory Physiology, New York: Academic Press.

109. Riesen, A. H. (1982). Two-way streets of the mammalian cerebral cortex. In: J. Orbach, (Ed.), Neuropsychology after Lashley. Hillsdale, New Jersey: Erlbaum, pp. 181-205.

110. Riesen, A. H., Dickerson, G., & Struble, R. (1977). Somatosensory restriction and behavioral development in stumptail monkeys. Annals of the New York Academy of Sciences, 290, 285-294.

111. Riesen, A. H., Sonnier, B., Lehr, P., & Struble, R. (In press). Branching differences in stellate cells related to cortical areas and rearing environments of monkeys. In: J. Prescott (Ed.), Consequences of Social Isolation Upon Primate Brain Development and Behavior. New York: Academic Press. (Abstracted in Agressive Behavior, 5, 199-200.)

112. Rosenzweig, M. & Bennett, E. (1978). Experimental influences on brain anatomy and brain chemistry in rodents. In: G. Gottlieb (Ed.), Studies on the Development of Behavior and the Nervous System. Early influences, New York: Academic Press.

113. Ruiz-Marcos, A. & Valverde, F. (1969). The temporal evolution of the distribution of dendritic spines on the visual cortex of normal and dark raised mice. Experimental Brain Research, 8, 284-294.

114. Ryugo, R., Ryugo, D., & Killackey, H. (1975). Differential effect of enucleation in two populations of layer V pyramidal cells. Brain Research, 88, 554-559.

115. Ryugo, D., Ryugo, R., & Killackey, H. (1975). Changes in pyramidal cell density consequent to vibrissae removal in the newborn rat. Brain Research, 96, 82-87.

116. Sanes, P. & Constantine-Paton, M. (1983). Altered activity patterns during development reduce neural tuning. Science, 221, 1183-1185.

117. Sanides, F. (1969). Comparative architectonics of the neocortex of mammals and their evolutionary interpretation. Annals of the New York Academy of Sciences, 167, 404-423.

118. Schade, J. & Baxter, C. (1960). Changes during growth in the volume and surface area of cortical neurons in the rabbit. Experimental Neurology, 2, 158-178.

119. Schade, J., Backer, H., & Colon, E. (1964). Quantitative analysis of neuronal parameters in the maturing cerebral cortex. Progress in Brain Research, 4, 150-175.

120. Schneider, G. (1973). Early lesions of superior colliculus: Factors affecting the formation of abnormal retinal projections. Brain and Behavioral Evolution, 8, 73-109.

121. Shepherd, G. (1979). The Synaptic Organization of the Brain (Second Edition). New York: Oxford University Press.

122. Sherman, S., Hoffman, K., & Stone, J. (1972). Loss of a specific cell type from the dorsal lateral geniculate nucleus in visually deprived cats. Journal of Neurophysiology, 35, 532-541.

123. Sholl, D. (1955). The Organization of the Cerebral Cortex. New York: Wiley.

124. Sholl, D. (1956). The measurable parameters of the cerebral cortex and their significance in its organization. In: J. Kappers (Ed.),Progress in Neurobiology, Amsterdam: Elsevier.

125. Sonnier, B. J. (1981). Quantitative analysis of the development of cortical stellate cells: Differences related to rearing environments of monkeys (M. Arctoides). Ph.D. Dissertation, University of California, Riverside (Dissertation Abstracts, Ann Arbor, MI, University Microfilms 82-07, 729).

126. Sonnier, B. J., Villablanca, J. R., Gomez, F., & Burgess, J. W. (1984). Reduced reorganization of corticorubral and corticothalamic fibers in adults versus neonatally hemispherectomized cats. Presented at Annual Society of Neuroscience Meetings, Anaheim, CA.

127. Spear, P. & Ganz, L. (1974). Effects of visual cortex lesions following recovery from monocular deprivation in the cat. Experimental Brain Research, 23, 181-201.

128. Sperry, R. (1963). Chemoaffinity in the orderly growth of nerve fiber patterns and connections. Proceedings of the National Academy of Sciences (USA), 50, 703-710.

129. Stewart, D. L. & Riesen, A. H. (1972). Adult versus infant brain damage: Behavioral and electrophysiological effects of striatectomy in adult and neonatal rabbits. In: G. Newton & A. H. Riesen (Eds.), Advances in Psychobiology, Vol. 1. New York: Wiley, 171-211.

130. Struble, R. & Riesen, A. H. (1978). Changes in cortical dendritic branching subsequent to partial social isolation in stumptail monkeys. Developmental Psychobiology, 11, 479-486.

131. Timney, B., Mitchell, D. & Cynader, M. (1980). Behavioral evidence for prolonged sensitivity to effects of monocular deprivation in dark-reared cats. Journal of Neurophysiology, 43, 1041-1054.

132. Tolman, E. (1949). Purposive Behavior in Animals and Men. Berkeley: University of California Press.

133. Tsumato, R., Eckart, W., & Creutzfeldt, O. (1979). Modification of orientation sensitivity of cat visual cortex neurons by removal of GABA-mediated inhibition. Experimental Brain Research, 34, 351-365.

134. Tuchmann-Duplessis, H., Auroux, M., & Haegel, P. (1974). Illustrated Human Embryology, Vol. 3, Nervous System and Endocrine Glands. (Trans.: S. Hurley). New York: Springer-Verlag.

135. Valverde, F. (1967). Apical dendritic spines of the visual cortex and light deprivation in the mouse. Experimental Brain Research, 5, 274-292.

136. Valverde, F. (1968). Structural changes in the area striata of the mouse after enucleation. Experimental Brain Research, 5, 274-292.

137. Valverde, F. (1971). Rate and extent of recovery from dark rearing in the visual cortex of the mouse. Brain Research, 33, 1-11.

138. Valverde, F. & Ruiz-Marcos, A. (1969). Dendritic spines in the visual cortex of the mouse: Introduction to a mathematical model. Experimental Brain Research, 8, 269-283.

139. Villablanca, J. R., Burgess, J. W., & Sonnier, B. J. (1984). Neonatal cerebral hemispherectomy: A model for post-lesion reorganization of the brain. In: C. R. Almli & S. Finger (Eds.), The Behavioral Biology of Early Brain Damage, Vol. 2. New York: Academic Press, 179-210.

140. West, R. (1976). Light and electron microscopy of the ground squirrel retina: Functional considerations. Journal of Comparative Neurology, 168, 355-378.

141. Windle, W. (1971). Origin and early development of neural elements in the human brain. In: E. Tobach, L. Aronson, & E. Shaw (Eds.), The Biopsychology of Development. New York: Academic Press.

142. Zamenhof, S. & Marthens, E. (1978). Nutritional influences on prenatal brain development. In: G. Gottlieb (Ed.), Studies on the Development of Behavior and the Nervous System. Early influences, New York: Academic Press.

ANIMAL MODELS OF PLASTICITY AND SENSORY SUBSTITUTION

B. J. Sonnier

University of California, Riverside

At the conference on spatial prostheses, which provided the stimulus for the current volume, it became clear that the interests and goals of participants went beyond simply developing effective technology for sensory substitution devices, and that some of the research objectives might be met through the development of animal models to study both the effectiveness and the effects of use of sensory substitution devices. Sensory substitution research is rapidly becoming a multidisciplinary effort to understand the nature of brain and behavioral relationships subsequent to sensory loss, the mechanisms underlying CNS plasticity, and the principles of perceptual development, with the goal of directing or manipulating sensory plasticity to produce functionally effective compensation for a sensory deficit. This comment considers the use of sensory substitution devices as research tools in the development of animal models of the basic processes underlying brain and behavioral plasticity, particularly those properties which are related to sensory processing.

Plasticity

Although there are probably some invariant aspects of brain and behavioral processes, they appear to be flexible or plastic, with a general capacity for variability in response to changes in stimulus conditions. We know of some forms of plasticity because of the altered brain and behavioral patterns observed in a number of species in a variety of research paradigms. Plasticity has been demonstrated in response to changes in environmental stimulus conditions, traumatic insult, genetic dysfunction,

and sensory deficits. We also know that some plastic responses
are aberrant, and that behavioral deficits often accompany some
CNS alterations. However, we do not have any real understanding
of the mechanisms underlying the changes that we attribute to
plastic processes, or even more importantly, of the way in which
these changes affect behavior.

Sensory substitution usually involves providing sensory
information through an alternate modality so that an organism
will be able to perceive features of the environment that would
normally be processed through another modality, e.g., presenting
auditory or tactile stimuli to provide information about the
spatial environment that is ordinarily obtained through the
visual system. In these examples, the substitution does not
replace vision, but increases the amount of information available
about the environment through other modalities such as audition
or touch. This intervention should make it possible for the
organism to compensate for the lack of access to visual stimuli,
and develop better spatial-motor skills. If compensation is
effective, then some reorganization of old brain and behavioral
response patterns and/or some development of new ones is to be
expected. Sensory substitution devices that are currently available can be used to manipulate and limit the type and content of
stimulus information available to an organism at any given time.
This makes these devices uniquely suitable tools for developing
productive animal research paradigms, or animal models, for
studying CNS and behavioral plasticity, and for learning how to
bring about the plastic changes that are necessary for adaptive
compensation.

Determining the role of plastic processes in brain and
behavioral response organization subsequent to sensory deficit is
not going to be an easy task even with the use of sensory substitution devices in animal research. For instance, mechanisms
underlying adaptive or compensatory changes in response to sensory
deficits probably differ between immature and adult organisms in
a variety of unknown dimensions. While we think that an immature
organism can learn to use a sensory substitution device more effectively during the initial acquisition of spatial-motor skills,
rather than after acquisition or as an adult, there may also be
some unknown, detrimental effects of such early device use. For
example, rather than being integrated with or supplementing
natural cues, device-generated cues may interfere with or eliminate the ability to use natural spatial cues. It is also possible
that some aspects of device-generated stimuli could result in
aberrant plastic changes in the CNS that might not be reflected
in behavioral responding until much later in life, such as changes
in sensitivity to sound or pressure, alterations in inhibitory
interactions, or development of aberrant cortical rhythms, any of
which could affect spatial-motor interactions.

Some human developmental issues related to device use could be examined in animals, which would help us learn how to avoid those aspects which are detrimental and to optimize those which prove positive in nature. For instance, systematic studies of device use in animals at different developmental stages are needed to determine if there are critical or sensitive periods when learning will be more efficient and effective, and when most impact on brain developmental processes is likely to occur. The periods for these two processes are likely to be correlated, or perhaps, even coincide and there may be only certain periods when device-generated stimuli can precipitate aberrant development. Time of day and number of hours per day of device use may prove to be important factors in learning effectiveness. For example, a device that becomes operational when a subject is awake, and nonoperational during sleep, may prove to be necessary for use in infant subjects.

There are several reasons for thinking that important alterations will occur in cortical association areas, and in their connectivity relationships with primary input areas, especially in primates. One reason for thinking these areas will play an important role in compensation for a sensory deficit is the sheer volume of associative regions available in primates. These regions are thought to occupy 20% of the cortical surface in rabbit, and with increases as one approaches the primate line, associative areas reach 70% in the human species (1). Another reason is that integration and effective use of both device-generated and natural cues about the spatial environment to compensate for a sensory deficit will require the formation of new attentional hierarchies, the learning of different ways to interpret and associate spatial stimulus cues, and active use of the cues in motor interactions with the environment. It does not seem likely that all these things can occur without extensive involvement of cortical association areas.

Animal Models

Because of the prolonged nature of human developmental processes, the extreme variability in human environments, and the lack of technology for performing many types of invasive CNS observations in human subjects, animal models provide the most feasible approach to studying the effects of sensory substitution on brain and behavioral interactions during development. Systematic testing of device-generated stimulus input effects in the brain and behavior of animals would provide an efficient way of obtaining information relative to the types and amount of supplementary cues necessary for acquisition or improvement of spatial-motor skills in blind persons. Even if one does not consider the effects of device-generated stimuli on brain development, think about how long it might take, using human subjects, to find out whether or not the information necessary for the initial learning of spatial-motor skills is the same as that needed for improvement of these skills later in life.

Animals models also provide a more practical means for examining behavioral hypotheses that imply some sort of response plasticity. One of these hypotheses is that an immature blind subject given prolonged experience with a sensory aid will show more effective use of it as an adult and be more adept at negotiating the spatial environment than a person who receives it only as an adult. Immature subjects may also be able to learn to use device-generated spatial cues more readily in conjunction with learning to use those cues that are naturally available. Study of device use in animals could also help us to find out whether or not natural cues interfere with learning to use sensory substitution devices introduced after the acquisition of spatial-motor skills.

On the other hand, prior visual experience appears to assist the ability of the blind to integrate some forms of spatial information (2). When a visually-experienced person learns to use a device, the perception of space may be enhanced because some object identification may be integrated with visual memory of spatial objects. In fact, those objects for which there is no visual memory to supplement or verify device-related identification, i.e., unfamiliar objects, may prove to cause disruption of effective device use in persons with prior visual experience. It may be that early device use in immature blind subjects will result in the development of a device-related memory that serves a purpose similar to that of visual memory in sighted or late-blinded persons.

Primate Models

Within the context of animal models, nonhuman primates provide the most practical approach to sensory substitution research because of the similarity of nonhuman to human primates in terms of brain size and structure, socio-spatial behavior, capacity for associational learning, ability to vary adaptive behavior and comparability of general physical characteristics such as the use of forepaws, resting posture and spatial orientation. Other species are useful in basic research on neurophysiological effects and plastic processes related to sensory deficits, however they are too far removed from the human species to provide much information useful in the clinical sense.

The biggest trade-off in hypothesis testing in animal experiments is usually between the normality of the experimental
environment and the degree of control over the stimulus information made available to the animal. Stimulus control is very
difficult to achieve in normal social rearing environments but
without precise stimulus control, we will not be able to determine
the differential impact of various forms and content of spatial
information that can be generated by sensory substitution devices.
Admittedly, animal social deprivation techniques, now necessary
in conjunction with long term studies of currently available devices, are not ideal. Nevertheless, because of the environmental
control possible in the social deprivation situation, data from
use of the different devices in these types of experiments will
be useful to examine interactions between plastic processes and
stimulus information content. Data from these types of animal
experiments should also prove useful in the design of sensory
substitution devices: For example, compensation for some sensory
deficits, like blindness, may require input of spatial stimuli in
a combination of forms, such as auditory and tactile combined,
rather than either one alone.

Conclusions

Our primary goal in sensory substitution research is to
develop sensory substitution devices that can be used effectively
by human subjects with sensory deficits. This means we have to
learn how sensory substitution devices can be used to enhance
those plastic responses or associations that promote compensation
and prevent those that do not. The use of animal subjects will
be necessary to test some of our hypotheses in sensory substitution research, but even if this were not so, the use of animals
is much more practical than the use of human subjects in terms of
potential risk, experimental control, and investments of time and
money. In view of the urgent need to compensate for sensory
deficits, I suggest that we consider the use of animal models
whenever possible to examine questions related to sensory substitution device use and design.

ACKNOWLEDGEMENTS

    This work was supported by NIH Grants 1 RO1 EY05224-01
and 5 RO1 HD10408, and by the Center for Social and Behavioral
Science Research, University of California, Riverside.

REFERENCES

1.   Tuchmann-Duplessis, H., Auroux, M., & Haegel, P.   (1974).
     Illustrated Human Embryology, Volume 3, Nervous System and
     Endocrine Glands. New York: Springer-Verlag.

2.   Warren, D. H. (1984). Blindness and Early Childhood Develop-
     ment (2'nd Ed.) New York: American Foundation for the Blind.

REHABILITATION ISSUES

INTRODUCTION

The papers by Freedman and Spungin, who are both with the American Foundation for the Blind, consider the use of spatial sensory aids from the perspective of rehabilitation and the rehabilitation agency. Rehabilitation issues include the questions of training, perception, and cognition raised elsewhere in this volume. However, when the technology is refined and the behavioral research issues are resolved, rehabilitation personnel and agencies must actually incorporate the use of such devices within the range of other services to the blind. Thus the interest of the rehabilitation agency extends more broadly into sociological and political factors which have a bearing on the delivery of services generally.

Freedman's paper deals with emotional aspects of space perception and visual loss. It adds another dimension to a problem which is generally treated by the research psychologist purely in terms of the provision of sensory information to allow the blind person to perform specific perceptual-motor spatial tasks. Drawing in part on the work of Carroll, he discusses the anxiety created by the diminished ability to feel a part of the environment and the loss of anonymity which results from the sense of being on display to the sighted community and not knowing when one is being observed by others. Of great importance to the acceptance of visual prostheses what is known about the resistance shown by many blind persons to regaining visual capabilities by electronic or surgical means (e.g. 1). The reasons for this are varied: The blind person may be unfamiliar with the concepts of visual sensing brought about by electronic prostheses and may feel threatened by the need to relearn modes of perceptual-motor activity or by the prospect of loss of social and institutional support available when he or she was blind.

Spungin's article gives an overview of sensory aid research, placing the problem within the perspective of the demographics of the population of the blind in the United States. Like Freedman, she draws attention to the need for a better understanding of the overall needs of the blind person in the rehabilitation process and notes several less obvious human factors influencing aid use and acceptance. Her section "Corridors of Insensitivity" provides a provocative listing of the problems of interaction among the research and professional groups involved with sensory aids. Issues of interdisciplinary co-operation are at times as much problems to be overcome as the purely scientific and rehabilitation issues. For perspective, it should be noted that these problems are generic ones in rehabilitation research and engineering, and are not restricted to the area of spatial sensors.

The Editors

REFERENCE

1. Valvo, A. (1971). Sight Restoration After Long-Term Blindness. New York: American Foundation for the Blind.

VISION PROSTHESIS AND AIDS: READINESS OR APPROPRIATENESS

Saul Freedman

American Foundation for the Blind

If given the opportunity to speak openly after trust is gained, many individuals seeking rehabilitative assistance because of vision loss have said words very close to "I'd give anything to be able to see again, even my right arm" or "Without my sight I feel dead" or "If only I could keep what little I have." Each individual's perspective upon loss of vision is appropriate for himself and honestly reflects his perception of himself and the impact he feels regarding vision loss. These expressions are consistent with the statements made by so many individuals who, when asked about their purpose in entering into a rehabilitation setting, state simply, directly, and immediately "to see a little better" or "to get glasses that might help me."

For those concerned with the restoration of sight through medical means or the scientific creation of prosthetic devices and aids that might help the individual enhance or regain his or her sight, the above statements should come as no shock. However, we must understand and accept the fact that many people who have become blind, while almost universally hoping to regain their sight, are ambivalent, fearful, suspicious, and sometimes reject-ing of a prosthetic or aid approach. It might be noted that in the process of assessing congenitally blind adults referred for rehabilitation purposes, I have observed an almost universal rejection of a prosthetic approach to give sight for the first time, especially if some form of surgery is involved. This point will be discussed later in this paper.

Most individuals who are blind lose their sight during adult-hood. Our understanding of what the individual may experience in terms of losses and possible changes in self perceptions may be crucial to the creation of a more effective rehabilitation process, of which prostheses, aids, and appliances are a vital part. Father Thomas J. Carroll (1) has done this most effectively in his book <u>Blindness, What It Is, What It Does, and How To Live With It</u>.

Although each of the 20 types of losses discussed by Father Carroll has a different impact for each individual, the first grouping, entitled "Basic Losses to Psychological Security," is particularly germane.

The Loss of Physical Integrity

In expressing his thoughts concerning loss of sight in adulthood, Father Carroll stressed repeatedly the multiplicity of handicapping conditions, with much attention on self perceptions. He described what he called "a loss of wholeness" in a most sensitive way, calling attention to the unique manner in which each person experiences alterations in the self image and the unique adaptive resources that are brought into play by each person. While Father Carroll placed an emphasis on loss as "maiming physically or emotionally" (and this phrase still causes readers, lay and professional, much discomfort), he spoke of each individual as having a certain self image--a body image--which now experiences a drastic unanticipated change that threatens the entire life style. He went on to say that "interwoven in the feelings of the newly blinded man are all the feelings that he turned on blind persons when he had his sight." In essence, Father Carroll pointed out the importance for all concerned, including the person who has become blind, of how that person felt about blindness prior to loss of sight. He suggested that we consider how to use that information--how we can help the person articulate his or her feelings--so that we can utilize this for the person's advantage.

The Loss of Confidence In the Remaining Senses

Father Carroll wrote that "When seeing is no longer possible, then for many people believing becomes difficult, if not impossible. They (the persons who have become blind or lost extensive sight) tend to doubt the information gathered by the other sources to support its validity...We use sight to test the information from some of the other senses." One of the stereotypes that flourishes concerning the blind is that they possess super-sensitive senses of hearing, touch, taste, and smell, and that the facility for recall of events, names, and voices is equally uncanny. Father Carroll also discussed the mistaken mythology of automatic compensation for the loss of sight by the "natural

phenomenon" of this sensory development. There is gross disap-
pointment, almost shocking surprise, that accompanies the individual realization that this extraordinary development is not
happening. Quite often, rather than expressing concern, the
individual internalizes these fears and silently concludes his or
her "failure" to develop according to the pattern of preconceived
notions held regarding "the adjustment to blindness."

Loss of Reality Contact With Environment

While there are many sensory modalities with which to maintain reality contact with the environment, blindness or severe
visual impairment, with its multiple handicapping losses, erodes
the confidence and consequent skill level necessary to maintain
such contact. This was part of Father Carroll's thrust when he
stated that "the loss of reality contact (the ability to affirm
and confirm) with the tangible world in which we live, is one
that easily leads to panic or that makes still more numb the
numbness of the stage of shock." He elaborated further by stating
"For those who have grown up with the use of it, sight is the
great source for contact with the concrete world of things as
they are." Apart from our capacity to use sight to orient us to
our environment, Father Carroll pointed out that sight is especially important in conveying the feeling that we are in control
of our environments, or at least of our ability to react to them.

The Loss of Visual Background

Much of our knowledge is based upon our visual perceptions
and capacity for imagery and recall. We are constantly bombarded
by stimuli, many of which are never recorded in memory. Much
visual background is like the radio music we hear while absorbed
in some task. The loss of such visual background, as described
by Father Carroll, "holds the emptiness, the loneliness of what
might be called visual silence." Perhaps because of the additional losses sustained that are physical, emotional, social, and
economic, the loss of visual background is translated into a
diminished ability to feel part of an environment as well as a
diminished ability to control it with confidence.

Rehabilitation training should provide the blind person the
means to compensate for the loss of visual background and the
many cues that it contains. Success in such training offers
confidence in the ability to recognize and utilize these cues and
offers the possibility of greater involvement, feelings of per-
tinence, and a measure of greater control of the person's life.
It is the constant threat of loss of control and/or greater
dependence upon others that is so emotionally debilitating. This
threat, however, can be arrested and perhaps reversed.

Loss of Light Security

In speaking of "light" and "dark," Father Carroll drew upon the popular myth that "blindness is darkness." He indicated that our specialized service field may add to this stereotype by giving so many facilities names such as "Lighthouse." Apart from the inappropriate use of the words light, dark, darkness, and lighthouse for the obvious purposes of sympathy and fund raising, he pointed out that such terms perpetuate public and professional ignorance regarding eligibility for service and availability for training. Many who are "blind" are able to distinguish light from dark and more. According to our accepted definition of blindness, most people eligible for assistance and training have useful light perception.

Another one of the 20 losses deserves particular attention. "Obscurity" is the ability to lose oneself unnoticed into the crowd. Loss of Obscurity essentially is "the loss of the ability to fit in among one's fellows without being marked out as strangely different." Loss of Obscurity has impact on the whole personality. Unless attention is to be focused upon us for some form of accepted, approved, or positive recognition of skills, attributes, or virtues, each of us would for the most part prefer to be part of the crowd. Anonymity can convey much comfort especially when we are not in the position of controlling how much or little exposure we want. The stigma that many sighted individuals possess about being a blind person is sometimes carried over and exacerbated in the event that they become blind. With appropriate interventions, support, education, and rehabilitation, these negative images can and do diminish.

There is another important aspect to the loss of obscurity. Chevigny (2) summed it up when he expressed his concern about "being observed without knowing it" without the comfort of being able to check out for himself and verify "how I look." The quiet remarks of sympathy addressed to another person of the public, the anxiety-ridden but well-meaning crowd on a bus that yells "somebody give that blind man a seat" or the constant choral chant "doesn't she have a beautiful dog" tends to confirm for most blind individuals the loss of obscurity.

Let us understand that for most people, blindness or severe vision loss is a gradual process. Degrees of denial are appropriate until other forms of assistance, hopefully rehabilitative or restorative in nature, can be offered. While professionals who wish to be of assistance take the prescription of canes or dog guides as appropriate standard practice, such a recommendation has deep meaning for the person who is to use the assistance. It is more than symbolic. It is another person's affirmation, and a

professional person's at that, that the assistance is now necessary. Much the same can be said of people who are able to profit
from the use of low-vision aids. Appearance of normality as well
as appropriate and sensitive instruction in the use of such devices are critical factors in their continued usage. This is all
part of the support that is necessary to help the individual
become ready for the acceptance of that assistance. Each person's
needs are different, but virtually everyone needs some form of
support. One can speculate whether there will ever be a device,
prosthesis, or aid that will gain universal acceptance. That
should not be the goal--but providing a person with the choice of
assistive techniques might be.

     The use of dog guides, while widely accepted now, was viewed
with much skepticism when first introduced in the late 1920s.
Koestler (5) commented that "It was the self denigrating belief
that blindness should be made as inconspicuous a possible, and
that the use of a dog guide or a distinctive cane attracted
undesirable public attention." She quotes Robert Irwin, Director
of the American Foundation for the Blind at the time, that he
personally "would not be caught using one of the blooming things."

     Rather prophetically in 1969, Shaw (6) wrote "As one glances
through contemporary literature in the subject of blind mobility
one is impressed by the ingenious technological advances which
are being suggested or used to help the blind become more fully
mobile. So intricate do the various aids become (the long
cane, of course, excepted) that one is tempted to imagine the
blind person of the future as an antennaed robot, emitting bleeps,
clicks, and pings. But before we reach that stage, it is perhaps
timely to remind ourselves that, whatever new mobility methods
lie ahead, we learn to use them well only if our attitudes are
right. In learning blind mobility, by old methods or by new,
attitudes are of prime importance... The cane, however, is of
some value to all blind people, no matter what their visual
standards may be, and it is rejected, ordinarily, not because it
is an aid which can be done without, but because it is a symbol
of abnormality" (p. 31).

     The concept of the person's readiness or the appropriateness
of the device is not an issue exclusive to work with people who
are blind or visually impaired. Comfort, security, utility, and
appearance are prerequisites regardless of the device. Proper
preparation, support, and self image play a role regardless of
the type of disability. In describing the high "rate of success"
of prosthetist Jan Stokosa, Director of the Institute for the
Advancement of Prosthetics, Gorski (3) spoke of the attention to
detail, the achievement of physical and emotional comfort for the
patient. The patient controls the artificial limb, not the other

way around. Limbs are made to match shape, color, shoes (including exposed toes). Patients are made to feel and act as they did
prior to the amputation.

Wright (8) stated that "no matter how good the quality of the
prosthesis, all too often the performance remains inadequate or
the prosthesis is discarded entirely because the patient, once
fitted, was left on his own to manage as best he could. It is
being recognized that there is a tremendous amount of know-how to
be acquired before a patient can cope with the varied conditions
of life. The desirable skills can be facilitated by teaching and
supervised practice" (p. 106).

Earlier in this paper, reference was made to the almost
universal rejection, by congenitally totally blind adults, of
artificial sight through the use of prosthesis. While initially
this finding may be surprising, even shocking to some, it is in
actuality an appropriate response. The congenitally blind adult
has never experienced the loss of sight. He or she has experienced
the negativism and lack of knowledge of a sighted public, and has
made adjustments to the total life situation every day. The
presentation of the possibility of sight is a very real threat
to the continuity of everyday functioning that the person has
learned. There can be the implication that they cannot function
effectively without such assistance, when perhaps they have
learned to function very well. A major issue, simply put, is
"What is sight?" How do we explain it to a person who has never
seen? How do we relieve his or her appropriate anxiety about the
process of having to relearn so many concepts while also acquiring
new ones? The issues are many, including ones of appearance. No
one, adventitiously or congenitally blind, wants to appear like a
robot, although some will say "if I can see I don't care what I
look like." It should be noted that in discussions with congenitally blind adults regarding the presentation of such a prosthesis
as part of an extensive re-educational process, the attitudes of
almost universal rejection turn to guarded willingness and interest in most situations.

The concept of normal appearance cannot be overemphasized.
Kleck and DeJing (4), in a recent study at a summer camp, found
that boys with obvious physical handicaps are less well-liked
than their able-bodied peers. Judgments of attractiveness by
peers were found to be strongly associated with the presence or
absence of a physically handicapping condition. Physical handicap
or limitation is associated with a generalized reduction in
attractiveness. The same was found in a study of young girls.
It may be assumed that able-bodied adults have similar attitudes.

The development of prostheses and aids that might enable people to see should be the interest and responsibility of every professional who has contact with a blind or visually impaired person. It must be recognized that the production of such devices will not be the end of an individual's rehabilitative process, but an important part of it. Individuals who have lost their sight may well worry about the integrity of the rest of their physical being. Most prospective users of such assistive devices are older. The issue of "user friendliness" must be dealt with as well as the availability and costs for people who may have limited financial resources or who are not candidates for return to the work marketplace. The issues of cost maintenance of devices and responsibility for them should be raised.

Congenitally blind children should be considered candidates for assistance. The impact upon learning would be profound. The involvement of family members, regardless of the age of the user, would be critical in order to assure maximal understanding and support for all concerned.

Siller (7) stated that "evidence suggests that people with disabilities have considerable control over how others respond to them. Their own behavior makes a difference; whether they present themselves as coping versus succumbing, what they say or don't say about themselves influences others' attitudes. Teaching people with disabilities specific ways to improve their interactions with other people can and should become a key element in the rehabilitation process" (p. 4). There are a number of key elements in a person's rehabilitation process, but perhaps the most important is helping the person learn that he or she has control and that choices are available. Hopefully prostheses and aids which will enable people to see better, which will enable people to see again, and which will enable people to see for the first time will be part of the process of choices in rehabilitation and education. We must look forward to the time when rehabilitation and education facilities will turn more and more of their attention and energies to teaching people how to see.

REFERENCES

1. Carroll, T. J. (1961). Blindness: What It Is, What It Does and How To Live With It. Boston: Little, Brown.

2. Chevigny, H. (1946). My Eyes Have a Cold Nose. New Haven: Yale University Press.

3. Gorski, R. (1982). To walk and work in comfort. Disabled U.S.A., Fall, 23-27.

4. Kleck, R. & DeJing, W. (1983). Attitudes toward disabled peers, Rehabilitation Psychology, 28, 32-37.

5. Koestler, F. A. (1976). The Unseen Minority. New York: David McKay.

6. Shaw, J. A. S. (1969). Attitudes in blind mobility. The New Beacon, 53, 31-32.

7. Siller, J. (1983). Rehabilitation Brief, 10, 3-4.

8. Wright, B. (1959). Rehabilitation Psychology. Washington: American Psychological Association.

NOTE

A version of this paper appeared in the Journal of Visual Impairment & Blindness, March, 1985.

TECHNOLOGY AND THE BLIND PERSON: CORRIDORS OF INSENSITIVITY

Susan Jay Spungin

American Foundation for the Blind

The past three decades have been no less than spectacular in terms of technological advances that have occurred and are occurring in enhancing the communication, mobility, vocational, and recreational opportunities of blind and severely visually impaired people.

Substantial accomplishments have been forged by a relatively small number of modestly supported scientists and engineers. Their achievements are even more impressive when viewed in terms of the various time spans and processes that are involved from the first emergence of an idea and throughout all the research, prototype development, evaluation, marketing, financing, manufacture, promotion, sales, maintenance, and distribution stages which must be accomplished before the original idea can become a practical reality in the blindness system. Most of us tend to overlook this long time span because manufacturers often do not inform us of a new product until it is about ready to go on the market. Nevertheless, the grapevine in our field and the news media never seem to tire of spreading the word about some miraculous new "proposed" device that will, at last, be the ultimate answer to the reading problems, the mobility problems, or some other problem facing blind people.

Happily, though, leading developers in technological development have come to recognize several factors peculiar to the visually impaired population:

1. Visual impairment is often merely one problem in the context of other chronic conditions or limitations, as for example, in the case of the multiply handicapped.

2.   Devices primarily designed for totally blind people are not necessarily relevant to those with limited vision.

3.   Only a fraction of the visually impaired will probably use any one, single kind of device, thereby making it invalid to assume that the visually impaired population in general is a universal market for a particular technologically-based product.

4.   The most likely market for sophisticated technical aids presently lies among the singly handicapped blind of school and working ages.

Technology for the blind was a virtually non-existent field less than 30 years ago. Since then, we have witnessed the start-up of a promising industry whose development has been admittedly painful for the researchers and the manufacturers, as well as for the user population. This is because technological development is a highly involved process. It is one with a time frame that more often than not starts with just an idea. That idea next has to be defined in concrete terms, and criteria and then solutions have to be generated, tested, and proven. Only then can one move toward the manufacture and distribution of the ultimate device or product. Seldom had this been easily or readily achieved.

CHARACTERISTICS OF THE PROBLEM

The Population

The legally blind population in the United States is expected to increase by 12% by 1990 - from about 522,000 in 1980 to about 585,000 - assuming the current prevalance of legal blindness and the projected population growth. Within the legally blind population, the number of individuals under age 5 and over age 65 should increase by 19% and 17%, respectively, whereas the number between the ages of 5 and 19 will decline by 6%. On the other hand, within the legally blind population changes in the age distribution should be relatively minor. The number of individuals in the 0 to 20 age group should decline by approximately 1%, and the number 65 and older should increase by about 2% (8).

People presently using Orientation and Mobility (O&M) services are in effect the potential consumers of technological aids for mobility, those aids being defined in the broadest sense.

Data from several sources make it possible to evaluate the current situation in O & M and to hypothesize about the year 1990 (3,8).

Today the number of people who receive O & M services is about equally distributed between individuals under and over age 22. However, current estimates indicate that 92% of all legally blind individuals are over age 20, and projections for 1990 indicate that this percentage will remain virtually constant. The age distribution of recipients of O & M services in 1980 is shown below.

Age	Number	Percentage
0-22	7,353	41
23-44	3,810	21
45-64	3,467	19
65 +	3,465	19

No data are available to document how many children under age five are currently being served by O & M specialists in the public schools. However, a small number of children in this age group are currently served by O & M specialists in schools and agencies that serve blind and visually impaired individuals (schools, 3%; agencies, 2%). Most individuals younger than 22 who receive O & M services from agencies and residential schools are between the ages of 6 and 21. And the people age 22 or older who receive these services from agencies are almost equally distributed among the following age categories: 22-44, 28%; 45-64, 26%; and 65 and older, 26%.

Today, the distribution of people in ages 22-44 and 45-64 who receive O & M services is about the same as the distribution of all legally blind people in these age groups. This is not the case for service recipients who are under 22 or 65 and older.

Legally blind individuals who are under age 22 represent approximately 8% of the legally blind population. Yet they represent 41% of all those who receive O & M services (most of these young people are between the ages of six and 21). On the other hand, people who are 65 and older represent 54% of the legally blind population but only 19% of them receive O & M services (8).

Cost Factors - An Historical Perspective

Although the annual expenditure from the public sector for research and development in technology for all disabled individuals during the first half of this decade ranges from 1.00 to 2.92 dollars per handicapped person, the technological development of devices has enjoyed, over the long haul, greater financial support. In the mid 1940s the federal government set up a Special Group Committee on Sensory Devices of the Office of Scientific Research and Development, chaired by Dr. George W. Corner. In January of 1944 their role was to focus on the needs of the blinded veterans specifically for devices for reading ordinary print and guidance for ranging and obstacle finding.

Dr. Corner wrote of the work of the Committee on Sensory Devices: "In each case...we come up against the question of the ability of the human user to make practical use of the sense-stimulation afforded by these instruments.... Whatever missteps the Committee made arose chiefly from insufficient realization of this fact or from disregard of it" (2).

In the succeeding decades there were engineering triumphs that worked in the laboratory and failed at the critical level of consumer use. The estimate in 1968 of what the federal investment in blindness technology had been during the past 20 years was 8 million dollars.

The Committee on Sensory Devices disbanded in 1954. The concept of the committee resurfaced in 1964 and reorganized and came together again under Dr. Robert Mann's leadership as Chair of the Subcommittee on Sensory Aids (2).

THE DEVELOPMENT OF ELECTRONIC TRAVEL AIDS

With heavy expenditures since World War II, one sees at least two dozen attempts at Electronic Aid development over 25 years. The partial list of devices reads as follows: G5 Obstacle Detector, Sonic Torch, Pathsounder, Binaural Sensory Aid (or Sonicguide), Lightprobe, Mowat Sonar Sensor, Nottingham Obstacle Detector, FOA Laser Cane, Bionic Laser Cane, MIMS Infrared Mobility Aid, Single Object Sensor or Bui Device, Canterbury Child's Aid, and AFB's Computerized Travel Aid.

Of that list, four ETAs are actively being pursued and refined; namely, the Pathsounder, the Mowat Sensor, the Laser Cane, and the Sonicguide. These electronic travel aids assist in obstacle detection and simple environmental surveillance. Russell (5) found the Pathsounder (an ultrasonic chest-mounted aid) to be a go-no-go device useful for:

1. Collision avoidance in pedestrian traffic.
2. Protection against overhangs.
3. Advance warning of obstacles and restricted openings.

Armstrong (1) found that, in general, hand-held ultrasonic devices can be used to assist in:

1. Simple location of landmarks and/or obstacles
2. Detection and negotiation of ascending stairs.
3. Shoreline monitoring.
4. Clear path indication (including restricted openings).

In the Laser Cane, laser beams built into a cane are directed forward, upward, and downward. To a varying degree, the Laser Cane offers many of the functions of the chest-mounted and hand-held ultrasonic aids. It is important to note that the Laser Cane is the only available device that provides dropoff detection. Additionally, because of its narrow beam, the Laser Cane allows for the user to detect obstacles and openings that are clustered close together.

The Sonicguide, which is mounted in spectacle frames, is an ultrasonic aid that displays information to both ears simultaneously. In contrast to the previously mentioned devices, the Sonicguide displays a large amount of information. In addition to information about the distance and direction of objects and openings, it provides information about surface textures to assist in object identification. A subsequent version, the Trisensor, is described by Kay (this volume).

As exciting as these four devices for mobility are, Dr. Eugene Murphy's comments made in 1971 when serving as chief of the Research and Development Division of the VA's Prosthetic and Sensory Aids Service are still applicable today:

> "It is not enough to say that the devices are
> accepted or rejected by certain percentages of
> users. Rather, it is necessary to discover
> types of users for whom it is most appropriate
> ....one needs an armamentarian of devices from
> which selection can be made" (2, p. 362).

It is in that spirit that the American Foundation for the Blind entered into a project in 1980 (7) to develop a computerized travel aid (CTA). In effect, it was an attempt to combine the best from the Laser Cane (drop offs excluded), the Pathsounder, and Sonicguide, and allow the blind consumer to select what type of feedback was needed under what circumstances.

The AFB's CTA is designed to be used as a secondary aid to the long cane or guide dog for travel in either indoor or outdoor environments. However, in familiar indoor environments, the CTA can be used as the primary aid. The device uses an ultrasonic transducer to locate environmental features, such as path obstructions, door openings, and environmental landmarks. It conveys information through audible tones.

Depending on the requirements of the environment and the travel task, the user can control either:

1. the type of audio presentation
2. the sensing range
3. the shape of the sensing beam.

Additionally, the user has the option of using the CTA as a chest-mounted aid, a hand-held aid, or a cane-mounted aid.

Looking ahead to the future, we must continue to take pains to ensure that technological developments for blind people will be tied directly to their needs. Some visually impaired persons simply do not need a great deal by way of technological aids or gadgets. Yet, others do and view their employment futures as dependent on technological advances if they are to compete on near equal terms with sighted people.

Only if our technological leaders have a clear sense of what blind people are doing, how they manage their lives, and the way they are integrated into their families and communities, can these experts develop intelligent solutions to their needs. We need to foster more respect for the wisdom, the values and insight of blind and visually impaired persons themselves, and, more particularly, of those least served by the present level of technology, namely the lesser skilled, the multi-handicapped, and the deaf-blind.

I would like to encourage engineers and perceptual psychologists to pay more attention to the organism they are trying to help and less attention to the tools they are using. To put it perhaps more succinctly let me quote a blind student who said "I walk with my head as well as my feet" (2).

There is no doubt that technology creates opportunities, but who prepares individuals for those opportunities? Overlooking the preparedness of the blind client, adult or child, is symbolic of society's fascination with high tech solutions to the neglect of low tech applications (4).

> "Despite important problems related to developing technologies, the more serious questions are social ones - of financing, of conflicting and ill defined goals, and of isolated and uncoordinated programs" (6).

What I am really saying is that in order to insure the purchase and use of an aid by the blind individual, of any age, one
really needs to understand, first, that single individual and how
he or she deals with the disability of blindness. I really don't
believe that the engineering community has done that yet, in any
real sense, and until that happens the success and/or wide use of
technological aids, of any sort, will remain limited.

UNDERSTANDING THE BLINDNESS SYSTEM IN THE U.S.A.

In addition to understanding the effects of blindness on the
individual, one must also understand the blindness system. It
has become very well organized over the past decade, and by understanding the network one can more easily infuse new ideas and
gain support and acceptance.

In the area of special education programs for the blind,
there are some five organizations: the state vision consultants,
representing some 75% of the school age population attending
neighborhood schools (more than 45,000 legally blind children);
the superintendents of the 53 residential schools for the blind
(more than 15,000 legally blind), representing some 25% of the
more severely disabled multiply handicapped population; the approximately 14 Instructional Material Centers for the Visually
Handicapped; about 50 large vision programs; and 30 to 35 university training programs training professionals in work for the
blind either in education, rehabilitation teaching, or O & M. In
addition to these five associations there are two more: The National Association of State Agencies of Blind and Visually Impaired serves children as well as adults and represents 50 state
agencies for the blind, and the National Association of Private
Agencies for the Blind and Visually Handicapped (NAPVI) represents
some 200 private agencies for the blind.

The blind consumer is no less organized, with a parent group
formed some five years ago, the National Association of Parents of
Visually Impaired, representing some 1500 families and growing.
The National Federation of the Blind and American Council of the
Blind are well known to you, I'm sure; they too have parent
groups but with greater emphasis on blind parents rather than
NAPVI's focus on parents of blind children. And last but not
least, there is the Blinded Veterans Association organization to
which we are all indebted not only for spearheading technological
development but for many training programs as well.

That is the system, consisting of individual members of the
newly formed professional organization of the Association of
Educators of Visually Handicapped and the American Association

of Workers for the Blind - Association of Education & Rehabilitation for Blind and Visually Impaired (AERBVI). To know these
organizations and their respective leadership is to begin to
infiltrate not only the potential consumer market, but to begin to
expose oneself to the many issues surrounding the complex problems
of vision loss. Perhaps in this process, collective input from
all concerned and interested parties can yield one or more usable
and affordable devices for blind people.

IDENTIFYING AND ANALYZING CHARACTERISTICS OF TECHNOLOGIES FOR THE
BLIND

For each of the technologies considered, the following characteristics should be analyzed:

. its availability;
. its simplicity of operation;
. its initial cost, including installation if applicable;
. its reimbursement or financing status;
. its future adaptability (add-ons, cost, flexibility);
. its repair record (including ease and time);
. the extent and quality of performance or evaluation data;
. its cost of operation, if any; and
. its ability to provide desired functions to the necessary
  level.

These are examples of characteristics; other certainly can
be added to the list. For each technology, the traits above
should be compared to the following characteristics of the potential users and their needs, desires, and capabilities. Again the
list is illustrative, not exhaustive:

. the functional limitations of the user--blind or multiply
  handicapped;
. the physical and mental capabilities of the user to apply
  the technology: child, adult, or aging person; born blind
  or recently become blind;
. the user's affinity or preference for the various types of
  technology: tactile or auditory learner; attractive looking aid or not; age-related problems; adolescence;
. the user's desire for independence: the loneliness of the
  elderly (sighted guide means more than mobility);
. the physical location of the user: geographic and environmental, rural or urban; school, home, or work setting;
. the occupation or potential occupations of the user;
. the vocational and avocational aspirations of the user;
. income or other funds available, if the aid is not work related;

. any ways in which the above characteristics might change
  over time; and,
. the specific performance level requirements of the activ-
  ity/environment in which the individual will be involved
  (6).

The major question is, then, what can the blind person do
with the aid that would be unique, different, and better than
he/she could do without the aid? Even if the benefits are apparent there remain at least three additional problems when attempting to assimilate a technological aid into any system, be it
educational, vocational, or recreational. There is the cost, the
availability of training and software, and the fast pace of technological development, which tends to make existing aids obsolete.
A fourth and overriding fear for many in the blindness field is
that technology will infringe on the individual blind person's
motivation to learn basic skills, be they in braille or mobility.
This attitude of the provider is most easily seen in the reading
skill area as far back as the talking book program and as recent
as the Optacon.

CORRIDORS OF INSENSITIVITY: PERCEIVED ISSUES AMONG GROUPS

Perhaps a productive way to proceed would be to seek an ability to understand more clearly how the various groups involved in
technological development of aids are perceived by each other,
particularly the three groups of engineers, perceptual psychologists, and the blindness field in general -- professionals as well
as consumers. The following lists are only suggestive and may
serve to break down areas of non-communication in order for all
involved to work more closely together.

Engineers are perceived as:

. goal-free versus goal-based in development efforts;
. not sufficiently knowledgeable about blindness and blindness field;
. interested in high tech development to the disregard of low
  tech application;
. unwilling to see professional intervention techniques,
  which are at least equally important if not a prerequisite
  before introduction of technological aids;
. unable to believe that an aid is not a stand-alone device;
. unable to accept evaluation of aids, too personally involved; and,
. interested in input from others but then ignoring it and
  going in their own direction.

<u>Perceptual Psychologists</u> are perceived as:

- using sighted subjects, even O & M instructors, with blind-folds inappropriately as subjects for research; using small numbers of subjects in research;
- disregarding age of onset and demographics of blindness;
- lacking knowledge on psychosocial effects of blindness;
- lacking knowledge of early childhood development of blind children;
- lacking understanding of adjustment or non-adjustment to blindness;
- using the "superblind" as subjects;
- unable to bridge from research to practice;
- locked into experimental paradigms as a protection from making decisions about application; and,
- regarding those working in non-research oriented fields as having little valuable information.

The <u>Blindness field</u> is perceived as:

- lacking cooperative spirit: concepts using technology are foreign to human service professionals;
- being insensitive to a need for a "profit" for technology in order to exist, instead having a "do gooder" mentality;
- clinging to turfdom for client/student ownership, protecting it from the "evils" of research;
- being impatient with those out of the blindness field, who have no experience, no union card; being a clique of professionals in the blindness field;
- feeling threatened by change;
- lacking appreciation for complexities of technological development;
- asking for the world and using very little offered in technology; and
- afraid to lose jobs due to technological advances: aids replace need for professionals, especially orientation and mobility specialists.

TRAINING AND DISSEMINATION

I would like to conclude my discussion with the Optacon project because I believe it serves as a good model for the training and dissemination component of technology, which is the third and final phase of a three level effort of technology working for the blind person. The Optacon project had, for the first time, taken a technological device off the shelf and put it into the hands of a relatively large number of blind children.

During the day when Dr. Edwin Martin was director of the Bureau of Education of the Handicapped (later the Office of Special Education), a very large dissemination grant was given to Telesensory Instruments and the University of Pittsburgh under the direction of Dr. Mary Moore, to insure that the Optacon would become a common device available to every blind child in the U.S. The University of Pittsburgh trained all of the teacher educators from some 35 universities in order that they in turn could teach their teachers in training not only the mechanics of learning how to use the Optacon but more importantly how to teach blind children using the Optacon. Millions of dollars were spent in this program, so that virtually every eligible blind child had an Optacon of his or her own which followed them through high school.

This model, stressing the training of teachers as well as the development of training materials specific to the needs of the target population to be served, is paramount to insure the life and utility of any device. It indeed used the blindness system in a very effective way. For without these two components, professional training and software development, we will continue to see the shelves of all programs servicing the blind buckle under the weight of unused devices.

Cost, of course, is critical. Any of these aids do not come cheap -- either in their purchase, cost for training, or development of material to effect their use. With the federal government continually pulling back, one truly wonders how we can do more with less. So I am not going to suggest that as a viable option. Instead, I ask you to consider that we do more with what we have -- namely, the use of the consumer, the blind people themselves, from the early stages of developmental work, even at the idea of conceptual stage of development. The blindness profession, the special educator, the O & M specialist, the rehabilitation teacher -- we need their input, especially as it relates to training and material development. The professional organization in the field of blindness, AERBVI, can help fight for legislative change and federal financial support for our efforts.

Let us not see technology sessions or seminars without consumer panels and presentations on educational and rehabilitational concerns separated out from discussions on technological development. With consumers, engineers, psychologists, and professionals in the field of blindness all working together from the idea stage on, perhaps many more than the 30 aids introduced since World War II would be with us today and, more importantly, doing what we are all in this business want to do -- improve the quality of life for blind people everywhere.

REFERENCES

1. Armstrong, J. D. (1977). Mobility aids and the limitations
    of technological solutions. New Beacon, 61 (721), 113-115.

2. Koestler, F. (1976). The Unseen Minority. New York: Amer-
    ican Foundation for the Blind.

3. National Society to Prevent Blindness (1980). Vision Prob-
    lems in the U.S. New York.

4. Perlman, L. G. & Austin, G. F. (Eds.) (1984). Technology and
    rehabilitation of disabled persons in the informational age.
    A report of the Eighth Mary E. Switzer Memorial Seminar.

5. Russell, L. (1964). Travel path sounder. Rotterdam: Pro-
    ceedings of the Mobility Research Conference.

6. Technology and Handicapped People   (1982). Office of Tech-
    nology Assessment.

7. Uslan, M., Smith, R. W., Schreibman, K., & Maure, D. (1983).
    AFB's computerized travel aid: Two years of research and
    development.   Journal of Visual Impairment & Blindness, 77,
    71-75.

8. Uslan, M. (1983). Provisions of O & M: Services in 1990.
    Journal of Visual Impairment & Blindness, 77, 213-214.

NOTE: A version of this paper appeared in the Journal of Visual
Impairment & Blindness, March, 1985.

PERCEPTUAL AND COGNITIVE CONSIDERATIONS

INTRODUCTION

The traditional concern of those who have been involved in issues of electronic spatial sensory aids for the blind and visually impaired has been with the technological and engineering side of the question: What devices can be created and produced that will deliver to the visually impaired traveler information about the structure of the spatial environment and the location of obstacles? More recently, there has been recognition that the characteristics of the potential user of such devices may have as much bearing on the successful use of such devices as the engineering and technical aspects. These user characteristics include important questions of perceptual and cognitive capability.

One of the major roles of spatial sensors for the blind is to assist independent travel. However, travel by the sighted person does not just involve the motor activity itself; it involves, as well, perceptual activity in sensing the environment, although the perceptual aspects of travel occur so naturally and quickly that they are difficult to dissect and therefore to study. Perceptual issues are no less important, and no less difficult to study, in the visually impaired traveler.

Several papers in this section address perceptual issues. Lie presents an analysis of the visual system and its functions, as a guide to specifying what characteristics a device would have to have to simulate visual functioning. Lie concludes that the quest for such simulation is unrealistic at the present time, and suggests that the search for the "single best" mobility device be abandoned. Instead of seeking the ideal visual simulation device, we should concentrate on the functional problem-solving characteristics of mobility aids. Lie's paper is useful, too, in calling attention to the need to take non-perceptual factors into account in the rehabilitation process. In his paper in another section, Freedman addresses this issue focally.

Jansson's approach is broader, addressing aspects of other sensory modalities than vision in their potential involvement in

electronically-aided mobility. Jansson analyzes some basic segments of the mobility task, such as moving toward a perceptible
goal, moving along a guideline, and moving around an obstacle.
He proceeds to discuss the implications of various potential
device characteristics for the perceptual mediation necessary for
those segments. In some respects his treatment is analogous to
that of Foulke (see below), whose approach however is oriented
more to the cognitive than to the perceptual issues. Jansson
defines a number of issues that require perceptual research for
their resolution, such as the relative utility of simple vs
complex information, the nature of appropriate coding by an ETA,
whether a continuous flow of information is necessary and useful
for mobility, and the like.

The chapter by Epstein is more theoretical in its orientation.
Epstein addresses the issue of modality-specificity of information
and perception, using the term transmodal perception to refer to
the equivalence of perceptual function across different sensory
modalities, such as spatial location or surface texture. The
term amodal, correspondingly, is used to refer to the information
that is available for transmodal perception. This concept is
potentially important for the design of spatial sensors, since if
there are natural equivalencies of function across sensory modalities, they may usefully be taken into account in designing the
display of the spatial sensor. Whether making use of such natural
equivalencies is an actual benefit, however, is a question which
must be addressed empirically: it is not necessarily the case that
points of theoretical logic translate into practical implications
(for examples of such counter-intuitive findings, see papers by
Easton and by Warren and Strelow in this volume).

The task of mobility involves cognitive as well as perceptual-
motor processes. Cognitive processes are involved in at least
two important ways.

First, travel is a goal-directed behavior. Often the eventual
goal is not perceptually detectable from the outset; furthermore,
there are often alternative routes possible to reach the goal.
It is clear that some type of cognitive representation of the
spatial environment is important to allow travelers, whether
blind or not, to deal with alternative routes to initially non-
perceivable goals. These issues of cognitive representation are
no less important for the travel of the blind than of the
sighted (1).

Second, while travel often occurs in novel environments, it
also occurs in familiar settings. What is it about experience
that changes a novel environment into a more cognitively based
familiar one? That is, what is learned about a space upon first

encounter, and how does repeated encounter with the space change the nature of the demands on the perceptual and cognitive systems? The available literature is not satisfying on this issue, as indeed the psychological literature generally tends to be less satisfying on issues of process than of product. Nonetheless, it is critically important that we seek to understand the process of acquisition of spatial information in the blind both by the use of spatial sensors and as a natural, unaided process. This is a classic problem of cognitive psychology, and the issue demonstrates the need for researchers in the field of travel in the blind to transcend issues of perception.

Haber addresses a problem in spatial behavior that has been largely unexplored, and that is of considerable importance for the mobility of the blind, although the empirical work that Haber reports is with a sighted sample. The problem of "layout" has to do with the person's understanding of the relationships of things in the environment, i.e., the geometric relationships of objects to each other. This problem is relatively understudied, compared for example to the question of the egocentric perception of radial direction and distance. The perceptual experience of layout may also be a very different process than the cognitive understanding of layout. The perception (and conception) of layout is important for the blind even without the issue of mobility aids, since evidence indicates that the spatial conceptions of the blind are relatively egocentrically based. Whether this necessitates the use, for guidance of mobility, of a spatial system that provides egocentric information is unclear. The study of layout may provide clues about how to encourage spatial conceptions that are not egocentrically based.

The question of layout is also importantly related to ETAs, however: It is important to understand the blind person's conception of spatial layout in order to determine how best to present information about spatial relationships via an ETA. The approach to studying layout that is illustrated in Haber's paper, if appropriately adapted for use with the blind, should prove to be a useful addition to our set of methodologies.

Foulke is concerned with the development of a theory of mobility, and in his paper he addresses the nature of the cognitive processes which must go into such a theory. Mobility necessarily depends on perceptual information, but particularly for the blind, successful mobility also rests heavily on stored information about the environment. Foulke argues that this stored information is necessarily of a limited nature, that memory is selective with respect to the information that is retained, and that this information is organized in what may be called spatial schemata. Foulke's approach is to outline the cognitive processes that are involved, not as a specific theory of mobility for the blind, but as a general theory that would, with appropriate varia-tion, be applicable to the issue of sighted travel as well. Of course there are major differences in the nature of the perceptual and conceptual guidance of mobility for the sighted and the blind, such as the lack or degradation of visual information for the latter, but Foulke suggests that these differences should, in the initial stages of theory building, be considered as quantitative rather than as qualitative differences. We can expect that further refinement of theory will gradually show whether a general theory can be maintained that is also capable of accounting for the mobility of the blind (1).

In his Comment, Foulke goes on to address a number of im-portant issues of the suitability of non-visual modalities for mobility aids, and the implications of the characteristics of these modalities for aid design.

In the final paper in this section on perceptual and cognitive issues, Brambring reports studies about the nature of the informa-tion that blind and sighted travelers have about the routes that are well-known to them. In his paper, Foulke stresses the impor-tance of "landmarks" in spatial schemata: Brambring presents the frequencies of reports of landmarks in the subjects' accounts of routes, as well as of obstacles, directions, and distances, and concludes that landmarks are indeed frequently reported, and, together with items in the other categories, are reported more frequently by the blind than by the sighted. He concludes that the blind may require more information for travel than the sighted. Whether this conclusion is justified on the basis that the blind report more information may be questioned, but it is evident that much can be learned about the person's knowledge about routes and spatial structure by this reporting approach.

The Editors

REFERENCE

1. Strelow, E. R. (1985) What is Needed for a Theory of Mobility - Direct Perception and Cognitive Maps - Lessons from the Blind. Psychological Review, 2, 226-248.

ON REPLACEMENT AND PROBLEM SOLVING POTENTIALS OF SPATIAL AIDS
FOR THE BLIND

Ivar Lie

University of Oslo

The functional usefulness of prosthetic aids is of ultimate
interest for rehabilitation. However, the simulation of visual
processing and the use of strategies for solving practical problems represent two alternative approaches to evaluation and
development of technological aids for the blind. Some basic
problems associated with both approaches are briefly outlined and
discussed.

Information Processing Characteristics of the Visual Field

The simulation approach may be argued for "on the grounds
that the visual system has evolved to process the most effective
control stimuli in our typical spatial environments", to cite
Strelow and Brabyn (7). This approach would be an obvious choice
if a full-scale simulation of the visual system were possible.
However, only partial simulations seem realistic and, unfortunately, we do not know much about the functional usefulness of
reduced visual systems. The replacement potential of such partial
simulations are, therefore, not easily predicted.

Although few devices have been designed with the explicit
purpose of simulating visual experience, the use of words like
visual substitution, visual prostheses, and computer vision suggests that visual simulation is of main interest among scientists
and designers. It seems important, therefore, to consider the
implications of a simulation approach by explicit descriptions
of visual functioning. As a first step, some basic principles
of information processing in the visual field will be outlined
on the basis of visual discrimination and eye-movement data.

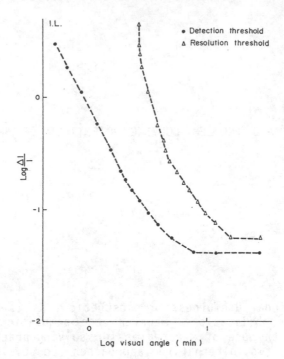

Figure 1. Area-threshold curves for detection and identification (From 2).

Experiments on area-threshold functions, using single test targets, indicate two basic resolving processes of the visual system: (a) a detection mechanism by which luminance differences are detected, and (b) an identification mechanism underlying shape discrimination and object identification. Different area-threshold curves are obtained for the two mechanisms (Figure 1) and different parametric effects of retinal location and back-ground luminance are shown in Figures 2 and 3. When the test field is increased beyond a certain size, the two thresholds coincide, staying nearly independent of retinal location and illumination conditions (background luminance). The functional significance of this coincidence and invariance is that the contours of large objects, making up the boundaries of the per-ceived layout, are maintained in the whole visual field, as well as down to the extreme limits of night vision. When the test field is reduced below a certain size, form discrimination becomes impossible, although the same test field can be detected at smaller sizes if the contrast is sufficiently increased.

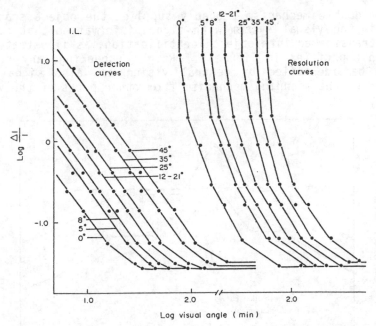

Figure 2. Area-threshold curves for detection and identification as a function of retinal eccentricity (From 2).

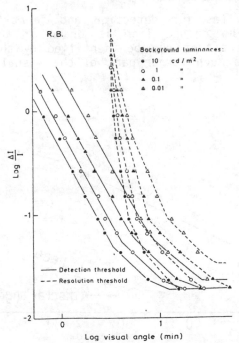

Figure 3. Area-threshold curves for detection and identification as a function of background luminance (From 3).

This double mechanism probably supplies the object scanning program in the visual system with signal information that can be readily transformed into object identification, as illustrated by the retinal profiles in Figure 4. Roughly speaking, any object that can be identified by central vision can also signal its existence to the scanning mechanism from other parts of the visual field.

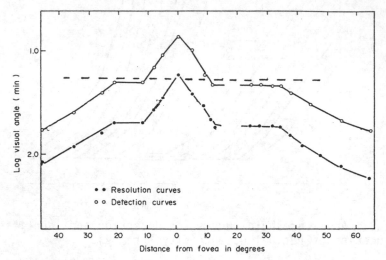

Figure 4. Retinal profiles for detection and identification thresholds (From 2). The dashed line is drawn in order to illustrate that any object that can be identified by the fovea can be detected within a much larger part of the visual field.

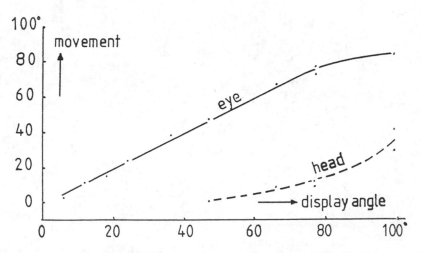

Figure 5. Eye and head movements as a function of display angle (From 4).

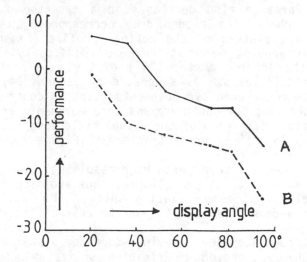

Figure 6. Performance (reaction time to visual discrimination)
tasks as a function of display angle and discriminability. Task
B is more difficult than task A (From 4).

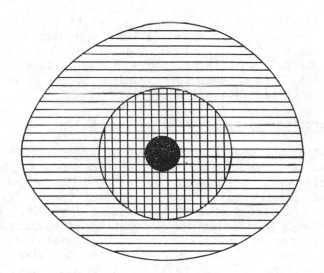

Figure 7. Illustration of the functional visual fields. See
explanation in the text.

Scanning involves eye and head movements, as shown in Figure
5. The area covered by eye movements alone is about 80°, corresponding closely to the outer diameter of the plateau of the
binocular perimetric visual field. Beyond this area, eye and
head movements are involved in combination with eye movements.

Scanning performance also decreases in a two-step fashion from fovea to periphery, the second drop corresponding to the outer diameter of the plateau of the retinal profile (Figure 6). The first drop, depending somewhat upon task difficulty, corresponds roughly to the inner diameter (20°) of the same plateau in the case of difficult tasks. As suggested by Sanders (4), the first drop seems to occur when eye movements start to control scanning, and the second drop when both eye and head movements are involved. The information efficiency of the visual field appears, therefore, to be divided into three concentric areas (Figure 7):

1. A small central area with high resolving power, where objects can be seen at one glimpse, thus avoiding any information delay caused by fixation shifts. The actual size of this area depends somewhat upon the task difficulty;

2. An intermediate area, having moderate visual acuity that needs to be improved by fixation shifts generated by eye movements;

3. A peripheral area, requiring both eye and head movements to perform fixation shifts.

The fixation shifts reflect the operation of scanning strategies, as indicated by the so-called "scanpaths," i.e., repetitive sequences of saccades during visual inspection of the physical world. When inspecting a hidden figure, for example, the scanpaths show changes corresponding to the alteration in the subject's cognitive state (Figure 8).

Basic Characteristics of Perceived Layout

"On-line" processed boundaries of the perceived layout are maintained as long as luminance differences can be detected. Illumination can, therefore, be reduced to night (scotopic) levels and visual acuity can be reduced toward "light vision" before the boundaries of the visual scene drop out. The significance of these boundaries for locomotion is obvious. Any small object that can be identified by central vision is perceptible at a detection level in the rest of the perceived layout, and can be transformed "upon call" into object identification by scanning. Object identification is of primary interest in situations requiring shape and object discrimination such as reading and eating. However, object recognition is also required when goal-directed locomotion is performed. When detection information is sufficient to avoid obstacles, object identification is required to orient oneself in the geographical surroundings.

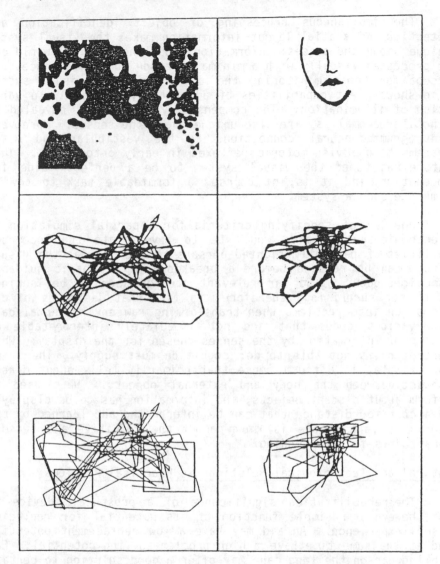

Figure 8.   Upper left shows fragmented figure and upper right fragmented figure with outline drawing of face superimposed to help reader to recognize hidden figure. Middle left represents eye movements during 75 seconds preceding identification, middle right represents eye movements during 75 seconds following identification. Lower left shows fixation regions before identification (From 5).

The simultaneous processing of object identification and detection and spatial layout information makes the visual system unique among the senses: Information about the physical world can be processed visually with a minimal load on cognitive processes, except for those monitoring the scanpaths. The visual system also shows great capabilities of adaptation, especially to variation of illumination. The compensatory properties, revealed by binocular anomalies, are also unique among the senses. Moreover, preprogrammed neural connections to the vestibular and motor systems become visuomotoric reflexes in early ontogenesis. Thus nature has tuned the visual system to be a perfect guide for locomotion, and it is, of course, a formidable task to try to simulate such a system.

One way of specifying criteria for a partial simulation of electronic spatial aids would be to investigate the locomotor abilities of partially sighted persons to see how far the visual system can be reduced before a breakdown of its basic guidance functions occurs. So far relevant studies seem to be lacking. It is not surprising, therefore, to find that designers of devices run into problems when transforming raw environmental data into various codes that are not immediately interpretable as locomotor information by the senses chosen for the display: What perception is not able to do, cognition must supply. The skin, for example, is a touch sense that primarily tells about direct contact between the body and external objects. When used to inform about distant objects, the information has to be displayed in a code for distance that can be interpreted and learned by the user. So far, little is known about the cognitive and sensory constraints for such coding.

Natural and Technological Solutions to Practical Problems

The rehabilitation significance of a prosthetic device is not, however, a simple function of its potential for replacing visual experience. An aid may have a low replacement potential and at the same time have a high problem-solving potential. For a blind person the long cane may offer a good solution to certain mobility problems, in spite of the fact that the long cane gives only a limited replacement of the visual guiding functions in locomotion.

The practical problems of everyday life suggest an alternative, and perhaps a more realistic reference, for the future development of technical aids for the blind. When sight is lost, the person is left with some kind of internal model of his environment, built up by previous visual and tactile experiences. This cognitive map (or schema) remains then as the primary subjective reference for the blind when interacting with the

physical environment. Without assistance of any aids, the blind
will employ more or less natural strategies of matching maps
and environments, such as stretching out arms and listening for
sounds. Attempts to analyze locomotor problems for technological
aid solutions should start with an analysis of the natural
matching strategies and the properties of the internal model of
the physical world. In other words, a theory of blind mobility
is needed in order to have a basis for systematical development
of problem-solving aids. Such a theory has to take account of
individual differences, such as age of onset of blindness, intellectual level, and kind of previous experiences (see 1,6 for partial analyses).

We are, so far, lacking a comprehensive theory of blind
mobility. This does not mean, however, that locomotor problems
cannot be classified and partly solved by the assistance of
technological aids. Bumping into obstacles, for example, represents an obvious type of locomotor problem to solve by obstacle
detectors like the long cane, the Laser cane, Mowat Sensor,
Sonicguide, and others. Shoreline guidance and landmark identification represent two other types of locomotor problems where
the blind are in severe need of technical assistance. The
so-called environmental sensors, like the Sonicguide, Sonic
Pathfinder, and recent developments within computer vision, provide assistance in these cases.

Further improvements of current devices and the design of
new ones are expected to follow the same guidelines, but the
shortcomings are too obvious to leave us content with the present
approach. A technological aid that makes the blind person a safe
and efficient pedestrian in all kinds of environments has not
been provided to date.

The blind person often has to choose between safety and
efficiency, and there are psychological reasons to expect that
safety is usually preferred to efficiency. Risk behavior is not
easily predicted, however; it may be of only minor psychological
significance to have the risk for obstacle collisions reduced
from 80 to 20%. This may explain why the long cane is often
preferred to electronic obstacle detectors. As to efficiency,
the long cane may be preferred to electronic devices when locomotion takes place in familiar environments. The user undertakes
some kind of cost/benefit analysis when given the opportunity to
choose between possible aids. In many cases cost differences may
decide the matter. Obviously, this analysis is not always undertaken by the most relevent pro et contra arguments.

General attitudes towards technical aids, being deeply rooted in the user's personality, may also play a main role. A Sonicguide type of spectacles may, like telescopic attachments to spectacles for the partly sighted, be refused for cosmetic reasons. When technical aids are presented as general mobility aids, the subjective cost/benefit analysis may easily turn out negative. While all blind persons have mobility problems, these may be of varying character, requiring different types of aids for each individual. Current devices are not equally appropriate for all mobility problems, and they may differ greatly with respect to their psychological demands on the user. The first step toward providing a future spurt in the development of mobility aids seems to be that designers must realize the variety of mobility problems and the individual differences in needs and psychological requests. The search for the <u>one</u> best mobility aid should, therefore, be put aside for some time.

SUMMARY

Simulation of visual processing and the presentation of more limited but practically oriented information are discussed as alternative guidelines for evaluation and development of visual aids. Some basic properties of visual functioning are outlined to illustrate the formidable challenges of a simulation approach. So far this approach seems unrealistic and the low replacement potential of current devices is expected to remain for the near future. It is argued, however, that a technical aid having low replacement potential may at the same time have high problem-solving capabilities. For example, the long cane may offer a good solution to certain mobility problems in spite of the fact that the long cane provides limited visual guiding functions in locomotion. The need for a theory of blind mobility as a basis for classification of mobility problems into more basic strategies for technical aid solutions is pointed out and some elements of such a theory are discussed. Meanwhile, the traditional search for the <u>one</u> best mobility aid should be put aside and more account taken of the variety of individual mobility problems.

REFERENCES

1. Kay, L. (1974). Towards Objective Mobility Evaluation:
    Some Thoughts About a Theory. American Foundation for the
    Blind, New York.

2. Lie, I. (1980). Visual detection and resolution as a func-
    tion of retinal locus. Vision Research, 20, 967-974.

3. Lie, I. (1981). Visual detection and resolution as a func-
    tion of adaptation and glare. Vision Research, 21, 1793-
    1797.

4. Sanders, A. F. (1970). Some aspects of the selective
    process in the functional visual field. Ergonomics, 13,
    101-117.

5. Stark, L. & Ellis, S. R. (1981). Scanpaths revisited:
    Cognitive models. Direct active looking. In D. F. Fischer,
    R. A. Monty, & J. W. Senders, (Eds.), Eye Movements: Cog-
    nition and Visual Perception. Lawrence Erlbaum Associates,
    New Jersey.

6. Strelow, E. R. (1985). What is needed for mobility: Direct
    perception and cognitive maps--Some lessons from the blind.
    Psychological Review, 92, 226-248.

7. Strelow, E. R. & Brabyn, J. A. (1981). Use of foreground
    and background information in visually guided locomotion.
    Perception, 10, 191-198.

IMPLICATIONS OF PERCEPTUAL THEORY FOR THE DEVELOPMENT
OF NON-VISUAL TRAVEL AIDS FOR THE VISUALLY IMPAIRED

Gunnar Jansson

Uppsala University

The goal of work on the mobility problems of the visually
handicapped is that their locomotion should be as safe, effective,
and relaxed as that of sighted people. There are many different
strategies to reach this goal. One is to adapt the environment
to the needs of the visually handicapped. In many countries this
has been done, to some extent, for the orthopedically handicapped,
and there is a budding insight that it is possible to do so also
for the visually handicapped (34).

However, changing the environment is a long-term and expensive project, and we cannot expect all the problems to be solved
in that way. There may also arise conflicts between the needs of
the visually handicapped and those of other groups of handicapped
people as well as those of non-handicapped people. In a shorter
time perspective we have to rely mainly on adapting the visually
handicapped to the existing environment, or rather to adapt a
system consisting of a person equipped with perceptual aids that
compensate for his lack of vision.

Whether we try to adapt the environment or to increase the
perceptual capacities of the traveler, a solid knowledge of the
functioning of the perceptual system to be substituted as well as
of the substituting technological system is helpful. Unfortunately, most of the scientific study of perception has concentrated
on problem areas that are not directly relevant to mobility.
Investigations concerned with static objects observed by a stationary person, as in a majority of the studies, are difficult to
generalize to functional situations where, typically, many objects
are moving in the environment as well as the observer. However,

there is a growing interest in these closer-to-life aspects of perception (16), and hopefully more theoretical and empirical work will include those aspects in the future. The aim of the present report is to discuss some principles relevant to the construction of non-visual travel aids, the general theoretical background being the pioneering work of Gibson (7) and of Johansson (12,13).

THE ANALYSIS OF LOCOMOTION

It is important to remember that locomotion is a very basic activity developed over thousands of years. For a locomotor mechanism to insure the survival of the animal, it must be very effective. It must, in the great majority of cases, be correctly guided by perception during searching of prey or mate, and avoidance of predator. This makes a close coupling of perception and action very probable. In fact, it is true on all levels of biological development that the main function of perception is its guidance of action (33). The elegant landing of a house fly on the ceiling demonstrates that complex locomotor acts are also possible at low cognitive levels.

There is probably no disagreement about the importance of perception for locomotion. The role of cognition has been more debated. In man, cognition certainly is involved, especially when orientation is involved. There is in many situations a complex interplay among perceptual, cognitive, and motor components of a locomotor act. Examples of general problems are the extent to which cognition gets involved, and the way in which cognition interacts with other functions. There are, for example, good reasons to believe that the visually handicapped have to rely more on memory than the sighted, as there is much less immediate information available to them (cf. 6,29). That I prefer, in the present context, not to go any further into the cognitive aspects of locomotion does not mean a denial of their importance, but only a choice of some other aspects of locomotion for discussion.

Aspects of Locomotion

When one moves from a starting point to a goal it is often the case that one does not perceive the final goal from the starting place. The whole route can, for the purpose of description, be divided into successive stages, each having its own starting point and goal (Figure 1). In the present context, interest is focused on how these stages can be analysed from a perceptual-motor point of view.

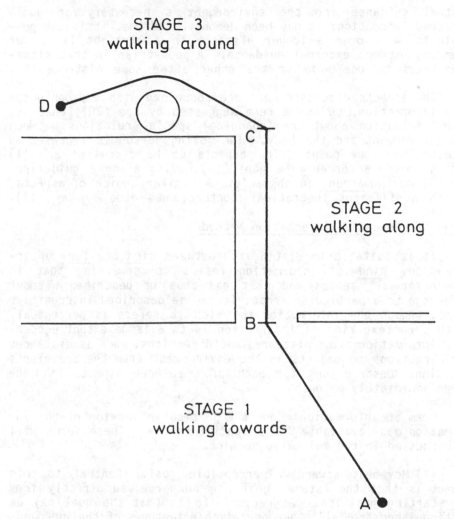

STAGE 3
walking around

D

C

STAGE 2
walking along

B

STAGE 1
walking towards

A

Figure 1. A route from A to D divided into stages exemplifying the three different aspects of walking. A is the start, D the goal, and B and C at the same time goal for the earlier stage and start for the later stage.

The maintenance of balance is crucial, of course, for effective walking. The role of non-visual travel aids for this aspect of locomotion will not be discussed here, but it should be noted that they contribute by providing information about the objects and the ground closest to the traveler (11). The aspects chosen for discussion in this paper are related to steering, the movement of the body toward a goal through a cluttered environment. Perceptual guidance from the environment is necessary for goal-directed locomotion; it has been demonstrated that it is not possible to walk over a longer distance in a straight line, for example, without external guidance. A pedestrian in that situation veers to one side or the other after some distance (4).

The aspects discussed here are concerned with exproprioceptive information, to use a term suggested by Lee (20), that is, with information about the (changing) spatial relations between the environment and the body. The moving person is represented here by just one point. The aspects to be discussed are (1) moving toward a perceptible goal, (2) moving along a guideline, and (3) moving around an obstacle. A similar choice of aspects, but in a different theoretical context, was made by Kay (17).

Kinds of Perceptual Information Needed

It is suitable to distinguish between kind and form of information. Kind of information refers to something that is common for all senses and that can thus be described without reference to a particular sense; it can be described in cognitive terms, though the information to which it refers is perceptual. In this context kind of information is to a large extent egocentric information about distances and directions, such as distances and directions to objects in the environment from the traveler's position. Descriptions for each of the three aspects will be given immediately below.

Form of information means the particular version of the information made available for a specific sense. These forms will be discussed in the following section.

(1) Movement toward a perceptible goal. Central to this aspect is that the (stage) goal can be perceived directly from the starting position. A prerequisite is that the goal may be distinguished from all other perceivable features of the surroundings. The goal may be an object or an opening; Gibson (7) treated the two cases separately because of the distinct differences in the corresponding visual stimulus patterns. These two kinds of goals also differ in the action suitable during the final approach: one can walk through an opening but should avoid bumping into an object.

In order to move properly toward the goal one needs information about the direction of the goal from the present position, about the direction in which one is moving, and, at least in the final approach, about the distance to the goal (Figure 2). One needs also to compare the two directions in order to be able to correct the direction of movement if it deviates too much from

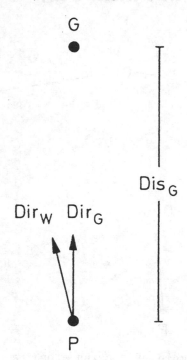

Figure 2. An example of "moving towards," P being present position, G goal, Dir_W direction of walking, Dir_G direction towards
goal, and Dis_G distance to goal.

the direction to the goal. The restricted range available to the
visually impaired, even with electronic travel aids, is a severe
limitation for their mobility, making this aspect of locomotion
possible only at short distances (8,30).

Information about the exact length of the distance to the
goal is probably not very important at longer distances; it may
be sufficient to get information about whether distance as the
goal is decreasing or not. At shorter distances the exact length
is more important, of course, although it may be that the necessary information is temporal (time-to-contact) instead of spatial,
as suggested by Lee (19).

(2) Moving along a guideline. When the (stage) goal is not
perceivable from the starting position it may nonetheless be
reached by perceptual guidance with the use of a shoreline or
guideline. The typical feature of a guideline is that it extends
from the starting position to the goal, whether it is a fence, a
wall, a handrail, or a wire with electric signals especially
built for the visually handicapped. "Moving along" is the aspect

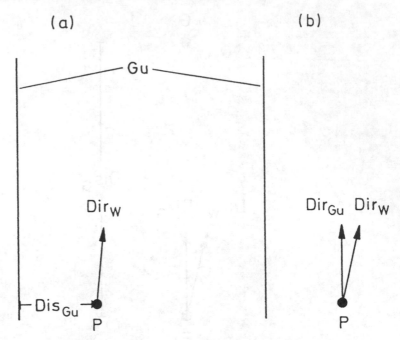

Figure 3. An example of "moving along" a staight guideline (Gu) with two different kinds of information about the guideline: (a) distance to it, Dis_{Gu}, and (b) its direction, Dir_{Gu}. P is present position and Dir_W direction of walking.

of locomotion most common for the visually impaired. In many cases, it replaces the sighted person's "moving toward" which may not be possible for a visually impaired person because of his restricted range (cf. above).

Even if the goal is not perceivable from the starting point when "moving along," there must be some information about the termination of the stage, for example that the guideline ends, or that some landmark appears. The information needed to follow a guideline may, typically, be in terms of the distance between the present position and the guideline (Figure 3a), constant distance indicating perfect moving along. If the distance from the guideline deviates too much from the desired distance, correction can be made by changing the direction of walking.

In the case of simple (e.g., straight) guidelines, the critical information may be the direction of the guideline and the direction of walking (Figure 3b). A comparison between these two directions gives information about the extent to which the guideline is followed, identical directions meaning perfect moving along.

(3) Moving around an obstacle. Usually, nobody wants to bump into obstacles, especially unexpectedly. This is probably the reason for the many efforts to produce travel aids that make it possible to avoid collisions. These aids have been called "clearpath indicators," a name which emphasizes the function of avoiding obstacles. What is not as often noted is that one of the problems with obstacle avoidance is to regain the initial direction after a deviation around the obstacle. In order to include this feature clearly, I prefer to talk about "moving around" instead of "avoiding" obstacles.

The visually impaired receive important information for this task from both traditional and electronic travel aids. However, the often very restricted preview due to the short perceptual range available is also an important problem in this context (1,30).

Moving around may be seen as a combination of moving toward and moving along. The traveler moves as directly as possible toward the goal and at the same time moves along the edge of the obstacle. To accomplish this he needs information about the directions to the goal and the obstacle, as well as the direction of his movement. An example of moving around an obstacle is given in Figure 4.

Forms of Perceptual Information

Even if the most basic problem concerning the construction of a perceptual aid is the kind of information to make available, the form of this information is also highly important. I have in some other contexts considered this problem applied to the travel aids developed so far (9,11), and I want here to discuss some general problems.

Available and useful information. It is seldom said plainly, but it seems sometimes to be implicit, when perceptual aids are discussed, that it is sufficient to make the perceptual information available via the aid. But of course that is not the case; the information must also have a useful form. For example, it is quite apparent that auditory frequencies presented in an aid must be within the range of frequencies the user can perceive. Even when the stimulation is within the audible range, it may not be presented in a useful manner. As an example, consider the efforts to make auditory form perception possible by presenting patterns of different frequencies; such efforts have not been very success-ful because of the problems of finding patterns that are easily perceivable. From the fact that a particular kind of information is available does not follow that it also is useful. The useful-ness has to be found out for each form of the information, by

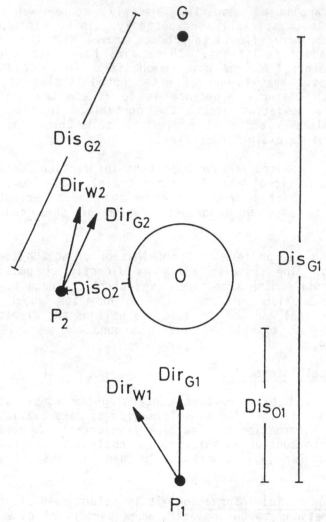

Figure 4. An example of "walking around" with two succesive psitions (P_1 and P_2) with direction of walking (Dir_W), direction toward goal (Dir_G), distance to goal (Dis_G), and distance to obstacle (Dis_O) given at each position. The figure 1 or 2 in the subscript indicates to which position the paramenter belongs.

referring to existing perceptual knowledge or by doing new experiments.

Analogic and coded forms of information. There is an interesting distinction between analogic and coded information (28). By analogic information is meant information that has a form that

is similar in some respect(s) to the information it replaces.
When vision is replaced by a device consisting of a TV camera and
a tactual display reproducing the visual picture, the device is
analogic; a well-known example is the Optacon. When the letters
of a visual text are replaced by Braille letters, the result is
given in coded form.

It is important to stress that what is or is not analogic is
the form of the information. What is given is the same information presented in different forms, be they analogic or coded. To
take an example from locomotion, the information "approaching an
object" has a visual form of several continuous changes in the
flow at the retina, e.g., increasing size of the portion of the
field containing the object and, in a more recent analysis, dele-
tion of texture outside the contour of the object (7). An analogic
tactual form of this parameter for a display consisting of a
matrix of point stimuli is an increase in the size of the tactual
pattern, i.e., the number of vibrators or electrodes representing
the object. A coded form of information about the event "approaching an object" is the change in frequency of an auditory
display, as in several travel aids for the visually handicapped.

It cannot be decided a priori if analogic or coded forms of
information are most useful. If there are sufficient similarities
between the substituted and the substituting perceptual systems,
analogic information may be very effective. But coded forms of
information may also be highly effective if they suit the functioning of the substituting perceptual system. It might be wise,
as Marks (23) put it, not only to look for similarities between
the senses but also to look for the particular strength of the
substituting perceptual system. One important aspect is if the
information has a form natural for this system.

Natural and artificial forms of information. It should be
observed that the natural-artificial distinction is different
from the analogic-coded one. A coded form of information may
very well be natural for the substituting perceptual system. A
form of information is artificial if man has not, by biological
evolution, developed a perceptual skill to utilize it. Distance
information given in the form of sound frequencies is an example
of such artificial information. This does not exclude it from
being a useful form of information, but it is less probable that
it is. However, nothing should be taken for granted. Humans,
with their great adaptability, can use many forms of information
that have no known usefulness from a biological point of view.
Technical development has provided us with many different forms
of information, e.g. those mediated by film and television, that
certainly are artificial but all the same can easily be picked
up. Again, empirical research has to decide (See Warren &
Strelow, this volume).

To utilize a natural form of information is, it seems to me, the first alternative to try. This is done, for example, when information about the direction to an object is given by inter-aural intensity differences, as by the Sonicguide. It is probable that less learning is needed when natural forms of information are utilized, and the compatibility between the perceptual and motor sides of performance can be expected to be better. However, there may be exceptions to this rule (35; Warren & Strelow, this volume).

Simple and complex forms of information. It is traditional in perceptual research to study stimulation that is simple to describe from a mathematical point of view. Such stimulation has been considered to be basic for the perceptual system. What has been studied is, to a large extent, the effects of stimulus parameters such as intensities of the stimulation, the size of the area stimulated, and simple forms such as the circle and the square. This is understandable from the point of view of the experimenter wanting a manageable experimental set-up. However, there is a risk that this tradition has obscured what the really important variables are.

Johansson (15) formulated a "law" which states that it might very well be the case that variables which are simple for the experimenter to describe are difficult to perceive, and variables that are simple for the perceiver are difficult to describe with the mathematical tools available to the experimenter. For example, the great discrepancy in the complexity of physically describing a simple sinusoidal tone and spoken language does not mirror a corresponding difficulty in perceiving them. Biological evolution has formed "smart" mechanisms (27) that are not necessarily congruent with simple mathematical models.

This means that the choice of form for the stimulation of the substituting perceptual system should not be based on the descrip-tion of it in physical terms. Stimulation that looks complex from this point of view might be simple to perceive, and mathema-tically simple stimulation may not be the best choice.

Amount of Information

It is sometimes suggested that the amount of information presented in a perceptual aid has to be small because of the restricted capacity of the substituting perceptual system. For example, the electronic travel aid that presents the most informa-tion of those developed so far, the Sonicguide, has sometimes been considered to give too much information. When making such a judgment it is important to contemplate not only the amount of information but also the naturalness of the form of the informa-tion (cf. above).

The perceptual systems are constucted to pick up large amounts of information. This is true not only of vision, but also of hearing and touch, the main potential substitutes for vision. If we manage to find natural forms of information, we can expect these perceptual systems to be able to handle large amounts of information when presented by perceptual aids. This means that there is no theoretical reason to restrict a travel aid to being a "clear-path indicator"; it might very well be possible to construct an "environmental sensor" (18). Even if the full richness of vision cannot be achieved, much more than what has been made available in present-day devices might very well be possible.

The importance of redundancy. Redundancy in information can compensate for lack of attention. A blind person, even with the best available travel aids, has to be more attentive than a sighted person; missing one version of some important piece of information may for a blind person mean that this information is totally lost, whereas a sighted person with the same unattentive-ness may still get the information in some other way. This may be a very important difference between visual and non-visual guid-ance of walking; as Leonard (22) put it: "it could be that sighted mobility is as good as it is because there would appear to be an awful lot of redundancy." The suggestion above, that it might be possible to present large amounts of information via a perceptual aid if it is in a suitable form, suggests the possibility of also presenting redundant information via a perceptual aid.

Is continuous guidance of locomotion necessary? The burden of presenting continuous information to the traveller may seem formidable. A series of experiments performed by Thomson (32) suggests that it may not be necessary. He found that subjects were able to perform some locomotor tasks very well without vision within a time limit of about eight seconds. Even if it is not yet clear how far this result can be generalized to other kinds of tasks, it is an interesting alternative to consider for the designer of perceptual aids for locomotion, that it might be possible to present information at particular intervals.

THE COMPLEXITY OF THE VISION SUBSTITUTION TASK

It is evident that the task of substituting vision in the guidance of locomotion is an enormously difficult one. Even if the task may be reduced by use of intervals in the information flow, the richness of vision, especially in the information for the guidance of action, makes the task very complex indeed. Some examples of recent relevant research will be given below to demonstrate this.

The Hypothesis of Two Visual Systems

The hypothesis of two visual systems (24) may have important implications also for substitution problems, especially as one of the visual systems it suggests, the ambient system, has special relevance for locomotion. This system, or this mode of processing spatially distributed information, involves mainly peripheral vision, and it functions at low levels of consciousness, even totally without consciousness. It is also interesting that this system does not demonstrate a systematic decrease in efficiency when luminance and optical quality taper off. The ambient mode works at maximum efficiency as long as anything can be seen at all.

A device presenting substituting auditory and/or tactual information picked up in such an automatic way would of course simplify the perceptual burden of the visually impaired person considerably. Typically, the devices developed so far require considerable conscious attention, even if training can be expected to decrease this necessity.

The Perceptual Analysis of Optic Flow

A main impression of the studies of the perceptual analysis of optic flow is how a tremendously complex task is elegantly performed by vision. From the optic flow the visual system extracts information about the static environment as well as about motions of objects in this environment and movements of the observer (13). Even if hearing and touch are highly developed senses, it does not seem probable that they can take over more than a minor fraction of these tasks for which nature has educated vision over millions of years.

For visual substitution, a main interest is to try to find out what the most important aspects of visual guidance are and to get ideas for a substituting device from an analysis of how vision solves those aspects. The information in the optical flow is not available in the substituting senses; at least nobody has been able to identify something that is as useful for the guidance of action.

Robot Vision Studies

In the present context artificial intelligence studies are especially interesting when they analyze the "perceptual" information necessary for the guidance of the movements of a robot. Even if a majority of the "seeing" robots made so far are stationary (3,26), there are also mobile robots which share some of their problems with locomoting human beings, such as updating their own location and avoiding obstacles (25).

The limitations of many robots in guiding themselves properly demonstrate, in an interesting way, how complex the functions are that are involved. One of the important but difficult tasks is to identify and locate the goal, a task which does not seem to have been addressed very much in robot vision studies. The Robot Rover, for example, has its goal defined internally in terms of location coordinates (25), not perceptually as is the case with humans and other animals.

There is one effort to utilize knowledge about robotics for the construction of a travel aid for the visually impaired, the guide dog robot (31). It is interesting to note that the problem of walking toward a perceptible goal is not solved in this aid. Instead, the perceptual guidance is based on following along a specially built guideline. Again, identifying the goal is a main unsolved problem.

From a theoretical point of view there are many challenging differences between most robot vision studies and much event-perception/locomotion research. For example, the starting point of a matrix of points of a static image proposed by Marr (24) is emphatically opposed by Johansson (14), who argues that the optic flow is a starting point much closer to real life.

THE DESIRABILITY OF INTERDISCIPLINARY COOPERATION

The primary mobility aids for the visually impaired, the long cane and the guide dog, were developed by dedicated people closely working with the rehabilitation of the people concerned (for the history of these efforts, see 2,36). The electronic travel aids (5, also Brabyn, this volume), so far only considered as secondary aids, have mainly been developed by people with engineering knowledge. From one point of view this is natural; technological knowledge is necessary in order to make an aid. However, engineering expertise is not sufficient to produce a useful aid, as the aid is only one part of the system formed by the user and the aid together. The aid must be adapted to the functioning of human perceptual-motor systems in order to be really helpful.

I think that, in principle, there is agreement about this among people working seriously on aids. However, in practice, I see a tendency sometimes to forget about the perceptual-motor aspects of the user-aid system with a concentration on the engineering problems. In particular, I think it is important that the perceptual-motor problems are considered very early in the process of designing an aid (10). Typically, non-engineering people are included in the discussions relatively late in the development of an aid, when there is at least a prototype available. This has the potential drawback of time and effort being devoted to not very successful alternatives that might have been avoided if perceptual-motor aspects had been considered at an early stage.   Interaction between engineering and perception-action experts might also, hopefully, lead to efforts that might not be tried without that interaction.   The complexity of the task of sensory substitution is a powerful reason for a close interdisciplinary cooperation.

ACKNOWLEDGEMENTS

My work on these problems was made possible by research grants from the Bank of Sweden Tercentenary Foundation (project no. 75/116, 79/149, 81/96), from the Swedish Council for the Humanities and the Social Sciences (project no. 926/78, 615/79, 453/80, 417/82) and from the Swedish Ministry of Health and Social Affairs, the Delegation for Social Research (project no. 82/117, 84/156).

REFERENCES

1. Barth, J. L. & Foulke, E. (1979). Preview: A neglected vari-
    able in orientation and mobility. Journal of Visual Impair-
    ment & Blindness, 73, 41-48.

2. Bledsoe, C. W. (1980). Originators of orientation and mobil-
    ity training. In R. L. Welsh & B. B. Blasch (Eds.), Founda-
    tions of Orientation and Moblity. New York: American Founda-
    tion for the Blind.

3. Casasent, D. P. & Hall, E. L. (Eds.) (1983). Intelligent
    robots: Third International Conference on Robot Vision and
    Sensory Control. Proceedings of SPIE - The International
    Society for Optical Engineering, 449.

4. Cratty, B. J. (1971). Movement and Spatial Awareness in
    Blind Children and Youth. Springfield, Ill.: Thomas.

5. Farmer, L. W. (1980). Mobility devices. In R. L. Welsh & B.
    B. Blasch (Eds.), Foundations of Orientation and Mobility.
    New York: American Foundation for the Blind.

6. Foulke, E. (in press). The role of memory in the mobility
    of blind pedestrians. In W. Hawkins (Ed.), Human Factors
    Application for Disabled People. Proceedings of 1981 Annual
    Symposium of Human Factors Society.

7. Gibson, J. J. (1979). The Ecological Approach to Visual Per-
    ception. Boston: Houghton Mifflin.

8. Jansson, G. (1984). Theoretical Reasons for Increasing the
    Range of the Next Generation of Electronic Travel Aids for
    the Visually Handicapped. Paper read at Symposium on Spa-
    tial Ability, University of Louisville.

9. Jansson, G. (1985). Perceptual theory and sensory substitu-
    tion. In D. Ingle, M. Jeannerod, & D. Lee (Eds.), Brain
    Mechanisms and Spatial Vision. The Hague: Nijhoff.

10. Jansson, G. (in press). Development and evaluation of mobil-
    ity aids for the visually handicapped. In P. L. Emiliani
    (Ed.), Communication Aids. Brussells: Commission of the
    European Communities.

11. Jansson, G. (in press). Perceptual information for orienta-
    tion and mobility. Proceedings of the XXIII International
    Congress of Psychology, Acapulco, Mexico, 1984.

12. Johansson, G. (1978). Visual event perception. In R. Held,
     H. W. Leibowitz, & H.-L. Teuber (Eds.), Handbook of Sensory
     Physiology: Vol. VIII. Perception (pp. 675-711). Berlin:
     Springer.

13. Johansson, G. (1982).Visual space perception through motion.
     In A. H. Wertheim, W. A. Wagenaar, & H. W. Leibowitz (Eds.),
     Tutorials on Motion Perception. New York and London: Plenum.

14. Johansson, G. (1984). Optic flow instead of retinal image.
     Unpublished manuscript.

15. Johansson, G. (in press). About visual event perception. In
     In W. H. Warren & R. E. Shaw (Eds.), Persistence and Change:
     Proceedings of the First International Conference on Event
     Perception. Hillsdale, NJ: Erlbaum.

16. Johansson, G., von Hofsten, C., & Jansson, G. (1980). Event
     perception. Annual Review of Psychology, 31, 27-63.

17. Kay, L. (1974). Towards Objective Mobility Evaluation: Some
     Thought About a Theory. New York: American Foundation for
     the Blind.

18. Kay, L. (1974). Orientation for blind persons: Clear path
     indicator or environmental sensor. New Outlook for the
     Blind, 68, 289-296.

19. Lee, D. N. (1976). A theory of visual control of braking
     based on information about time to collision. Perception,
     5, 437-459.

20. Lee, D. N. (1978). The functions of vision. In H. L. Pick,
     Jr. & E. Saltzman (Eds.), Modes of Perceiving and Process-
     ing Information. Hillsdale, NJ: Erlbaum.

21. Leibowitz, H. W. & Post, R. B. (1982). The two modes of pro-
     cessing concept and some implications. In J. Beck (Ed.),
     Organization and Representation in Perception. Hillsdale,
     NJ: Erlbaum.

22. Leonard, J. A. (1971). The Concept of the Minimal Informa-
     tion Required for Effective Mobility and Suggestions for
     Future Non-Visual Displays. Nottingham, England: University
     of Nottingham, Department of Psychology.

23. Marks, L. E. (1983). Similarities and differences among the
     senses. International Journal of Neuroscience, 19, 1-12.

24. Marr, D. (1982). Vision. San Francisco: Freeman.

25. Moravec, H. P. (1981). Robot Rover Visual Navigation. Ann Arbor, Michigan: UMI Research Press.

26. Rosenfeld, A. (Ed.). (1982). Robot vision. Proceedings of SPIE - The International Society for Optical Engineering, Vol. 336.

27. Runeson, S. (1977). On the possibility of "smart" perceptual mechanisms. Scandinavian Journal of Psychology, 18, 172-179.

28. Sherrick, C. E. (1975). The art of tactile communication. American Psychologist, 30, 353-360.

29. Strelow, E. R. (1985). What is needed for a theory of mobility: Direct perception and cognitive maps: Lessons from the blind. Psychological Review, 92, 226-248.

30. Strelow, E. R. & Brabyn, J. A. (1981). Use of foreground and background information in visually-guided locomotion. Perception, 10, 191-198.

31. Tachi, S., Tanie, K., Komoriya, K., Hosoda, Y., & Abe, M. (1978). Study of guide dog (seeing eye) robot (I). Bulletin of Mechanical Engineering Laboratory (Japan), No. 32.

32. Thomson, J. A. (1983). Is continuous visual monitoring necessary in visually guided locomotion? Journal of Experimental Psychology: Human Perception and Performance, 9, 427-443.

33. Turvey, M. T. & Remez, R. E. (1978). Visual control of locomotion in animals: an overview. In L. Harmon (Ed.), Proceedings of Conference on Interrelations of the Communicative Senses. Asilomar, California,

34. Wardell, K. T. (1980). Environmental modifications. In R. L. Welsh & B. B. Blasch (Eds.), Foundations of Orientation and Mobility. New York: American Foundation for the Blind.

35. Warren, D. H. & Strelow, E. R. (1984). Learning spatial dimensions with a visual sensory aid: Molyneux revisited. Perception, 13, 331-350.

36. Whitstock, R. H. (1980). Dog guides. In R. L. Welsh & B. B. Blasch (Eds.), Foundations of Orientation and Mobility. New York: American Foundation for the Blind.

AMODAL INFORMATION AND TRANSMODAL PERCEPTION

William Epstein

University of Wisconsin, Madison

In common with other forms of knowing, the act of perceiving involves processing of information. In this paper I have two objectives: First, I will offer a number of observations concerning the nature of information for perception with the emphasis on amodal information. In this portion of my presentation the influence of J. J. Gibson's (7,8,9) ideas will be obvious. Second, I will raise a number of questions suggested by these observations concerning the potential of vibrotactile stimulation to substitute for visual stimulation.

Transmodal Perception and Amodal Perception

Egocentric location can be given by vision, audition, and for nearby positions by touch and in some instances by olfaction. Surface texture can be given by vision and by touch and the same is true for a number of geometric properties although not necessarily with the same degree of accuracy in all sense modalities. I would like to refer to this class of percepts as transmodal. Transmodal percepts are functionally equivalent perceptual descriptions secured through application of different sense modalities. The descriptions are equivalent because they contain the same information about the source.

The facts of transmodal perception suggest an interesting hypothesis: that some of the information for perceptual systems is amodal. Used as a prefix, the first letter of the alphabet indicates without, as in amoral. In the case of amodal the prefix is used to indicate information that is not specific to a particular modality.

It may seem that the facts of transmodal perception establish the hypothesis of amodal information. Doesn't the fact that different modalities afford the same information about environmental states and events confirm the hypothesis that stimulation in the different modalities carries identical information? The answer is only a weak affirmative. The facts of transmodal perception show that functionally equivalent perceptual descriptions are provided by stimulation in different sense modalities, but these facts do not establish that the form of the information in stimulation is identical across different modalities. It is this latter claim that is theoretically significant: the claim that amodal information is a higher-order spatio-temporal pattern of stimulation which is not specific to a modality, but is invariant over different modalities.

To summarize, the following are conjoint attributes of amodal information.

(1) Information in stimulation is amodal if the information is carried by spatio-temporal patterns of stimulation which exhibit the same form of change across modalities.

(2) Information in stimulation is amodal if the information affords different perceptual systems with equivalent descriptions of environmental states or events.

Both of these attributes must be exhibited to qualify as amodal information. It follows that to assess the hypothesis of amodal information in the latter sense, first we must identify the relationships in stimulation which afford information for functionally equivalent perceptual descriptions in the various modalities; next we must determine whether these patterns are isomorphic.

The Distinction Between Stimulation and Information

The hypothesis of amodal information for perception is only plausible if one is willing to distinguish between stimulation and information. This distinction is central to Gibson's theoretical work. Stimulation is that portion of the energy capable of activating receptors. In the case of vision, stimulation is the portion of the radiant light which enters the eye to activate the photoreceptors. Stimulation is for receptors and as such, stimulation cannot sustain the perceptual representation of the world. Structured ambient light is visual information in the sense that temporal and spatial variations of structure stand in a one-to-one relationship with behaviorally significant properties of the environment. Presumably, the perceptual system of an organism has evolved neuronal structures that are selectively responsive to the variables of stimulation that carry information. The process of perceiving is the process of detecting or picking up the information in stimulation.

Commentary on Gibson's Concept of Information

Before proceeding I would like to comment on the implications of this notion of information for theorizing about perception.

1. Notice that information is carried by stimulation because higher-order spatio-temporal patterns stand in a one-to-one relationship of correspondence with significant attributes or events. The correspondence may be analogic or iconic as in the case of a photograph and the pictured scene, or it may be coded or synthetic. No theoretical importance attaches to this distinction; in fact, Gibson and the neorealists (e.g., 19) have argued that references to retinal pictures, images, and icons have tended to mislead investigators.

It is an empirical question whether correspondences involving analogic and coded representations are equally accessible to a perceptual system. In the case of vibrotacticle stimulation, one study which compared pictorial and coded vibrotactile patterns found the two forms of correspondence to be equally useful for letter discrimination. In this study, Craig (3) compared letter identification for cutaneously presented stimuli under two conditions, one in which the spatial relations among various parts of the optical patterns were preserved; the other in which the vibratory stimuli did not retain the spatial relations of the optical patterns. No large differences were found in sighted observers' abilities to identify letters, or in the rates of acquisition of letters, or in the confusion matrices for the 'pictorial' and the coded nonpictorial condition. Of course, while the coded vibratory patterns did not resemble their corresponding visual patterns, the coded patterns were instances of one-to-one correspondence between photocells and vibrators. Consequently, the coded vibrotactile stimulation carried information. Inasmuch as it was information which supported discrimination, it is not surprising that discrimination was exhibited when perturbed abstract vibratory patterns were used. Furthermore, Craig reported that observers could switch from a pictorial to a coded presentation with little decrement in performance. This finding reinforces the impression that analogic or iconic correspondence does not confer a special advantage. It is not pictures at the fingertips which are needed, only potential information.

2. Upon reflection, it is plain that Gibson's discovery of information in stimulation cannot stand in for a theory of perception. As noted earlier, Gibson insists that while stimulation is for receptors, information is for perceptual systems. But Gibson does not tell us how the information becomes available to the perceptual system. Information, in Gibson's thinking, is a relationship between the environment and structured stimulation. These relationships between descriptions of the environment and events at the receptor surface may be indisputable objective facts of the matter, accessible to the scientist, but we need to know how these relationships become facts for a perceptual system. For example, how do geometric constraints which inhere nomically, i.e. in virtue of certain natural laws, in optical stimulation become perceptual constraints? It will not do to impute knowledge of these constraints to the perceptual system. The neorealists (e.g., 18,19) have been very quick to charge constructivist theorists with this form of a priorism and they would not wish to stand similarly charged.

Although this point is clear once made, an example may be useful. The following rule seems to be a regulative principle, something inherent in the ordinary notion of information: If A carries the information that B, and B carries the information that C, then A carries the information that C. Fred Dretske, my colleague in philosophy at the University of Wisconsin, calls this rule the Xerox principle (5). The Xerox principle most certainly seems inherent in Gibson's conception of information. Applying the principle we may assert the following: If vibrotactile patterns carry the information that specific optical patterns have been generated, and if these optical patterns carry information that particular distal configurations are present, then vibrotactile patterns carry information about distal configurations. This assertion is indisputably correct; it is a statement of the objective state of affairs given Gibson's definition of information in stimulation. But the statement does not compel conclusions about vibrotactile perception; it is obvious that the assertion does not say anything about the capability or propensity of the perceptual system to use the information in vibrotactile stimulation to secure knowledge about distal sources.

3. Once we recognize that the task of a theory of perception is twofold: (a) to identify the information available to the perceptual system, and (b) to describe the processes for exploiting this information, another conclusion emerges. In the debate between constructivists and direct realists it has been customary (e.g., 6,10,14,15,18) to note that the constructivist theory draws inspiration from the premise that stimulation is inherently and intractably equivocal. It is true that con-

structivist theorists beginning with Bishop Berkeley commonly
have placed this claim at the head of their argument. Nevertheless, if the force of the preceding observation is granted, it
matters less whether one subscribes to the initial premise of
inherent equivocality or not. Nor is the constructivist edifice
undermined if stimulation is shown to be informative in the sense
intended by Gibson. Whichever position is adopted, the task of
providing a description of the processes that utilize the potential information afforded by events at the receptors will remain
as one of the two chief tasks for perceptual theory.

Is Perception of Three Dimensional Structure Transmodal?

I would like to return to consideration of transmodal perception and amodal information. The modalities I propose to
examine are the visual perceptual system and the vibrotactile
perceptual system. The latter obviously is a contrived system.
Vibrotactile stimulation is not often provided by normal commerce
with the environment and it seems unlikely that neuronal structures in the brain have evolved for selective processing of
variables of vibrotactile stimulation. Nevertheless, there are
reasons for examining the commonalities between visual perception
and vibrotactile perception. One reason is that the deployment
of prosthetic devices such as the Optacon and the devices in-
vented by Paul Bach-y-Rita and his colleagues (1; Bach-y-Rita &
Hughes, this volume; Collins, this volume) show that vibrotactile
stimulation can substitute for vision in certain tasks. These
successes and their implications for enriching the perceptual
world of the blind person provide one motivation for comparing
visual and vibrotactile perception. Another reason is that an a
priori case can be made that patterns of vibrotactile stimulation
are formally similar to the patterns of optical stimulation which
carry information for visual perception.

The testing ground which I have elected to stake out is the
recovery of three-dimensional structure from motion. Since the
early 1950s, J. J. Gibson and Gunnar Johansson (11,12,13) have
insisted that dynamic changing patterns of optical stimulation
which accompany movement in the environment or movement of the
observer are uniquely informative concerning spatial layout and
three dimensional configurations. Prompted by the theoretical
and empirical precedents in the work of Gibson and Johansson,
investigators have set out to provide quantitative descriptions
of the information carried by dynamic patterns of changing stimulation and to examine the visual system's exploitation of this
information to arrive at useful descriptions of three dimensional
structure and spatial layout. Fine exemplars of this work have
been supplied by Braunstein (2), Lappin (4), Todd (17), and
Ullman (20). It now seems indisputable that Gibson's and

Johansson's insistence on the importance of structured patterns of optical change was not misplaced.

Granting that the visual system recovers structure from motion, what of vibrotactile perception? Can the vibrotactile perceptual system exploit patterns of change in vibrotactile stimulation to arrive at perceptual descriptions of three-dimensional structure? Is the perception of three-dimensional structure transmodal, and if the answer is affirmative, will it prove to be the case that the information which supports these descriptions is amodal? (See also Bach-y-Rita & Hughes, this volume.)

In order to avoid entanglement in a new variant of Molyneux's question, I will stipulate that the subjects are sighted persons. In addition, assume that these persons have completed a period of familiarization with the Optacon Camera system with the result that they are able to discriminate vibrotactile patterns and that distal attribution becomes routine. By distal attribution, I mean that vibrotactile stimulation is attributed to an environmental source other than the array of vibrotactile stimulators, more specifically to the presence of an object in the 'visual field'. In the absence of familiarization it seems implausible that a subject would make an attribution to a source more remote than the vibrating array. Quasi-epistemological concerns have a way of intruding: one wonders what sort of experience, if any, disallowing explicit tuition concerning the facts of the matter, could induce an originally naive subject to make a distal attribution? I look at this question as concerning the nature of the evidence which would activate the hypothesis of distal attribution and favor this hypothesis over other competing accounts for the experienced vibrotactile events. In an experiment currently in progress we have created a variety of conditions which present vibrotactile stimulation contingent on optical registration of movement of an object into the camera's field, and other contrasting conditions which present vibrotactile stimulation uncorrelated with optical registration of the distal object. The set of conditions comprise a set of operations which, in principle, should converge on the hypothesis of distal attribution.

Returning to the proposed study of recovery of structure through motion, having prepared the subjects, we are ready to put the question: If the vibrotactile correlate of a spatiotemporal optical pattern that normally elicits perceptual descriptions of three-dimensional structure is presented, what will the subject report? Suppose we program the following pattern for the Optacon's vibrotactile display: a single linear arrangement of vibratory elements is caused to undergo two concurrent changes, oscillation about its center accompanied by systematically correlated changes of length. The rates of change and the correlation between the changes are chosen so as to mimic the optical trans- formations associated with a rod of constant length oscillating in a depth plane. Indeed, when this optical pattern is displayed on a monitor in the absence of strong conflicting cues it does appear to be of fixed length and turning in depth (16,21). The effect can be compelling even in the less than ideal punctiform visual display of the Optacon.

How will the subject respond to this pattern of vibrotactile stimulation? I would like to focus the experimental question more sharply. Suppose two other types of vibrotactile displays are included in the experiment: (a) <u>Changing angle display</u> - the sequence of angular changes exhibited in the first display is reproduced but no changes of length are introduced; (b) <u>Changing length display</u> - the line retains a constant orientation but it undergoes a cyclic pattern of length change, continuous shrinking from one end to a fraction of its original length then growing to restore the original length. The displays are illustrated in Figure 1.

It is reasonable to suppose that the descriptions of the latter two vibrotactile displays will attribute the first vibro- tactile pattern to a rod oscillating in a plane perpendicular to the vibrotactile display and the second vibrotactile pattern to a rod behaving like Alice in the Looking Glass World. How will the first display be described? One possibility is a description which simply combines both descriptions elicited by the single- change displays, that is, a rod which oscillates in the plane per- pendicular to the vibrotactile and changing length at the same time. Another possibility is that the higher-order invariant inherent in the concurrent changes of length and angle will elicit a very different description. The subject may attribute the vibrotactile pattern to the presence in the field of the camera of a rod of constant length oscillating in depth. Plainly, it is the latter description which would excite interest. This descrip- tion would be a prime candidate for membership in the class of transmodal percepts. Of greater significance is the fact that the information supporting this description might fairly be considered to be amodal.

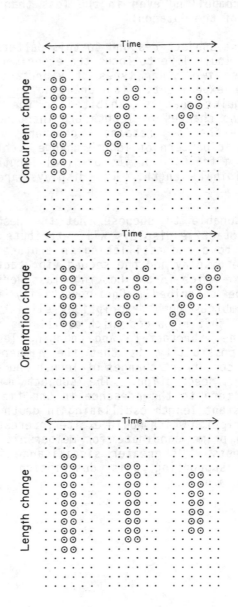

Figure 1. The upper panel depicts a segment of the transformation in the concurrent change display involving the optacon vibrotactile surface. The middle panel depicts a segment of the transformation in the orientation change display. Note that the orientation changes over time are not accompanied by changes of length. The lower panel depicts a segment of the transformation in the length change display. In this case length change is not accompanied by changing orientation.

REFERENCES

1. Bach-y-Rita, P. (1972). _Brain Mechanisms in Sensory Substi-
    tution_. New York: Academic Press.

2. Braunstein, M. (1976). _Depth Perception Through Motion_.
    New York: Academic Press.

3. Craig, J. C. (1974). Pictorial and abstract cutaneous dis-
    plays. In F. H. Geldard (Ed.), _Conference on Vibrotactile
    Communication_. Houston, TX: Psychonomic Society, 78-83.

4. Doner, J., Lappin, J., & Perfetto, G. (1984). Detection of
    three-dimensional structure in moving optical patterns.
    _Journal of Experimental Psychology: Human Perception and
    Performance_, 10, 1-11.

5. Dretske, F. (1981). _Knowledge and the Flow of Information_.
    Cambridge; MA: MIT Press.

6. Epstein, W. (1977). Historical introduction to the constan-
    cies. In W. Epstein (Ed.), _Stability and Constancy in Visual
    Perception: Mechanisms and Processes_. New York: Wiley.

7. Gibson, J. J. (1950). _The Perception of the Visual World_.
    Boston: Houghton Mifflin.

8. Gibson, J. J. (1966). _The Senses Considered as Perceptual
    Systems_. Boston: Houghton Mifflin.

9. Gibson, J. J. (1979). _The Ecological Approach to Visual
    Perception_. Boston: Houghton Mifflin.

10. Hochberg, J. E. (1978). _Perception_ (2nd ed.). Englewood
    Cliffs, NJ: Prentice-Hall.

11. Johansson, G. (1950). _Configurations in Event Perception_.
    Uppsala: Almquist and Wiksell.

12. Johansson, G. (1977). Spatial constancy and motion in
    visual perception. In W. Epstein (Ed.), _Stability and Con-
    stancy in Visual Perception: Mechanisms and Processes_. New
    York: Wiley.

13. Johansson, G., von Hofsten, C., & Jansson, G. (1980).
    Event perception. _Annual Review of Psychology_, 31, 27-63.

14. Michaels, C. F. & Carello, C. (1981). _Direct Perception_.
    Englewood Cliffs, NJ: Prentice-Hall.

15. Rock, I.   (1984).   The Logic of Perception.   Cambridge,   MA:
    MIT Press.

16. Rock, I. & Smith. D.   (1981). Alternative solutions to kine-
    tic stimulus   information.   Journal of Experimental Psycho-
    logy: Human Perception and Performance, 7, 19-29.

17. Todd, J. (1982). Visual information about rigid and nonrigid
    motion: A geometric analysis. Journal of Experimental Psy-
    chology: Human Perception and Performance, 8, 238-252.

18. Turvey, M. T. (1974). Constructive theory, perceptual sys-
    tems and tacit knowledge. In W. B. Weimer and D. S. Palermo
    (Eds.), Cognition and Symbolic Processes.   Hillsdale, NJ:
    Lawrence Erlbaum Associates.

19. Turvey, M. T. (1977). Contrasting orientations to the theory
    of visual information processing. Psychological Review, 84,
    67-88.

20. Ullman, S.   (1979).   The   Interpretation   of Visual   Motion.
    Cambridge, MA: MIT Press.

21. Wallach, H. & O'Connell, D. N.   (1953).   The kinetic depth
    effect. Journal of Experimental Psychology, 45, 205-217.

UNDERSTANDING PERCEIVED SPATIAL LAYOUT OF SCENES:
A PREREQUISITE FOR PROSTHESES FOR BLIND TRAVELERS

Ralph Norman Haber

University of Illinois--Chicago

When normally sighted people observe a natural scene, their perceptions include seeing the supporting ground surface and the arrangements of the objects on that surface, where each object is in relation to the others, to the ground surface, and to themselves. Seeing this arrangement is what is meant by the visually perceived layout of a scene. It is the major source of information to the visual system that provides control of locomotion through natural settings. Blind travelers have no comparable visually perceived layout, and must acquire information about the arrangements of the objects and the ground plane of the scene from vastly degraded visual sources, and more typically from non-visual sources, and from special devices designed to provide layout information. In the development of these prosthetic devices for blind travelers, designers have had to make ad hoc decisions both about how information of the physical layout of scenes is to be represented to the blind traveler and what information to represent, ad hoc because the designers do not know which sources of information are necessary, how that information is normally represented for sighted travelers, or whether blind travelers optimally use the same information.

There are many questions that need to be asked. For example, how many dimensions are necessary to represent the information about a scene for a sighted traveler? What are the relative saliences of those dimensions? What accuracy is necessary for each dimension? Are nearby objects represented in a perceived layout more accurately than more distant objects? Do certain arrangements or properties in the physical scene lead to systematic distortions of perceived layout? And so forth.

The analysis of perceived layout is not included in current theories of space perception (in contrast to perceived radial distance from observer to object), so there is little research currently directed at the study of perceived layout. Further, while theories of spatial cognition have analyzed spatial representations based on memory for previously viewed scenes, and so can tell us something about the dimensionality of remembered or constructed scenes, such analyses rarely contrast those representations to ones made while the scene is actually on view. This means that we cannot determine how much the distortions that are found in spatial cognition research are due to memory, and how much to initial perception. Consequently, neither theories of perception and cognition, nor research in perception and cognition, have provided any knowledge of the properties of perceived layout of scenes, the way a scene looks to an observer. (See also 18).

The purpose of this paper is to provide an analysis of visually perceived spatial layout, and to contrast visually perceived layout with other kinds of spatial representations about the scenes we look at and move through. From this theoretical base, the relationship between the visually perceived layout available to the sighted person and possible layouts available to blind travelers is discussed. My aim is to show that we must understand the nature of visually perceived layout in the normally sighted before we can hope to design fully successful prosthetic devices for the blind traveler. Following these more theoretical sections, I show how visually perceived layout can be measured and assessed, and then report empirical data pertaining to the dimensionality and accuracy with which normally sighted observers can perceive to the layout of scenes. Finally, from the data, I will return to the problems faced by blind travelers.

What are the Properties of Visually Perceived Spatial Layout?

Visually perceived layout concerns the perception of the locations of the objects in a scene. This includes seeing the ground surface supporting the objects, the location of each object on that ground surface, the relations of the objects to one another, the relationships of the objects to the boundaries of the scene, and the relationships of the objects to the observer who is doing the perceiving. For normally sighted persons, visual stimulation provides virtually all of the information about the locations of objects in a scene, so that perceived layout is typically synonymous with visually perceived layout. Audition may make a negligible contribution if there are important sound emitting objects in the scene, but rarely does any information come from smell, taste, or even touch.

Visually perceived layout requires a three-dimensional representation to convey the layout information in a natural scene, with a fourth dimension of time needed when some of the objects in the scene move. Consequently, perceived layout is much more than simply perceiving how far away each object is located from the observer. This perceived "radial" distance, as it is typically assessed in current research, can be displayed in one dimension, since the direction of the object from the observer is usually not important or manipulated. If all we knew about a scene was derived from such a one-dimensional representation, it could be of little use as a guide to locomotion, since it does not include differences in the direction of the various objects from us, and it does not include information about distances between objects, or potential pathways and routes. Further, a one-dimensional representation certainly does not represent the richness that most normally sighted perceivers feel they achieve when looking at natural scenes.

Unfortunately, current perceptual theories of space perception have focused almost exclusively on the determinants of radial distance perception--the apparent distance of an object from the observer. Rarely does this research ask questions concerning the relationship of one object to another. While it is sometimes useful to perceive the distance of an object at a particular moment in time, usually we need to know the patterning of the locations among all the objects in the scene.

There have been no experiments that ask observers, while looking at a scene in front of their eyes, to report on what they perceive about the arrangements of the objects in the scene, the relation of the objects to the supporting ground plane, the nature of the ground plane itself, or any other aspect of perceived layout. The reasons for this absence are complex, and not relevant to this discussion (see Haber [7] for a detailed discussion). The end result is a lack of theoretical description of perceived layout, and a lack of data about the properties and the determinants of perceived layout. I will provide some data in a later section of this paper.

Visually Perceived Spatial Layout Contrasted to Spatial Cognition and Remembered Layout

While perceptual theories have virtually ignored the study of visually perceived layout, more general cognitive theory has begun to include knowledge of spatial arrangements under the rubric of cognitive maps, or spatial cognition. A number of recent volumes (e.g., 5,9,14,15,16) attest to the interest shown in how we represent the spatial arrangements of the objects in scenes we have encountered. Almost without exception, however,

this research on cognitive maps is concerned with the representations of scenes that have been <u>previously</u> perceived, or imagined
by the subject, or have been described to him. It has not been
concerned with the concurrent perception of scenes. The operational definition for perception is the physical presence of the
scene visible to the eyes, audible to the ears, and so forth. To
describe the events internal to the observer as visual perception,
there must be a scene on view before the eyes. Using this distinction, almost all of the research on cognitive maps has been
post-perceptual research, since invariably, subjects are asked to
make responses concerning the layout of scenes that are not presently on view.

There are a number of different kinds of representations of
spatial layout, remembered layout, constructed layout, and imagined layout.

For a blind person, auditory stimulation can provide some
information about the layout of objects in a scene, an auditorily
perceived layout, but only under restricted conditions. Unlike
vision, which provides continuous stimulation to the visual
system (as long as illumination remains present and the eyes are
open), audition is useful only to locate sound-emitting objects
while they are noisy, or for echo location of objects with appropriate observer-generated or environmental noises. In either
case, the objects "disappear" when quietness prevails. The
comparable circumstance in vision occurs when the illumination of
the scene occurs only intermittently, interspersed between periods
of darkness, so that the objects in the scene also "disappear."
In addition to continuity, visual stimulation also provides far
more precise information about layout, compared to what we can
learn through audition. Sound localization is only marginally
accurate for the judgment of the distance of objects, especially
unfamiliar ones, in contrast to visually perceived distance estimates. Human echo location is also not very accurate, and only
so over short ranges of distances, and only for relatively large
and dense objects (20). Finally, an auditory perceived layout
can specify nothing about the ground surface on which the objects
in the scene rest. Not only are irregularities on the ground
surface absent in auditory stimulation, but even the overall slope
and extent of the scene is not signalled. For all these reasons,
the content of an auditory perceived layout is vastly impoverished, compared to one derived from vision.

Memory layout is a much more general concept, and comes
closest to what is studied in most of the cognitive map research.
In the narrowest sense, if after becoming familiar with a scene
through visual inspection, an observer is asked about the arrangements of the objects in the scene, those questions pertain to a

representation of the layout of the scene contained in memory. The memory could have been based on a variety of inputs and combinations of inputs. Much of the research on cognitive maps has used scenes which are never completely on view at any one time. For example, I may have a reasonable cognitive map of the town in which I live, even though there is no place where I can stand and see all of the town in a single glance, or even a succession of glances without walking considerable distances. Clearly, by my definition, such a map is based on memory. There has never been a single percept of the scene itself.

There is yet another sense in which a remembered spatial layout may not have a perceived spatial layout as an antecedent. When normally sighted observers are given verbal or conceptual information about a scene they have never seen, such as being told directions of a route to follow, then they presumably develop some kind of cognitive map of the scene (or at least the route), in the absence of ever having seen it. By definition, there has been no perceived layout, since there had been no physical layout providing stimulation to the eyes, but there certainly is some variety of conceptual layout, which may or may not have similar properties to the other types of layout already described.

While there are many theoretical differences between perceiving and remembering, this operational definition of the conditions under which observation occurs is critical in the study of spatial layout. The research on spatial cognition has already identified a number of variables that affect cognitive maps: familiarity of the scene; the frequency and conditions of original observation; the interplay between visual information, other sensory information and nonsensory knowledge about the scene; the relevance of the scene to the subject; the cognitive developmental level of the observer; and the conditions of testing and the response measures used. Generally, the cognitive maps produced by the subject, or constructed from the subject's responses, are evaluated against a physical description such as a geographer's map of the original scene, with the similarity between the two being interpreted as a measure of the accuracy of a cognitive map. The failure to distinguish between perception and memory means that this research is incapable of determining which kinds of inaccuracies result from perceptual processes that occur during the viewing of the scene, and which inaccuracies in the cognitive maps result from memorial processes.

For example, Kosslyn, Pick and Fariello (10) distributed 10 objects in a 17 foot square scene, bisected by an opaque barrier perpendicular to the line of sight and a transparent barrier parallel to the line of sight. Objects separated by the opaque barrier were remembered as farther apart than they really were, and this was true for the transparent barrier for children as well. However, since the experiment did not have a perception condition, this distortion in layout might be only an effect of memory, and had the subjects been assessed while looking at the scene, the presence of the fences would have made no difference. Without the perception condition, we cannot determine whether the distortions are present in perceived as well as remembered layout, or only in remembered layout.

As another example, Bradley and Vido (4) did contrast perception with memory, but unfortunately only for measures of radial distance. They asked subjects to make magnitude estimates of the radial distance of 15 objects from themselves as they stood on a hilltop. The objects ranged from 20 feet to 14 miles in the distance. The estimates were made either while looking at the objects or from memory of the scene. The authors found that both sets of distance judgments underestimated the far distances, in relation to the nearer ones, but this effect was much more pronounced for the estimates made from memory. This suggests that memory for radial distances undergoes a distortion during the memory process, in which far objects are brought in closer than they really are. This distortion is similar to one that also occurs during perception of radial distance itself, and is added onto the perceptual distortion.

Consequently, it is at least theoretically possible that the perceived layout of space is highly accurate, and that all discrepancies between the physical layout and subjects' cognitive maps are due to changes that occur during retention or retrieval. In contrast, it is also possible that even while the scene is on view, an observer's perceived layout is distorted in just the ways the spatial cognition research suggests. Without the measurement of perceived layout, while the scene is on view, we can never learn where between the two extremes the answer lies.

Layouts of Space Available to Blind Travelers

These distinctions between the different kinds of spatial layouts become particularly important when we contrast sighted and blind travelers. For an unaided blind traveler with no useful vision, any information about the locations of objects in a scene must come either from natural audition (from the return of self-generated sounds and from sound-emitting objects), and from expectations and prior experiences with the same or similar scenes. Foulke (this volume) has discussed the development of memory for routes, and has suggested that such memory structures are similar to those that would be developed by a sighted person. However, while his assumption is plausible, and consistent with the analysis presented here, it is not very helpful, since we do

not know very much about how sighted people structure and represent routes in memory. Strelow (18) reviews what literature
there is on the structure of layout information. His conclusion
also is that we know next to nothing about the structure and
properties of such non-visually perceived and remembered layouts.
It seems most likely that the blind operate more on cognitive
layout, constructed from their cumulative experiences, rather than
on perceptual layout based on their modest sensory capacities.

To explore this question, the category of blind traveler must
be defined more precisely, in terms of severity of blindness, age
of onset, and type of travel. A person can be classified as blind
with no useful vision at all, or with some intensity discrimination, and even with some detail acuity. Legal definitions restrict acuity to less than 20/200 (being able to recognize a
pattern at 20 feet or less when the normally sighted can recognize
the same pattern at 200 feet). A level of 20/200 acuity is not
adequate to read normal sized print, though some reading is
possible for enlarged print or with the use of magnifiers. This
degree of visual functioning permits some gross object recognition, and certainly permits discriminating the presence of large
contrasting objects in the line of sight. Obviously, this range
of the severity of blindness means that not all blind travelers
are equally impaired.

Age of onset is another variable of importance. The vast
majority of blinding occurs after childhood, with much of it in
middle age and beyond. The number of infants born blind is a
very small percentage of the population of blind persons. Many
persons being considered for prosthethic devices have only been
recently blinded, although some have been blind for ten or twenty
years.

Finally, when considering the question of mobility, a variety of tasks needs to be considered, ranging from full independent
travel in pedestrian environments to limited travel over highly
familiar routes. We must have a careful analysis of these
environments, and the tasks required to travel in them, in order
to understand the kinds of layout structures that are needed, and
the kinds of devices that might offer assistance.

Given the obvious superiority of vision, compared to our
other senses, for the pickup of information about spatial arrangements in scenes, it seems likely that normally sighted people
develop representations of spatial relationships in scenes that
are closely based on the information that comes from vision.
Said another way, visually perceived layouts are the norm. This
reliance on vision for our representations of the world around us
could be developed in each child during the course of its normal

interactions with the world over the first year or two of life. It is likely, however, given the long course of evolution in which the visual sense has been so dominant for spatial perception, that specialized neural structures have evolved precisely for the purpose of representing visually perceived spatial arrangements. If this is the case, then the role of development for each infant is not for the learning of such structures, but only to acquire sufficient visual experience to permit the fine tuning of prewired systems.

Following the same line of reasoning, it is likely that representations of spatial relations in the world around us that go beyond the visual information available are based on the same structural characteristics as the visually perceived layouts. If the first representation of scenes available to an infant is a visual one, with specific properties of dimensionality, scaling, viewpoint, orientation, perspective, and intrinsicality, then these same structural properties are likely to underlie the other kinds of cognitive representations developed in the natural course of interaction with scenes. It is for this reason that the criticism of the research on cognitive maps is important: we must know about the visual perceived layout as well as remembered layout in order to evaluate the properties and distortions in the latter.

To the extent that these assumptions about the anchoring of perceived layout in vision are correct, then blind people have structures for the representation of scenes with similar properties to those possessed by normally sighted people. Even infants born blind may begin with the same structures, though without visual experience those structures may degenerate over time and be replaced by others. This means that to understand how blind people represent space, we must begin with what is known about the kinds of representations available to sighted people as a baseline. Further, it may mean that the alternative layouts required by blind people, because of the absence of adequate visual information, will follow the same structures found in visually perceived layouts, possibly even for blind persons who never have had visually perceived layouts in the first place.

Just as important, the design of a sensory substitution device to provide information about layout must incorporate knowledge about the way in which layout information is represented. Given the myriad of ways in which the properties of spatial relations can be represented, and given the likelihood that most blind persons who can potentially use such aids already have neural structures designed for such representations, it would be unwise to map the spatial characteristics of the scene onto the stimulus dimensions of a device simply because it is technologically feasible or convenient (see also 17). The study of visually

perceived layout in the normally sighted should help the design
of the display for visual substitution devices. This study should
also help the development of training programs for the use of such
devices, and for the development of better spatial awareness in
the blind.

THE ASSESSMENT AND MEASUREMENT OF THE PERCEIVED LAYOUT OF SPACE

Physical and Perceived Layout

     Before we can analyze perceived layout, it is necessary to
define physical layout. The easiest way to describe the physical
location of objects in a natural scene is to posit a three-dimensional Euclidean coordinate system, with an arbitrary origin
placed either in the middle of the scene, or off along one edge.
The basic supporting ground surface is then defined as a plane,
on which are attached the objects of the scene, each intersecting
the ground surface at defined XYZ coordinates. Euclidean coordinates can completely specify a scene even if the ground is uneven
and unlevel, and even if the objects have some mass so that their
intersections with the ground cover some substantial area. Further, scenes can have free-floating objects, such as a swing
hanging from a branch. A Euclidean three-dimensional space can
locate all of these, fixing each part of each surface of each object. Figure 1 is an example, with a few coordinate locations
indicated. Objects can also be located while in motion, by
integrating the three dimensions over time, creating a fourth
dimension. I call this geometrical description the physical
layout of a scene.

     The above description is sufficient to provide a physical
definition of a scene in terms of the locations of its ground and
all of its objects. When observers look at a scene, part of
their perception includes seeing the locations of the objects in
relation to each other, to the ground, and to themselves. But
while we can use the same geometrical measuring sticks to describe
perceived layout, we cannot assume the same measurement scales,
or even that there is a necessary relationship between appearance
and physical reality. Consequently, we must contrast the above
physical description of the layout of the scene with a perceptual
description of what observers see while looking. The latter is
what I call the perceived layout of a scene. My concern is with
the specification of perceived layout, its measurement, and its
psychophysical relationships to physical layout.

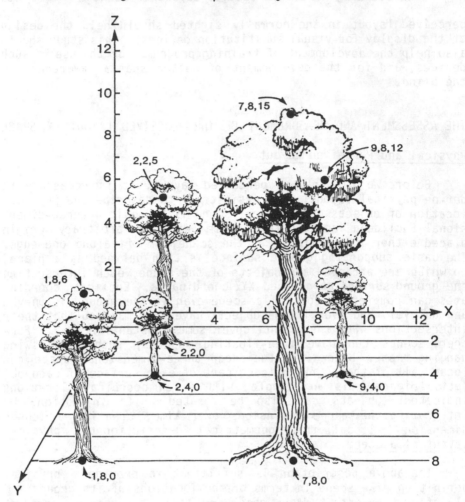

Figure 1.   A Euclidean three dimensional coordinate specification of a scene.   Several XYZ coordinate locations are indicated.

Strategy for Measuring Perceived Layout From Responses
About a Scene

I will describe in detail the results of an experiment by
Toye (21,22), working in my laboratory (see [7] for more background). This is the first experiment I know of that has provided a direct assessment of perceived layout.

The most direct way that has been used to assess the location
of objects as perceivers see them in a scene is to have them draw

a map. This procedure has been used extensively in the spatial cognition research concerned with memory for scenes. We also wanted data based on a very different response indicator, and chose one in which we asked subjects to estimate the distances between every pair of objects in the scene. We asked them to do this in two different ways: first as an absolute distance in feet, and second, as a relative judgment between subsets of distances. While these interobject distance estimates are not themselves a layout of space, when we submit the matrix of all the estimates to a multidimensional scaling program, that program constructs an n-dimensional arrangement of the objects that satisfies all of the interobject distance estimates made by the observer. This n-dimensional construction can then be evaluated as a measure of an observer's perceived layout of the scene, through a psychophysical comparison between the constructed layout and the geometrical description of the actual scene. Thus, while the construction might seem like an indirect measure, by comparing it to the geometric structure of the real scene, we can examine the psychological reality of these constructions.

Since we have constructions based on three different kinds of input data (absolute distance estimates, relative distance judgments, and distances between points drawn on a map), we can also examine the resulting perceived layouts in terms of the properties of the input data themselves, such as their stability, consistency, scaling characteristics, and the like.

Four different kinds of tests are used for this evaluation process. First, do the interobject distance estimates produced by the observers bear a lawful relationship to the actual distances in the scene? Second, are the distance estimates internally consistent with themselves, so that the regression equation can locate each object without stressing any of the interobject distance estimates? Consistency does not imply anything about accuracy: to be consistent, an observer has to provide distance estimates that are derived from some possible n-dimensional space. It does not necessarily have to be observed. Third, does the n-dimensional space constructed from the multiple regresson analysis resemble the real scene in predictable ways, in terms of its dimensionality, scale size, and accuracy and shape? And fourth, how sensitive is the perceived layout of space constructed by the scaling program to changes in the viewing position of the observer? Physical layout of space is, by definition, independent of the position of any potential observer, but we do not know anything about whether perceived layout differs depending on the position of the observer.

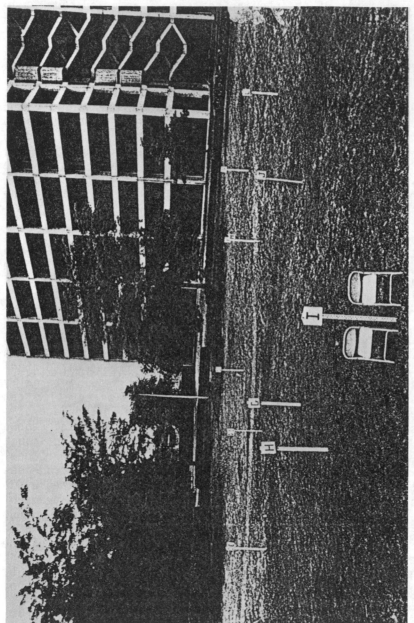

Figure 2. Photograph of the stake scene used by Toye (21), showing the location of the 13 stakes, the ground, and the boundary areas beyond the scene. The camera is elevated and behind the scene more than were the subjects, whose positions can be seen by the sets of chairs on two sides of the scene.

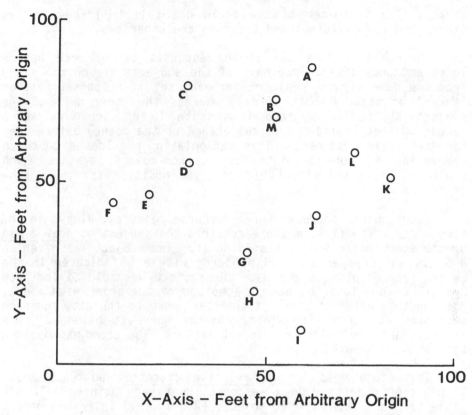

Figure 3. A plan view map drawn of the stake scene, as viewed from above. The X and Y axes are in feet. The subjects sat either next to stake F or stake I while making their responses.

Experimental Procedures to Measure Perceived Layout

To demonstrate the appropriate evidence on each of these four evaluations just described, Toye (21) tested eight subjects on a visually rich scene (see Figure 2 for a photographic view of the scene taken from one of the viewing positions used, though slightly elevated to show the scene better, and Figure 3 for a two-dimensional template of the scene). It was an open grassy field 250 feet on a side, in which Toye planted 13 identically sized metal stakes, in an area spanning a diameter of about 70 feet in the center of the field. Each stake was about an inch in diameter, and three feet tall. It was capped with a flag with an easily-read large letter drawn on it. He had his observers sit next to one of the outermost stakes (either stake I or F), and except for having to remain seated, the subject was free to make eye, head, and body movements while looking at the scene of stakes. The perimeter of the field had tall buildings on two sides, and low buildings and trees on the other two.

The subjects made all their responses twice, once before lunch and once after. One half of the subjects viewed the scene from the same viewing position for each set of responses (either stake I or stake F both times), whereas the other half of the subjects shifted 90 degrees from stake I to F or vice versa (about 50 feet around the circumference of the scene) before they repeated their responses. This manipulation provides a check on the reliability of judgments for the non-movers, against which can be assessed the effects of observer position for those subjects who moved.

Each subject produced three response measures, always in the same order. The first measure required the subject to draw a map of the scene while freely observing it. The subject was given an 8 by 10 white paper on a clip board, with a G indicated in the center (representing stake G). The subject was told to indicate his or her own location near the bottom of the paper with a dot, putting the letter of the adjacent stake next to the dot, and then to place each of the remaining objects where it belonged, each indicated as a dot with an adjacent letter. The drawn map measure took about 5 minutes.

The second measure was relative distance judgments among triplets of objects. On a response sheet were printed all possible triplets among the 13 objects (286 in all) in random order. For each triplet (e.g., BDH), the subject had to indicate which of the three interobject distances (i.e., BD, BH or DH) was the largest. This test took about 45 minutes with 13 objects.

The third measure asked the subject to estimate the absolute distance between all 78 pairings of the 13 objects. These 78 interobject distances were printed as letter pairs in random order on a response form. While looking at the scene, the subject wrote down an estimate of the distance in feet between the two stakes with those letters. No anchor values were provided, either as to the absolute size of the stakes, or to any of the distances in the scene. The absolute distance estimates took about 20 minutes to complete with 13 objects.

The three response measures provided three different kinds of inputs to the multidimensional scaling analysis. All three measures produced quite similar constructions, each of which met the evaluation criteria similarly. This increases our confidence that we were tapping the same underlying perceived layout of space with these responses.

The drawn map is already a two-dimensional construction of the scene of stakes. However, since each subject was free to fill up as much of the paper as he wished, the sizes of the drawn maps differed from one another. To facilitate comparison of the maps with the scaled solutions based on the distance estimates in which the axes of the scaled solutions were in standard deviation units (based on the standard deviation of the actual 78 inter-object distances), we also submitted the maps to the scaling routine. To do this, we measured each of the 78 interobject distances between the 13 dots drawn on a map to the nearest millimeter, and used this matrix of 78 scores as an input to the multidimensional scaling analysis. To scale the absolute distance judgments, we used the matrix of the 78 interobject distance esti-mates in feet as the input to the scaling program. With the relative distance judgments, we started by counting the number of times a subject selected each of the 78 interobject distances as the largest. This matrix of 78 frequencies was then used as an input to the scaling routine. Each of these inputs yields outputs of 13 points in an n-dimensional space. We also applied Procrus-tean rotations to the points to examine their relationships to the actual distribution of the points of the physical scene.

All multidimensional scaling analyses were carried out on the data from each subject separately.

Results of Empirical Measurements of Perceived Layout

The four evaluations of the subjects' responses, and the multidimensional scaled solutions based on them, are described below.

The lawfulness of distance estimation responses. Tradition-al analyses of the accuracy of distance judgments plot judged distance against true distance and examine the slope, intercept, and linearity of the resulting (Stevens) function. In this experiment, there are 78 distances to be estimated, one for each distance between each pair of objects in the scene. Each of the eight subjects provided six sets of the 78 estimates (48 sets in all), two each for the absolute distance, relative distance, and measured map distance. Figure 4 presents one of these sets, based on the absolute distance estimates of the first set of responses before lunch. For all of them, the functions are close to straight lines (the exponents average about 1.00), the slopes of the lines also average about 1.00, and the intercepts are about zero when the functions were extended through the origin. Similar data are found with the drawn maps. The zero intercept is consistent with a ratio scaling of the esimates, the unity exponent with an equal interval scaling of the estimates, and the unity slope implies that the subjects have an accurate sense of the absolute magni-

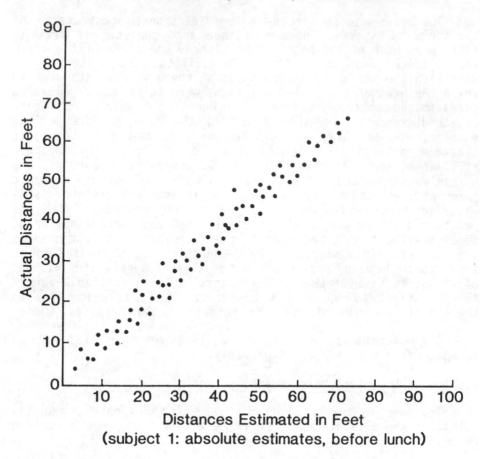

Distances Estimated in Feet
(subject 1: absolute estimates, before lunch)

Figure 4. A plot of the estimated absolute distance estimates
as a function of the actual distances in feet for each of the
78 interobject distances for Subject #1, based on his first set
of observations (before lunch). The plots of the other 7 subjects are very similar.

tudes of distances in feet. The properties of the relative
distance judgments are nearly as good as those of the absolute
and map indices, but are more consistent with ordinal scaling
properties, as of course they should be.

The consistency of the estimated interobject distances. When
a matrix of numbers, such as the interobject distance estimates
generated by our subjects, is subjected to multidimensional
scaling, the regression process attempts to find a location for
each object in an n-dimensional Euclidean space in such a way

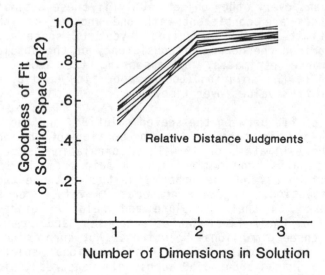

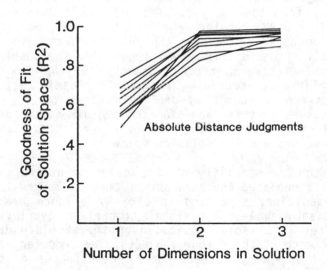

Figure 5. Plots of the amount of stress (R^2) in the scaled solutions of the multidimensional scalings for one, two and three dimensional solutions for each of the eight subjects, based on their first set of observations (before lunch), for the absolute distance estimates and the relative distance comparisons. No graph for the drawn map scaling is presented because R^2 must be 1.0 (less our error in measuring the interobject distances on the maps in millimeters) for two or more dimensions.

that its location simultaneously satisfies all of the judged distances between it and every other object. Only if these estimated interobject distances are consistent with one another can they satisfactorily estimate what a perceived layout of space might look like. We examined the degree of consistency of the absolute and relative distance estimates, by assessing the amount of variance explained by the solution (goodness of fit), and by the stability of the output values over time.

The goodness of fit between the scaled solutions and the input data is specified in terms of the proportion of variance explained among the estimates, or R^2. This correlation is based on the 78 distance pairs, one member of each pair from the subjects' distance estimates and the other from the distance taken from the scaled solution. Figure 5 presents R^2 values for the eight subjects based on their absolute and relative distance judgments, taken from their first set of responses, and computed for one, two, and three dimensional solutions. Not surprisingly, the amount of variance explained by a one-dimensional solution was quite low (R^2 averaged about 0.50 across all measures), since it attempts to reconcile all of the interobject distances estimates as if the objects had been arranged in a single straight row stretching away from the subject. The two-dimensional solutions had a mean R^2 = 0.92 (ranging from 0.78 to 1.00). Addition of a third dimension added no further explanatory power. The R^2 values were slightly though significantly higher for the absolute as compared to the relative distance judgments for the two (or more) dimension solutions. Kruskal (11), in his classifications of R^2 values taken from a number of different kinds of scaling problems, treats values in this range for the two-dimension solutions as excellent fits, showing a remarkable internal consistency between the input values and the solution space.

We also assessed the stability of the scaled solutions over time. Four subjects repeated the same set of three measures from the same viewing position, separated in time by a lunch break. Figure 6 provides an example of a visual comparison overlaying the before and after lunch solutions based on the absolute distance judgments of each of these four subjects. We computed, for each subject, the discrepancy between the XY coordinates of the first and second location of each object, as estimated by the multidimensional regression analysis, and averaged these across all 13 objects. We used as a metric for the X and Y axes the standard deviation of the 78 actual interobject distances, so that the average discrepancy measure is also in standard deviation units. We adapted a metric related to one proposed by

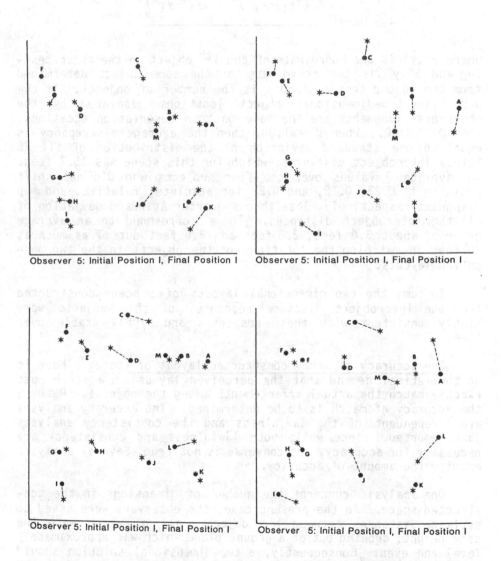

Observer 5: Initial Position I, Final Position I   Observer 5: Initial Position I, Final Position I

Observer 5: Initial Position I, Final Position I   Observer 5: Initial Position I, Final Position I

Figure 6.   Data from 4 subjects who did not shift positions,
showing the overlap between the position of each object estimated
by the scaling program based on data taken before and then again
after lunch. The dots represent the before lunch location and the
asterisk the after lunch location, with the dotted line indicating
the direction and amount of discrepancy. Data are from the subjects' absolute distance estimations.

Kruskal (12) in which:

$$D = \frac{\Sigma\sqrt{(x_i{'}-x_i{''})^2 + (y_i{'}-y_i{''})^2}}{k}$$

where x',y' is the coordinate of the ith object on the first test-ing and x",y" is the coordinate of the same object determined from the second testing, and k is the number of objects. If the underlying two-dimensional object locations generated by the observers' judgments are the same on both observation occasions, then D = 0.00. When D = 1.00, then the average discrepancy is equal to one standard deviation of the distribution of all 78 actual interobject distances, which for this scene was 15.7 feet. The average D values over the four subjects who did not shift position is 0.23, 0.18, and 0.23 for absolute, relative, and map responses respectively, less than a quarter standard deviation of all the interobject distances. These correspond to an average error of about 3.6 feet, 2.8 feet and 3.6 feet out of as much as 70 feet in matching the locations of the objects in the two per-ceived layouts.

In sum, the two dimensional layouts of a scene constructed from the interobject distance responses of the subjects were highly consistent with their responses and highly stable over time.

The accuracy of the constructed layout of space. There is no theoretical demand that the perceived layout of a scene must exactly match the actual arrangements among the objects. Rather, the accuracy of match is to be determined. The accuracy analyses are independent of the lawfulness and the consistency analyses just reported, since while both lawfulness and consistency are necessary for accuracy, the converse is not true. Several analyses examine the amount of accuracy.

One analysis concerns the number of dimensions in the con-structed space. In the present case, the observers were asked to estimate distances between the objects, all of which were the same height, growing out of a ground plane which was approximately level and even. Consequently, a two-dimensional solution should be found. The R^2 analysis of consistency provides an estimate of the number of dimensions needed in the scaled solutions to account for a particular proportion of variance. The proportion of variance explained is low for one-dimensional solutions, reaches a high asymptote (mean R^2 = 0.92) when two dimensions are used, and increases trivially for three or more dimensions. There is no statistical requirement that two dimensions would suffice, since 12 degrees of freedom exist in the scaling of 13 objects. That

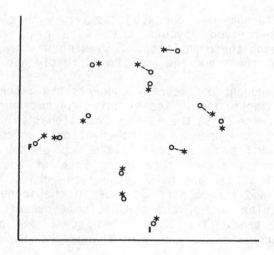

o Actual Layout
* Subjective Layout

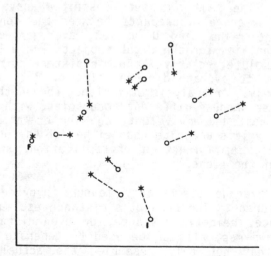

Figure 7. Examples from 2 subjects of the overlap between the actual positions of each object and the positions indicated by the two dimensional solution based on the absolute distance estimates. The first shows a very high degree overlap (D=0.15), while the second is an example of less overlap (D=0.40).

we found R^2 approaching 1.00 with only two dimensions lends credibility to the equation of the solution space with what the observer perceives when looking at the scene.

While we did not give our subjects very much choice, all of them produced perceived layouts that were plan views of the scene, even though their position of viewing was in perspective, from the edge of the scene and not from directly above.

Another component of accuracy concerns the match between the locations of objects in the constructed layout and the actual scene. To determine this, the 48 two dimensional solutions (eight subjects by three measures by two observation opportunities) were each rotated and fit to the coordinate map of the true scene, using a Procrustean factor rotation. Each of these rotations represents the best fit possible between the object locations in the real scene and the object location in the scene constructed from the particular set of the subject's responses. Being Procrustean, while the entire constructed scene can be shrunk or expanded, it cannot be elongated, or changed in shape.

Figure 7 shows two examples of a visual comparison made by placing a template of the real scene over a constructed scene. The first of these is an example of a very good fit, and the second of a very poor one. The remaining 46 fall in between these extremes. The same D measure described above can be used to describe the average discrepancy between the constructed and the actual scene. The mean D values, averaged over the two response opportunities for the eight subjects are 0.24, 0.22, and 0.32 for the absolute, relative, and map distances, respectively, which correspond to average discrepancies of 3.8, 3.5, and 5.0 feet, respectively. An analysis of variance showed that the three response measures produce different accuracies, with the two distance measures best and equivalent, and the drawn maps slightly but significantly less accurate than either of the others. There are no differences as a function of replication, shifting position, or view of the scene.

Even this average discrepancy measure provides impressive evidence of accuracy. The subject's distance estimates, whether absolute distance, relative distance, or even distances between points on a drawn map, all can be used to generate a two-dimensional layout that not only resembles the actual scene, but resembles it closely enough that the average discrepancy between the actual and the constructed locations of objects is only a quarter standard deviation of all of the interobject distances. (We cannot examine the discrepancy in locating each object independently. Such an analysis is not interpretable because of the nature of the scaling and rotation process that finds the best fit. The entire solution space is rescaled to minimize discrepancies, preserving only the relative positions of the objects along either axis. Consequently, the amount of mismatch for any single object cannot be determined. This problem was not appreciated by Kosslyn, Pick and Fariello (10), who tried to use a similar overlap analysis.)

The dependence of observer's position on perceived layout. If viewing position affects the perceived layout, then when subjects move, their first and second constructed layouts should be less similar to each other compared to subjects who made all of their observations from the same viewing position. The group of subjects who did not move already provided evidence for the reliability of spatial perception over time, as shown in Figure 6. If the D values for those subjects who moved are as low as those from subjects who merely repeated their judgments from the same viewing position, then moving is irrelevant, and the scene must look the same to the subjects regardless of the position from which they view it.

Figure 8 shows visually the discrepancies between the two sets of absolute distance estimates for the four subjects who moved. The same D measure yields means over these four subjects of 0.36, 0.26, and 0.47, for the absolute distance, relative distance, and drawn maps, respectively. While these values are still quite low, each of them is significantly larger for the movers, averaging about a two foot discrepancy increase over that of the non-movers. Therefore, viewing the scene twice from the same place yields more similar versions of the scene than if the observer views it from two different positions. This suggests that perceived layout is dependent on viewing position.

The D analysis does not indicate the nature of the dependence of perceived layout on viewing position. One likely possibility is that the distances between pairs of objects that are parallel to the observer's line of sight (radial distances) are underestimated, at least in relation to distances perpendicular (horizontal) to the line of sight. If these two kinds of interobject distances are perceived differently, then the observer's position, which defines the orientations of the interobject distances, becomes a determinant of the perception of the scene.

To test the relative accuracy of radial vs. horizontal distance estimates, we separately examined the magnitudes of those interobject distances that are roughly perpendicular to the line of sight of the observer when sitting at one location and also roughly parallel to the line of sight from the other position: these define a class of interobject distances that are radial when viewed from one position but horizontal from the other, and

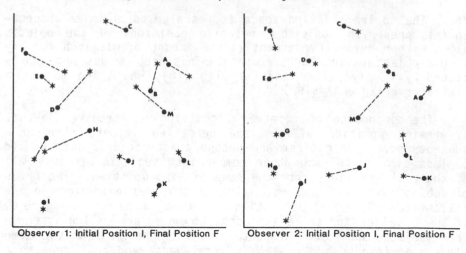

Observer 1: Initial Position I, Final Position F   Observer 2: Initial Position I, Final Position F

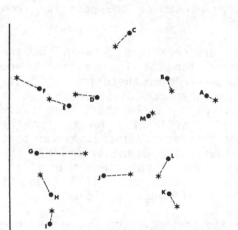
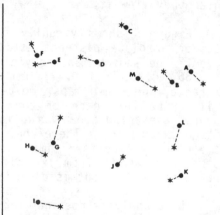

Observer 3: Initial Position F, Final Position I   Observer 4: Initial Position F, Final Position I

Figure 8. Data from the four subjects who shifted position between their first and second observations, showing the overlap
between the position of each object estimated from data taken
before and again after lunch. The dots indicate the before lunch
location and the asterisks the after lunch locations, with the
dotted line indicating the direction and amount of discrepancy.
Data are based on absolute distance estimates.

a second class that are just the reverse (see Figure 9). If any
overall systematic distortion occurs in the perception of one
direction of distance relative to the other, then contrasting the
estimates of the same distance when viewed from two different
positions should reveal a difference.

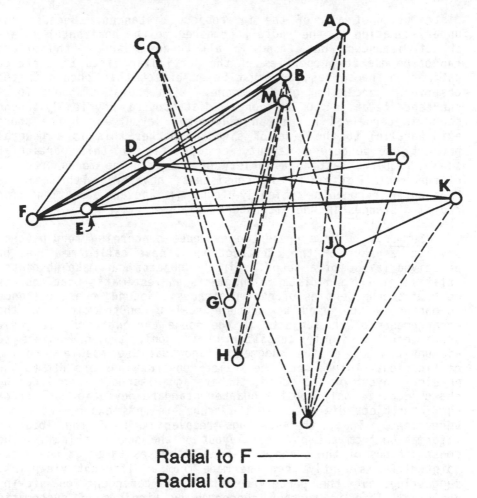

Radial to F ———
Radial to I — — — —

Figure 9.   A subset of the interobject distances from the stake scene.   The solid lines represent interobject distances that are radial to an observer when sitting at F and horizontal when sitting at I.   The dashed lines are radial to an observer sitting at I and horizontal when sitting at F.

We found a consistent significant difference for each of the three response measures, in which an interobject distance viewed as radial was estimated to be shorter than when the same inter-object distance was viewed as horizontal.   When this was analyzed with just the four subjects who shifted position, allowing a within-subject comparison, the average magnitude of the radial-horizontal difference was about seven feet for the absolute distance estimates, or nearly a half standard deviation of the

distribution of all of the interobject distances. Because the
underestimation of the radial, compared to the horizontal interobject distances, was found in all three measures, the effect
cannot be due to properties of the particular kinds of distance
estimation themselves, but must be an effect that occurs in the
observers' perception of the scene. With radial distance fore-
shortened relative to horizontal distance, a physically round
scene is perceived having an elliptical layout, with the short
axis parallel to the line of sight. Whether this is a general
property of perceived layout, or specific to this particular
scene, requires testing a variety of scenes. The foreshortening
of the radial distances is consistent, however, with the less
than unity exponents typically found in Stevens functions for
radial distances in the literature (13).

Summary. I have presented evidence concerning four psychophysical aspects of the constructions I have called measures of
perceived layout of a scene. First, subjects can make absolute,
relative, and drawn distance judgments and estimates that possess
most of the properties of real distances. Second, these distance
responses can be used to produce scaled constructions of the
arrangements of the objects in the scene currently on view that
are internally highly consistent using only two dimensions to
account for all of the judgments, and that are stable across a
replication. Third, when the scaled constructions are fit to the
physical layout of the scene, the average discrepancy in locating
the objects is only about a quarter standard deviation of all of
the interobject distances in the scene--in this experiment about
three feet. Thus, the scalings recover much of the location
information from the physical layout of the scene. Finally, the
constructions of the scene made from responses taken at one viewpoint differ slightly from one made from a different viewpoint,
suggesting that the perceived layout is dependent on viewing
position. This is further supported by findings of systematic
distortions in the shape of the scene, measured in terms of
differences in estimates of horizontal vs. radial interobject
distances.

The above conclusions are supported by data taken from each
of the three response measures. Two-dimensional constructions of
the scene, whether made by the subject directly as a drawn map,
or scaled as a multidimensional solution from the absolute or
relative interobject distance responses, all yield pretty much
the same information. Therefore, based on the above relationships and tests, all three of the constructions can be used as
measures of perceived layout of space. This evidence shows that
as measures of an observer's perceived layout of space, they
possess the minimum psychophysical properties that make them
usable as dependent variables in further research on perceived
layout.

CONCLUSIONS: VISUALLY PERCEIVED LAYOUT AND COGNITIVE LAYOUT IN
THE BLIND

The data just examined indicate a few of the properties of
a visually perceived layout in normally sighted observers. It is
obvious that unaided totally blind travelers have no comparable
"perceived" layout, because of the lack of any concurrent visual
information available to them during interaction with scenes,
coupled with the inherent inability of auditory and tactile information to replace the spatial information available from
vision.

Those concerned with the mobility of blind persons have
generally focused on the development of sensory substitution
devices capable of providing equivalent (or at least sufficient)
concurrent sensory information about the scene to replace the
missing visual information. The most ambitious project has been
Bach-y-Rita's and Collins' tactile sensory substitution system
(e.g., 1; Bach-y-Rita & Hughes; Collins, this volume) which
attempted to translate spatial information about a scene acquired
by a video camera located on the traveler's head into a vibrotactile stimulus on the skin. The limitations to this system are
not clear, though they do not seem to be due solely to a lack of
discrimination by the skin. One likely cause of failure is that
the display to the skin was a perspective rather than a plan view
of the scene, so that the user had to both learn to discriminate
among the complex patterns and also to translate each incoming
perspective view into a perceived layout of the scene as a whole.
Normally sighted observers, as the above data show, either automatically perceive the scene as a plan view, or make this translation easily. There is no evidence that the vibrotactile device
wearers were ever able to do so. Brabyn, Collins and Kay (2)
have provided the only report of a substitution device with a
plan view display. Little data are available on its use.

All of the other sensory substitution devices that have been
developed have been far less ambitious in what is displayed to
the user. From the long cane to the various ultrasonic devices
(See Brabyn, this volume, for a review), all of these provide some
kind of range and direction (and occasionally quality) information
about the objects in the path of the traveler. This information
is also perspective: it is only from the viewpoint of the device's
sensor, which is attached to the blind traveler, and it only signals when the traveler orients directly toward objects. In every
case except the plan-view device, the blind traveler is only being
given radial information.

The hope for these devices is that they can provide enough useful and usable information about the locations of objects to enable a blind traveler to move through the scene safely and effectively. Intuitively, knowing perspective (radial) information of range and direction would seem to be useful, but so far, the added mobility demonstrated with such devices, compared to just the long cane, has not been impressive (see various reports in this volume).

Many developers of these devices approach the problem as a technological one, such that when we discover how to increase the sampling angle of the device, increase the range over which it operates, and increase information leading to recognition and identification of the objects themselves, then performance benefits will be easier to demonstrate. It is likely that improving the information transmission of the devices will be helpful, but I do not expect any breakthrough in performance. My pessimism stems from the lack of attention being paid to how blind travelers represent the information provided by sensory substitution devices. Without knowing the nature of the representation, we cannot ask the proper questions about the kinds of information needed from a device, nor about how that information is to be presented (see Foulke, this volume; and 18).

For example, if a device only provides the range and direction of one object at a time while that object is being oriented, how does a blind traveler fit that information into a representation of what is likely to be a plan view of the scene being negotiated? Natural vision provides a continuity of perception of a scene, regardless of moment to moment shifts in eye and head position, and even shifts in attention and intention with respect to the scene. The entire scene continues to have a perceptual existence regardless of where a normally sighted observer orients. While there are many contributors to this achievement, the availability of nearly 180 degrees of viewing angle at every moment of time is undoubtedly a major source of the panoramic quality of scene perception. The substitution devices do not currently have this property at all, so that it is likely that only single objects have any perceptual salience at any one moment in time, much like normally sighted people would have if they viewed a scene in the dark with only narrow beamed flashlight.

Developing and maintaining an integrated plan view of a scene is compounded by the difficulty of extracting perceptual invariants from isolated radially oriented range and distance information about single objects. With normal vision, substantial information at the retina remains invariant with the properties of the layout of the scene, irrespective of the movements of the eyes, head, and body of the observer. It is from these invariances that the scene continues to look the same as we move while viewing it. Geometrical analyses suggest that invariances are not available in the light reaching the eye when only single sources of information are presented to the viewer (see 8 for a discussion), and substantial laboratory research shows that perceptual constancies break down under such impoverished viewing conditions (see 6 for a review). But these are exactly the conditions presented to a blind traveler receiving only range and direction information about single objects. With each step, or each movement of the sensor, the radial distance information changes, making the value from a moment ago obsolete. How does a blind person translate these continually changing values into a cognitive map that locates objects with respect to one another and to barriers and borders, and keeps those locations intact as the traveler moves about? When a traveler has such a cognitive map of the scene, then the incoming perceptual information from the device fits into an already represented display and is preserved, rather than being overlaid at each step of the foot and turn of the head.

This argument suggests that the design of sensory substitution devices must be coupled with a thorough understanding of how blind people represent scenes through which they move, an understanding that can only come through a prior understanding of how human beings in general represent the spaces around them.

ACKNOWLEDGEMENT

Parts of this paper are theoretical and parts empirical. Most of the research reported here was carried out by Rick Toye, as part of his Ph.D. dissertation (21,22). Rick also contributed several subsequent analyses, and was helpful in reading earlier versions of this paper. I have also been assisted by Bernadette Berardi and Janusz Przeorek, both graduate students at the University of Illinois at Chicago. Partial support for the research reported here was provided by the Office of Social Science Research, and by the University Research Board, both of the University of Illinois at Chicago.

REFERENCES

1. Bach-y-Rita, P. (1972). Brain Mechanisms in Sensory Substitution. New York: Academic Press.

2. Brabyn, J. A., Collins, C. C., & Kay, L. (1981). A wide bandwidth CTFM scanning sonar with tactile and acoustic display for persons with impaired vision. Proceedings of the Ultrasonic International 1981. Brighton, England.

3. Brabyn, J. A. & Strelow, E. R. (1977). Computer-analysed measures of characteristics of human locomotion and mobility. Behavior Research Methods and Instrumentation, 9, 456-462.

4. Bradley, D. R. & Vido, D. (1984). Psychophysical functions for perceived and remembered distance. Perception, 13, 315-320.

5. De Renzi, E. (1982). Disorders of Space Exploration and Cognition. New York: Wiley.

6. Haber, R. N. (1983). Stimulus information and processing mechanisms in visual space perception. In J. Beck, B. Hope, & A. Rosenfeld (Eds.), Machine and Human Visual Perception. New York: Academic Press, 157-236.

7. Haber, R. N. (1985). Toward a theory of the perceived spatial layout of scenes. Computer Vision, Graphics, and Image Processing, in press.

8. Haber, R. N. & Hershenson, M. (1980). The Psychology of Visual Perception. New York: Holt.

9. Hein, A. & Jeannerod, M.(1983). Spatially Oriented Behavior. New York: Springer-Verlag.

10. Kosslyn, S. M., Pick, H. L., Jr., & Fariello, G. R. (1974). Cognitive maps in children and men. Child Development, 45, 707-716.

11. Kruskal, J. B. (1964). Multidimensional scaling by optimizing goodness of fit to a nonmetric hypothesis. Psychometrika, 29, 1-27.

12. Kruskal, J. B. (1964). Nonmetric multidimensional scaling: a numerical method. Psychometrika, 29, 115-129.

13. Marks, L. (1974). Sensory Processes: The New Psychophysics.
     New York: Academic Press.

14. Olsen, D.R. & Bialystok, E. (1983). Spatial Cognition: The
     Structure and Development of Mental Representations of Spa-
     tial Relations. Hillsdale, N.J.: Lawrence Erlbaum Asso-
     ciates.

15. Pick, H. L., Jr. & Acredolo, L. P. (1983). Spatial Orien-
     tation: Theory, Research and Application. New York: Plenum.

16. Potegal, M. (Ed.) (1982). Spatial Abilities: Development and
     Physiological Foundation. New York: Academic Press.

17. Strelow, E. R. (1982). Sensory aids: Commercial versus re-
     search interests. Journal of Visual Impairment & Blindness,
     76, 241-243.

18. Strelow, E. R. (1985). What is needed for a theory of mobil-
     ity: Direct perception and cognitive maps--Some lessons from
     the blind. Psychological Review, 92, 226-248.

19. Strelow, E. R. & Brabyn, J. A. (1981). Use of foreground
     and background information in visually guided locomotion.
     Perception, 10, 191-198.

20. Strelow, E. R. & Brabyn, J. A. (1982). Use of natural sound
     cues by the blind to control locomotion. Perception, 11,
     635-640.

21. Toye, R. (1984). Judging the locations of objects in space:
     do we really know where things are? Unpublished Ph.D. Dis-
     sertation, University of Illinois at Chicago.

22. Toye, R. (1985). The effects of viewing position on the
     perceived layout of space. Submitted for publication.

THE COGNITIVE FOUNDATIONS OF MOBILITY

Emerson Foulke

University of Louisville

The primary thesis that I hope to develop in this chapter is that what humans are able to do in space depends heavily on what they remember about it. Humans are continually, but selectively, storing in memory the experience that they accrue in the course of living. This memorial representation of experience is in a sense an internal model of the world in which they live. However, because memory is selective in character (11), the model is not a facsimile. The model is characterized by the economy of a schematic representation, and exhibits a preference for the information that humans need to interact with their world, just as a map exhibits a preference for the information that travellers need for wayfinding. This schematic representation preserves both the spatial extention of relevant things and the temporal extention of relevant events.

By using such schematic representations, which I will call schemas, humans are able to escape the chrysalis of the present. They can manipulate memorial representation of things not present in space and time. They can, therefore, consider past experience, and, to the extent the future imitates the past, they can predict future experience. This ability allows them to imagine and compare the results of possible courses of action and, by such implicit behavior, to select a course of action without the necessity of engaging in overt behavior. To put the matter simply, they can make plans, and because they can plan behavior, they are then in a position to compare observed behavioral outcomes with expected behavioral outcomes, and to modify either plans or behavior as necessary. Thus, by taking advantage of their schemata, they promote the adequacy, the economy, and the safety of behavior.

SPECIAL OR GENERAL THEORY

In recent years, several writers, including myself, have called for a theory of mobility to account for the behavior of blind pedestrians (23,35,59), and the implication has been that it must be a special theory, pertaining only to blind pedestrians. Admittedly, the task performed by blind pedestrians is different from the task performed by sighted pedestrians, because it is performed without the benefit of the spatial information that can be acquired by vision, and because its performance depends on information supplied by other perceptual systems that sighted pedestrians generally have no reason to acquire. On the other hand, parsimony is a usual desideratum in theory-building, and one should maintain a more general theory until evidence forces one to make it more specific. In any case, the central nervous systems of blind pedestrians are not designed differently from those of the sighted, although differences may develop due to differing experience, and blind pedestrians do not have fundamentally different cognitive equipment. The mobility of both blind and sighted pedestrians depends on cognitive and perceptual processes common to all humans (61). Accordingly, hypotheses about the behavior of blind pedestrians will be developed within the same general cognitive and perceptual theory that must account for all informed behavior. To be sure, some details of a general theory of mobility will not be as functionally applicable to the sighted as they are to the blind; nonetheless, they may be retained in the theory on the grounds that while they may not be important for the sighted, they are also not wrong.

INFORMED MOVEMENT THROUGH SPACE

The Definition of Mobility

Mobility has been defined satisfactorily by a number of writers (5,23,24,38,59,62), and I will not dwell on its definition here. However, there are some essential criteria for successful mobility which should be emphasized in order to set the stage for the conception of mobility that I will present in the following pages.

Purpose

Mobility is movement through a (potentially complex) environment with the purpose of reaching a goal. The simple ability to avoid obstacles while moving aimlessly through space is not mobility in any meaningful sense.

Orientation

Furthermore, if pedestrians are to reach the goals they have in mind, they must know not only where their goals are, but also where they are. They must be able to orient themselves in space, and to maintain the currency of their orientation as they move through space.

CHARACTERISTICS OF THE MOBILITY TASK

Mobility is a clear example of what Poulton (51) has called an open skill. It is a task performed in a changing environment that is only partially predictable. The information needed to perform the task must be obtained from the space in which the task is performed, and that space contains irrelevant as well as relevant information. The pedestrian who performs the task must cope with irrelevant information as well as with stimulation that interferes with useful information. The requirements of the task are generally not sufficiently specified by the information that can be acquired while the task is in progress, and the needed information may arrive too late to give the pedestrian time to act upon it. Finally, mobility performance may be characterized by highly integrated sequences of behavior that make observation difficult (61).

THE MEMORIAL REPRESENTATION OF SPACE AND TIME

The memorial representations constructed by pedestrians as they gain experience with the spaces in which they operate are schematic in character. Just as a road map preserves the information needed by travelers to find their way through a network of roads, while omitting most of the detail that would be present in an aerial photograph of the territory described by the map, the memorial representations of pedestrians are hypothesized to preserve the information needed to move through space independently and to reach spatial goals, while omitting the abundance of irrelevant detail that is also available to the senses. These spatial schemas are thus selective.

However, there is more than one way to inform the behavior of a pedestrian performing a spatial task (48), and more than one kind of schema is possible as a result.

One extreme possibility is that a pedestrian might, with experience, simply build up a concatenation of S-R associations. Once this is accomplished, the stimuli present at choice points would elicit the correct responses, and the route would be tra-

versed without error. Although pedestrians programmed by experience in this manner would be able to perform the trips that
they intended to take, they would not be able to indicate, by
drawing maps or rendering verbal descriptions, the routes they
intended to follow. Travelers of this type would be inflexible.
They would not be able to retrace routes, and if their paths
were blocked, they would not be able to choose alternate routes.
If they strayed from a route, they would not know how to find
it again. Unlikely as it may seem, there are travelers whose
behavior suggests that they reach at least some of their spatial
goals in this way (37,40). Piaget and Inhelder (46) suggest that
such behavior is characteristic of young children.

As a variation of this model, some linguistic encoding could
be added. Travelers would behave more flexibly if the relevant
stimuli at choicepoints and the appropriate responses were represented in their schemata by linguistic symbols, because they
could manipulate symbols without actually traversing routes.
They should be able to retrace routes, tell others the routes
they intended to follow, give directions to others for getting
places, and so forth.

An alternative concept involves maps with representational
qualities. Tolman (64) referred to the memorial representation
of space as a cognitive map. For many, the metaphorical appeal
of this term is irresistable, and it has been widely accepted and
used. However, the term is not well defined, and some writers
(2,26) prefer not to use the term because it implies an unwar-
ranted assumption, namely that a picture-like image is stored in
memory. For example, consider Lynch's (40) and Tobler's (63)
use of the term. They seem to be proposing a "map in the head"
that resembles a graphic map. They allow that it may be a topo-
logical transformation of a graphic map that does not preserve a
Euclidian representation of space. Lynch (40), Beck and Wood
(9), and Appleyard (3) all suggest that a cognitive map may
contain several regions which, though internally well-defined,
are only loosely related to each other. Nevertheless, they propose a picture-like image that can be recalled from memory and
consulted in the same way one would consult a graphic map or a
natural scene. Although there is experimental support for this
view, a variety of experiments suggest that we do not store picture-like images of space in memory, but that rather spatial
knowledge is stored in the form of propositions about space (14,
52). Whether space is represented in memory by images or by
propositions may be an issue of the type that canot be resolved
by experiment. As Anderson (2) points out, we have not, so far,
been able to devise experiments whose results can decide between
these possibilities. In any case, it is safe to conclude that
spatial schemata consist of considerably more than S-R strings.

Even though experimental results are not conclusive in regard to the nature of the memorial representation of space, we may at least conclude with Appleyard (3,4), Evans, Marrero, and Butler (19), Lynch (40), and Shagen (58) that memory is selective in regard to the spatial information that is stored. It therefore appears reasonable to regard the memorial representation of space as a schema in the sense that only selected spatial information is retained in memory.

Information Available from the Schema

At the most general level, a spatial schema is a representation of some of the things that are in a given space and where those things are (5,24). In most of the spaces through which people move there are affordances; that is, movement along some courses is easy, while movement along other courses is difficult or impossible. These affordances are, simply, paths. The paths in a space usually intersect. Intersections are connected by path segments. The entire collection of path segments and intersections in a space constitutes its path structure. The path structure of a space is a pattern that can be learned and committed to memory. When people move along path segments, they arrive at choice points, where they must make decisions. I suggest that to learn a route is to learn a sequence of decisions that select the path segments needed to connect a starting place and a goal. Of course, the initial decision in such a sequence is a decision concerning the direction in which to start, and the final decision is a decision about when to stop. In the simplest case a route includes only one path segment, in which case the pedestrian has to make only the initial and the final decision. However, most routes include choicepoints, and when pedestrians follow such routes, they must also make decisions about which way to proceed and for how far. A route affords movement from a starting place to a goal, and in most spaces, more than one route is possible.

I will use the term feature to refer to any part of a space that can be distinguished from other parts and remembered. Objects can be features, curves in paths can be features, and irregularities in the surface can be features. I hypothesize that features may become landmarks, which allow pedestrians to locate themselves in the spaces through which they are moving, and by doing so to find out where they are. For features to serve as landmarks, it is necessary not only to remember them, but also to remember their relationship to other features, and to monitor their relationship to the moving observer.

Features that have become landmarks may be located in the spaces bounded by path segments, or on the path segments themselves. The large house with the distinctive roofline, the old hollow tree, the unusually sharp curve in the path, the distinctive smell of the bakery, and the bump in the path caused by the tree root underneath the sidewalk may all, with experience, become landmarks.

As already pointed out, routes, path structures, and landmarks are learned and incorporated, in varying degrees, in the schemata of pedestrians. I hypothesize that the proportional representation of these kinds of knowledge in the schema will depend on the strategies employed by the pedestrian for maintaining orientation, and that this, in turn, will depend, among other things, on the perceptual systems used by the pedestrian and the functional adequacy of those systems.

A Thought Experiment

Consider the following example, in which you are the subject in an imaginary experiment. Suppose that you are blindfolded and are traversing a route with a number of choicepoints. There are no irregularities in the route surface, no curves to be detected by proprioception, no distinctive sounds that reliably occur at fixed locations, and all the possible turns at choice points have angles of 90 degrees. Suppose, further, that you know only enough about the route to identify its beginning and its end. As your experience with the route accumulates, you will gradually learn the correct sequence of correct turns, and will finally be able to traverse the route without error. However, because your performance depends entirely on route knowledge, it will be limited in a number of ways. In order for you to know where you are at any point along the route, you must remember what turns you have made. If you have a lapse of memory, you will be lost. If, for some reason, you stray from the path, you will be lost, because your schema will not include any information about the spaces bounded by path segments, and no landmarks will be represented in it. If you find your path blocked, since you have acquired only route knowledge you will not be able to select an alternate route.

And now for the other condition of service in this imaginary experiment. You are still a subject in a wayfinding experiment, but this time you have prepared for service in the experiment by becoming visually familiar with the space in which your performance is to be observed, and thus not just with the route. You thus have a schematic representation of the space. You are then blindfolded, brought to some location in that space of which you are not informed, and told that your task is to reach the goal indicated by the experimenter. At this point, your blindfold is removed. As you look around you, you see a large building which, because of your previous familiarization with the space in which your task is to be performed, has been incorporated in your schema and is therefore what we call a landmark. Thus you know where it is in relation to other landmarks, and in the act of seeing it, you realize your relationship to it. Consequently, you know where you are. As a result of your previous experience in this space, you may have learned a route to a goal, and you may even have learned a path structure. However, it was not necessary for you to learn about routes and path structures in order for you to know where you are now. You have all of the information you will need to find your way through this space if a number of things in it have become landmarks. Once you find a landmark, you will have established your position in a frame of reference.

Spatial Generalization

When pedestrians are operating in spaces that have, with experience, become familiar, their schemata provide them with information about those spaces. But sometimes they find themselves in spaces that are not familiar. Of course, if current space is not represented in their schemata, they cannot consult their schemata for information about it. However, their schemata can often provide information about similar spaces that may be applicable. Most people spend most of their time in constructed environments, where certain patterns are likely to be repeated over and over again. For example, in cities, streets usually cross other streets, and they often intersect at right angles. Many of them have been given contours that promote drainage. From the center, they slope downward to either side. They are usually bounded by curbs, so that one must step up in order to pass from a street to the adjacent land. On both sides of the streets, one frequently finds sidewalks, and in residential areas, these sidewalks are often separated from the streets by grassy verges, on which trees, utility poles, and lampposts are occasionally to be found. Beyond the sidewalks, and parallel to them, are rows of buildings. The point to be made by this example is reinforced by the ease with which it could be extended. Because constructed environments exhibit extensive regularity, generalization is possible, and the schema is hypothesized to incorporate what may be regarded as spatial generalization (61).

FUNCTIONS MADE POSSIBLE BY THE SCHEMA

Cognitive Anticipation

Numerous experiments have demonstrated the dependence of skillful performance on the ability to anticipate behavioral requirements by observing the features of a situation in advance of the time at which some action will be required (7). It is useful to distinguish two kinds of anticipation--perceptual anticipation and cognitive anticipation (24,49). Perceptual anticipation is made possible by direct observation of the space in which the task is performed. The pedestrian who perceives in advance that a curb is coming up has time in which to prepare for the sequence of movements that, when executed with proper timing, will ensure that the curb is negotiated skillfully.

As pedestrians gain experience with the spaces through which they move, they gradually construct schemata of those spaces, and they are then able to obtain the benefits of cognitive anticipation by consulting their schemata. I hypothesize that in order for cognitive anticipation to be effective, pedestrians must be able to monitor the positions they occupy in their spatial schemata, and that this monitoring is made possible by reference to landmarks. When a blind pedestrian has had enough experience with a route to know that the curb is three steps beyond a particular bump in the sidewalk that has a distinctive feel underfoot, detecting that bump provides the cognitive anticipation that the blind pedestrian needs to prepare and time the sequence of movements that will be made when the curb is reached.

The degree of reliance on cognitive anticipation depends, in large measure, on the adequacy of perceptual anticipation. If, as in the case of the pedestrian who relies on vision for information about space, adequate perceptual anticipation is easily possible, there is little need to consult memory in order to anticipate. If, as in the case of the pedestrian who must rely on senses other than vision for information about space, it is not possible to stay well informed about the space in which the task of traveling is performed by observing that space while performing the task, the pedestrian must rely more heavily for anticipation on the schema that is the product of past experience.

The Detection of Errors

I hypothesize that when a pedestrian has had enough experience with a space to construct a schema of that space, it becomes possible to compare observed space with the schema, and that spatial errors can be detected by such comparisons. The information provided by detecting an error depends on the adequacy of the schema. For instance, blind pedestrians who have learned only a single route to a spatial goal may, by detecting a discrepancy between observed space and remembered space, discover that they have strayed from the route, but they may not know what action to take in order to regain the route. On the other hand, blind pedestrians who have schemata of the path structure of the space in which they are operating may discover, by detecting a discrepancy between observed space and the remembered route, not only that an error has been made, but also the corrective action required to regain the route.

Generalized Information

As already mentioned, because humans live, for the most part, in constructed environments which exhibit extensive regularity, I hypothesize that their schemata include spatial generalization and that these generalizations allow them to make predictions about what they will encounter in spaces not previously experienced. Of course behavior informed by such generalizations is more likely to result in spatial errors than behavior informed by direct observation of the space in which the task is performed, or by an accurate schema of that space, but in the absence of better information, these generalizations are useful. Blind pedestrians who enter new spaces can have no memory of them to consult, and the observations that they can accomplish on first encounter will not be sufficient to inform their behavior in a very precise manner. Their only recourse is to rely on the generalizations based on experience, and these generalizations, though not entirely trustworthy, may suffice until there has been enough direct experience to enable the construction of adequate schemata of the spaces in which their tasks are performed.

THE ROLE OF CONTEMPORANEOUS INFORMATION

Contemporaneous information is information that is acquired by observing the space in which the task of traveling is performed, while the task is in progress. I propose that its utility is determined by factors such as quantity, relevance, accuracy, and specificity, and that pedestrians put such information to several uses.

The Task at Hand

If pedestrians can gather enough contemporaneous information, if it is sufficiently accurate and specific, and if it can be acquired quickly enough to allow for the organization and timing of the behavior which depends on it, then it can control the tasks in which the pedestrians are currently engaged. The spatial information that can be acquired by visual observation generally meets these requirements.

Observation of Landmarks

Included in the contemporaneous information acquired by pedestrians is information about landmarks. I suggest that it is by landmarks that pedestrians maintain their orientation, and that for blind pedestrians, the detection of landmarks makes possible the substitution of cognitive anticipation for the visual perceptual anticipation they lack. They cannot see the crosswalk ahead, where a turn must be made, but they can learn that when the walk underfoot has a certain feel, or when they are abreast of the large tree, whose presence is discovered by echo location, it will be necessary to turn in approximately three steps.

Constructing the Memorial Representation

Informing the behavior of the moment is not the only use to which contemporaneous information can be put; it can also be remembered. Whether or not contemporaneous information is sufficient to specify the movements required for successful performance of the mobility task, it can be added to information already in memory, and as experience with a space accumulates, a representation of that space can be gradually formed in memory.

I suggest that the representation resulting from this piecemeal information acquired at many different times, as tends to occur tactually, is probably less accurate than the representation that results from information gathered on one, or at least a very few occasions, as it tends to be visually. For instance, because visual observers can observe a relatively large space on one occasion, they can observe not only the things in space, but also the spatial relationship of those things. Blind observers, perceiving tactually, must bring together spatial information gathered on different occasions and establish the spatial relationship of many things by inference. Of course, even representations based on piecemeal information can be evaluated and corrected by the feedback resulting from the behavior based on them, but it would still be worth knowing a good deal more about the differences between these representations and representations based on information acquired on one or just a few occasions.

The schemata of blind pedestrians may also be different from the schemata of sighted pedestrians in respect to the quantity of information they contain. Blind pedestrians can observe very little of the spaces bounded by the paths along which they walk. They learn very little, by observation, about the buildings, trees, fences, and so forth, commonly found in such spaces, and things not observed or remembered cannot serve as landmarks. It would be useful to know how much the task performed by sighted pedestrians is facilitated by landmarks not available to blind pedestrians.

A Conclusion

The schema, without which at least blind pedestrians could not maintain the orientation that makes purposeful travel possible in complex environments, is a cognitive edifice, constructed with the materials provided by perception. The utility of this cognitive edifice, which is of particular importance to blind pedestrians, is limited by the quantity, relevance, accuracy, and specificity of the information it contains.

COMPARISON OF PERCEPTUAL SYSTEMS

The perceptual systems of humans are obviously not equivalent in their ability to inform their users about space, and the skill with which the task of traveling independently can be performed will depend, in part, on the nature of the spatial information provided by the functioning perceptual systems. Accordingly, in order to know how well and in what way pedestrians can perform the mobility task using different perceptual systems, it will be necessary to examine and compare the idiosyncrasies and characteristics of various perceptual systems as processors of spatial information. This examination can be made by posing a number of questions to each of the perceptual systems.

What is the extent of view? How much of the space surrounding the pedestrian can be observed at one time and from one position? The answers to these questions have a bearing on whether spatial relationships are perceived directly or must be discovered by integrating piecemeal information acquired serially.

What selectivity of information is possible? The answer to this question indicates the vulnerability of a perceptual system to interference caused by competing information, noise, masking, and so forth.

Can the information in the stimulus pattern impinging on the receptors of the perceptual system be acquired by that system, and does the stimulus pattern contain the information that the perceptual system needs to acquire? Of what degree of resolution is the perceptual system capable? Where is the threshold below which the details of a pattern are too small to be discriminated? The better a perceptual system is in respect to pattern resolution, the more information it can acquire from a stimulus pattern. Human perceptual systems differ widely in this regard.

How much perceptual anticipation is possible? This question is answered partly by indicating the distance at which a thing can be perceived, because that distance determines the available time for preparing sequences of movements before they must be executed. However, in answering this question, it is necessary to consider the answers to the preceding questions, because the value of perceptual anticipation also depends on the quantity, relevance, accuracy, and specificity of the information that enables anticipation.

The Visual System

The visual system is said to be the spatial system par excellence (57). The stimulus patterns that impinge on its receptor surfaces are spatially extended, and it is well equipped to acquire spatial information from those patterns. It has both a large field of view and selectivity of regard. Because its use permits the observation of a large sector of space at one time, the relationships among events in space can be perceived directly. Its capacity for pattern resolution is much better than the capacities of the other perceptual systems that inform their users about space. Because physical contact with the thing perceived is not required for the excitation of its receptors, the visual system provides for perceptual anticipation (6,24,49). Since the visual system has these properties, visual observers are generally able to answer two kinds of questions about space-- "what?" and "where?" (5). They know what things are in space, and where those things are (29).

The Auditory System

The auditory system is well equipped for the analysis of temporal patterns (28). Consider, for instance, its ability to analyze the acoustic patterns that convey speech. The information in the acoustic energy that reaches the ears is discovered, for the most part, by interpreting temporal variations. As a consequence, acoustic energy can contain information about the sequence and timing of acoustic events (31), but only weak information at best about the shapes and sizes of objects. It is true that because they are capable of associative learning, auditory observers are often able to identify things, or, at least, categories of things, by the characteristic sounds they make. The sound of a car's horn will inform auditory observers who have learned to associate horn sounds with cars that a car is in the vicinity, but the sound of the horn contains no perceptual information about the size and shape of the car.

Physical contact with the thing perceived is not a requirement for stimulation of the auditory system, and its field of view is large. Sounds reach the ears from all directions, and auditory observers can estimate distance (8,12,21), direction (18,60), and the state of motion of sound sources (30,43), but none of these as accurately as visual observers can (29). Furthermore, many things in the auditory field of view are not sources of sound, and other things are so only part of the time (25). For these reasons, the auditory system is not able to acquire as much information about things and their positions in space as the visual system can. The auditory system is capable of perceptual anticipation, but the value of anticipation is limited for spatial events, because things and their positions are not as identifiable by sound as they are by sight.

Although auditory observers can, by turning their heads, favor the reception of some sounds over others (65), auditory selectivity falls short of visual selectivity (29). Auditory observers cannot, while listening to some sounds, exclude other sounds from auditory observation. The auditory system is thus more vulnerable than the visual system to interference.

In summary, the auditory system is less able than the visual system to answer "where" questions (41). The locations of some objects are indicated by the sounds they make, and if they are close, large, and dense enough, some objects can be found by echo location (1,15,32,33,36,53,54,55). However, most of the things with which space abounds generally escape auditory observation, and those things that do not are identifiable only indirectly by means of associated learning.

The Haptic/Proprioceptive System

Pedestrians who learn what the things are in the space around them, and where those things are, by walking to them, reaching for them, and feeling them are informed by both haptic perception and proprioception (47). The receptors on which haptic perception depends include the pressure receptors that are excited by mechanical stimulation of the skin, and the receptors in muscles, tendons, and joints, of which the kinaesthetic system is comprised. The proprioceptive system includes the receptors of the kinaesthetic system and the receptors of the vestibular system (30). Haptic perception provides information about the shapes, sizes, surface textures, and states of motion of things within arm's reach. Proprioception provides information about the relative positions of parts of the body, and the orientation

of the body in the gravitational field. (Proprioceptive information is also provided by the visual system, but visual proprioception will not be given further consideration in this
discussion.) Because receptors of the vestibular system are
excited by head motion, they can provide some information about
the space that is explored by walking (10,45). Because haptic
perception and proprioception depend on overlapping receptor
systems, and because they are employed cooperatively to acquire
information about the shapes, sizes, surface characteristics,
states of motion, and relative positions of things, and information about the shape and texture of the surface underfoot, I have
chosen, for present purposes, to treat them as if they were a
single perceptual system.

Because things must be touched by blind observers for their
sizes, shapes, surface characteristics, and states of motion to
be appreciated, the haptic/proprioceptive system's field of view
is small, and relatively little can be observed at one time. As
a consequence, haptic observers, unlike visual observers, are required to examine most of the objects in the space around them
serially, and unless they are small enough to be encompassed by
the hands, even single objects must be examined serially. The
results of serial examination must then be integrated to achieve
the perception of whole objects, and of their relative positions
in space. An obvious consequence of the haptic/proprioceptive
system's restricted field of view is that some things are too
large for their shapes to be appreciated by touch. Imagine
trying to discover the shape of an aircraft carrier by haptic/
proprioceptive observation!

Because physical contact with the thing perceived is a requirement for haptic/proprioceptive perception, little in the way
of perceptual anticipation is possible. Because the position of
the body must be changing in order for the receptors of the
vestibular system to make their contribution to the perception of
space, that contribution is realized as a function of time, and
the vestibular system is not able to provide perceptual anticipation of the features of space shortly to be encountered. Of
course, the information that travelers acquire about the relative positions of things in space may be incorporated in the
memorial representation of space that makes cognitive anticipation possible.

The haptic/proprioceptive system has more selectivity of
regard than the auditory system, and even the visual system, because it can perceive only those things with which it makes physical contact. On the other hand, there is nothing corresponding
to the peripheral vision that provides a minimal awareness of
events in the visual field outside the focus of attention.

The haptic/proprioceptive system cannot provide as much information about the composition of things in space as the visual system can because, in comparison to vision, its capacity for pattern resolution is relatively poor. Many details of things that are quite obvious to visual observers cannot be distinguished by touch, although it is also true that some kinds of surface irregularities can be better discerned by touch than by vision.

Many things which are readily observable visually are simply beyond the purview of the haptic/proprioceptive system. They cannot be reached, they are too fragile to withstand haptic/proprioceptive observation, or touching them is dangerous (22,25). For examples, consider the cloud, the spider web, and the wasp.

Nevertheless, in the absence of vision, the haptic/proprioceptive system may be the best system for acquiring information about the composition of space. Like the visual system, it is, by design, equipped for the appreciation of the spatial extension of things.

The remaining senses can provide some spatial information by way of associative learning (23,62). By feeling the heat of the sun on the cheek, and by taking into account the time of day, direction can be inferred. The aroma issuing from the doorway of a bakery can serve as a landmark. However, the remaining senses contribute relatively little to the perception of space.

THE FEASIBILITY OF ELECTRONIC TRAVEL AIDS

In the preceding sections, I have attempted an analysis of the cognitive and perceptual processes on which sighted and blind pedestrians are hypothesized to depend when they undertake purposeful movement through space. This analysis is certainly incomplete, and it may also, at some points, be wide of the mark. However, to the extent it is valid, it should suggest guidelines for the evaluation of existing electronic travel aids (ETAs) and the design of new ones.

A number of decisions are implicit in the design of any ETA. These decisions are about such matters as the kind of information needed by blind pedestrians, the sector of space in which the patterns of stimulus energy containing that information occur, whether the patterns of stimulus energy sensed by the ETA are to be displayed to the pedestrian directly or after preprocessing, what perceptual system is to be presented with the ETA's output, and what sort of display is to be used. These decisions should, of course, be based on information about the pedestrians who are to use the ETA, the task they are expected to perform, and the space in which that task is to be performed. However, much of this information is not yet available, and the designers of ETAs often find it necessary or expedient to base such decisions on assumptions which are sometimes only implicit.

A designer may, for instance, not be able to specify the spatial information that blind pedestrians need, and may not know with any certainty that the energy to be sensed by a proposed ETA contains the needed information. Furthermore, the designer may not specify (although he should be able to) how much of the information in the input to the ETA is preserved in its output. This problem can be particularly acute if the ETA receives patterns that exhibit spatial distribution and displays patterns that exhibit temporal distribution. If there is some correlation between changes in the input to the ETA and changes in its output, and if the output appears to exhibit enough complexity to suggest the presence of considerable information, the designer may simply reason that although human perceptual abilities are poorly understood, they are remarkable, and with experience blind pedestrians will find in the display the information that they need.

In any case, the functional characteristics of an ETA become fixed by the decisions the designer makes. The change in the performance of blind pedestrians that is made possible by an ETA with a given set of functional characteristics can be evaluated by treating it as an extension of the perceptual system to which it provides information, and by asking the same questions about the now-extended system that were asked earlier in this paper about the perceptual systems of pedestrians. Some of these questions, because of their implications, seem to me to be worthy of special comment.

The Information Blind Pedestrians Need

The designer who believes that blind pedestrians need, above all, the assurance that the path ahead is free of obstacles will design an ETA with a restricted field of view whose primary purpose is to detect obstacles directly ahead of its user. The ETA will enable some perceptual anticipation, but the value of the anticipation will be limited because the ETA is only a detector. Its display does not contain the information that would permit object identification. Because its field of view is restricted, many things in the space around its user will not be detected, and it will not be a very effective tool for learning about the spatial relationships of things. It will, therefore, be of limited value to its user in maintaining orientation. The Path-sounder (56) and the Mowat Sensor (44) are clear path indicators of this sort.

The designer who believes that meaningful mobility presupposes spatial orientation, and that in order to maintain spatial orientation, blind pedestrians must know not only about obstacles in the path ahead, but also about things in the space around them, will design an ETA with a large field of view, and will try to provide some means of informing the ETA's user of the positions of things detected by the ETA. The designer who believes that it is important for blind pedestrians to know not only where things are, but also what they are, will strive for a display that can provide at least some clues about the identity of the things it detects. An ETA of this type will enable perceptual anticipation, and to the extent it can assist in the identification of things, perceptual anticipation will be enhanced. If the field of view is too large, selectivity of regard may be a problem, and it may be necessary to provide some means of varying the size of the field of view. Kay's Binaural Sensor (34) is an ETA with a relatively large field of view. It provides some information about the direction, and less, but still some, information about the identity of the things it detects.

The designer who believes that blind pedestrians need most to know about the presence of things in the space above ground level (from knees to head, for instance) will design an ETA which examines that sector of space. An ETA of this type will provide the means for locating such things as trees, lamp posts, and walls. However, it will not give its user information about the surface ahead. It will not tell the user about step-downs, changes in surface texture, and so forth.

The designer who believes that the surface over which blind pedestrians walk is a source of important information will attempt to design an ETA that informs its user of the surface characteristics shortly to be encountered. To my knowledge, no ETA with this capability has yet been produced, partly because the importance of surface information has not been sufficiently appreciated, and partly because of limitations imposed by the current state of technology. A number of techniques for examining the space above ground level are known and can be implemented economically, but a practical way of obtaining information about the surface awaits discovery. (See Deering, this volume, for discussion of a system under development.)

CONCLUSIONS

Independent, purposeful mobility is not possible without spatial orientation. The maintenance of spatial orientation is accomplished by knowing what things are in space and where those things are. To maintain orientation, pedestrians, whether blind

or sighted, use information of two kinds, information they acquire as they move through the environment, and information
supplied by their spatial schemata. It follows, therefore, that
purposeful movement through space is both a perceptual and a
cognitive enterprise. The success of this enterprise depends on
the quantity, relevance, accuracy, and specificity of the spatial
information that is acquired and remembered. The visual system
is the only perceptual system that can fully support the mobility
task by providing the spatial information on which its performance depends. However, if the abilities and limitations of the
other perceptual systems are properly understood, and if the design of ETAs is guided by this understanding, it should be possible to bring about a significant improvement in the performance
of blind pedestrians.

REFERENCES

1. Ammons, C. H., Worchel, P., & Dallenbach, K. (1953). Facial vision: The perception of obstacles out of doors by blind-folded and blindfolded deafened subjects. _American Journal of Psychology_, 40, 519-553.

2. Anderson, J. R. (1978). Arguments concerning representations for mental imagery. _Psychological Review_, 85, 249-277.

3. Appleyard, D. (1970). Styles and methods of structuring a city. _Environment and Behavior_, 2, 100-117.

4. Appleyard, D. (1976). _Planning a Pluralistic City_. Cambridge, MA: MIT Press.

5. Armstrong, J. D. (1975). Evaluation of man-machine systems in the mobility of the visually handicapped. In R. M. Pickett & T. J. Triggs (Eds.), _Human Factors in Health Care_. Lexington, MA: Lexington Books.

6. Barth, J. L. (1979). _The effects of preview constraint on perceptual motor behavior and stress level in a mobility task_. Unpublished doctoral dissertation, University of Louisville.

7. Barth, J. L. & Foulke, E. (1979). Preview: A neglected variable in orientation and mobility. _Journal of Visual Impairment & Blindness_, 73, 41-48.

8. Batteau, D. W. (1968). Listening with the naked ear. In S. J. Freedman (Ed.), _The Neurophysiology of Spatially Oriented Behavior_ (pp. 109-133). Homewood, IL: Dorsey Press.

9. Beck, R. & Wood, D. (1976). Comparative developmental analyses of individual and aggregated cognitive maps of London. In G. T. Moore & R. G. Golledge (Eds.), _Environmental Knowing: Theories, Research, and Methods_. Stroudsburg, PA: Dowden, Hutchinson, & Ross.

10. Beritov, I. (1965). _Neural Mechanisms of Higher Vertebrate Behavior_. Boston, MA: Little, Brown, & Co.

11. Brewer, W. F. & Treyens, J. C. (1981). Role of schemata in memory for places. _Cognitive Psychology_, 13, 207-230.

12. Coleman, P. D. (1963). An analysis of cues to depth perception in free space. _Psychological Bulletin_, 60, 302-315.

13. Collins, C. C., Scadden, L. A., & Alden, A. B. (1977). Mobility studies with a tactile imaging device. Paper presented at the Fourth Annual Conference of Systems and Devices for the Disabled, Seattle, WA.

14. Corballis, M. C. (1982). Mental rotation: Anatomy of a paradigm. In M. Potegal (Ed.), Spatial Abilities: Development and Physiological Foundations. New York: Academic Press.

15. Cotzin, M. & Dallenbach, K. M. (1950). Facial vision: The role of pitch and loudness in the perception of obstacles by the blind. American Journal of Psychology, 63, 485-515.

16. Cratty, B. J. (1967). The perception of gradient and the veering tendency while walking without vision. American Foundation for the Blind Rsearch Bulletin, 14, 31-51.

17. Crossman, E. R. (1960). The information capacity of the human motor system in pursuit tracking. Quarterly Journal of Experimental Psychology, 12, 1-16.

18. Deatherage, B. H. (1966). Examination of binaural interaction. Journal of the Acoustical Society of America, 39, 232-249.

19. Evans, G. W., Marrero, D., & Burtler, P. (1981). Environmental learning and cognitive mapping. Environment and Behavior, 13, 83-104.

20. Fender, O. H. (1983). Reading machines for blind people. Journal of Visual Impairment & Blindness, 77, 75-85.

21. Fisher, H. G. & Freedman, S. J. (1968). The role of the pinna in auditory localization. Journal of Auditory Research, 8, 15-26.

22. Foulke, E. (1962). The role of experience in the formation of concepts. International Journal for the Education of the Blind, 12, 1-6.

23. Foulke, E. (1971). The perceptual basis for mobility. American Foundation for the Blind Research Bulletin, 23, 1-8.

24. Foulke, E. (1982). Perception, cognition, and the mobility of blind pedestrians. In M. Potegal (Ed.), Spatial Abilities: Development and Physiological Bases. New York: Academic Press.

25. Foulke, E. & Berla', E. (1978). Visual impairment and the development of perceptual ability. In R. D. Walk & H. L. Pick, Jr. (Eds.), Perception and Experience. New York: Plenum Press.

26. Hart, R. & Berzok, M. A. (1982). Children's strategies for mapping the geographic-scale environment. In M. Potegal (Ed.), Spatial Abilities: Development and Physiological Foundations. New York: Academic Press.

27. Hershman, R. L. & Hillix, W. A. (1965). Data processing in typing: Typing rate as a function of kind of material and amount exposed. Human Factors, 7, 483-492.

28. Hirsh, I. J. (1974). Temporal order and auditory perception. In H. R. Moskowitz, B. Scharf, & J. C. Stevens (Eds.), Sensation and Measurement. Dordrecht, Holland: D. Reidel Publishing Co.

29. Howard, I. P. (1973). Orientation and motion in space. In E. C. Carterette & M. P. Friedman (Eds.), Handbook of Perception: Vol. III. Biology of Perceptual Systems. New York: Academic Press.

30. Howard, I. P. (1973). The spatial senses. In E. C. Carterette & M. P. Friedman (Eds.), Handbook of Perception: Vol. III. Biology of Perceptual Systems. New York: Academic Press.

31. Julesz, B. & Hirsh, I. J. (1972). Visual and auditory perception: An essay of comparison. In E. E. David, Jr. & P. B. Denes (Eds.), Human Communication: A Unified View. New York: McGraw-Hill.

32. Juurmaa, J. (1970). On the accuracy of obstacle detection by the blind: Part 1. New Outlook for the Blind, 64, 65-72.

33. Juurmaa, J. (1970). On the accuracy of obstacle detection by the blind: Part 2. New Outlook for the Blind, 64, 104-118.

34. Kay, L. (1974). A sonar aid to enhance spatial perception of the blind: Engineering design and evaluation. Radio & Electronics Engineer, 44, 605-627.

35. Kay, L. (1974). Towards a mobility theory for the blind (Electrical Engineering Rep. No. 22). Christchurch, New Zealand: University of Canterbury.

36. Kohler, I. (1964). Orientation by aural clues. American Foundation for the Blind Research Bulletin, 4, 14-53.

37. Kuipers, B. (1983). The cognitive map: Could it have been any other way? In H. L. Pick, Jr. & L. P. Acredolo (Eds.), Spatial Orientation: Theory, Research, and Application. New York: Plenum Press.

38. Leonard, J. A. (1972). Studies in blind mobility. Applied Ergonomics, 3, 37-46.

39. Levin, H. & Kaplan, E. L. (1969). Listening, reading, and grammatical structure. Perception of Language: Part I. Annual Symposium Proceedings. Pittsburgh: Learning and Development Center, University of Pittsburgh.

40. Lynch, K. (1960). The Image of the City. Cambridge, MA: MIT Press.

41. Martinez, F. (1977). Does auditory information permit the establishment of spatial orientation? Experimental and clinical data with the congenitally blind. Annee Psychologique, 77, 179-204.

42. McLean, J. R. & Hoffman, E. R. (1973). The effects of restricted preview on driver steering control and performance. Human Factors, 15, 421-430.

43. Mills, A. W. (1972). Auditory localization. In J. V. Tobias (Ed.), Foundations of Modern Auditory Theory: Vol. 2.

44. Morrissette, D. L., Goodrich, G. L., & Hennessey, J. J. (1981). A followup study of the Mowat Sensor's applications, frequency of use and the maintenance reliability. Journal of Visual Impairment & Blindness, 75, 244-247.

45. O'Keefe, J. & Nadel, L. (1978). The Hippocampus as a Cognitive Map. Oxford, England: Clarendon Press.

46. Piaget, J. & Inhelder, B. (1967). The Child's Conception of Space. New York: Norton. (Originally published in French, 1948).

47. Pick, H. L., Jr. (1980). Perception, locomotion, and orientation. In R. L. Welsh & B. B. Blasch (Eds.), Foundations of Orientation and Mobility. New York: American Foundation for the Blind.

48. Pick, H. L., Jr., Yonas, A., & Rieser, J. J. (1979). Spatial reference systems in perceptual development. In M. Bornstein & W. Kessen (Eds.), Psychological Development from Infancy. Hillsdale, NJ: Erlbaum.

49. Poulton, E. C. (1952). The basis of perceptual anticipation in tracking. British Journal of Psychology, 43, 295-302.

50. Poulton, E. C. (1954). Eye-hand span in simple serial tasks. Journal of Experimental Psychology, 47, 403-410.

51. Poulton, E. C. (1957). On prediction in skilled movements. Psychological Bulletin, 54, 467-478.

52. Pylyshyn, Z. (1973). What the mind's eye tells the mind's brain: A critique of mental imagery. Psychological Bulletin, 80, 1-24.

53. Rice, C. E. (1967). Human echo perception. Science, 155, 656-664.

54. Rice, C. E. & Feinstein, S. H. (1965). Echo detection ability of the blind: Size and distance factors. Journal of Experimental Psychology, 70, 246-251.

55. Rice, C. E. & Feinstein, S. H. (1965). The influence of target parameters on human echo-detection tasks. Proceedings of the American Psychological Association.

56. Russell, L. (1971). Evaluation of Mobility Aids for the Blind, Pathsounder Travel Aid Evaluation. Paper presented at the National Academy of Engineers, Washington, DC.

57. Sedgwick, H. A. (1982). Visual modes of spatial orientation. In M. Potegal (Ed.), Spatial Abilities: Development and Physiological Foundations. New York: Academic Press.

58. Shagen, J. (1970). Kinaesthetic Memory, Comparing Blind and Sighted Subjects. Unpublished doctoral dissertation, George Washington University.

59. Shingledecker, C. A. & Foulke, E. (1978). A human factors approach to the assessment of the mobility of blind pedestrians. Human Factors, 20, 273-286.

60. Simpson, W. E. (1972). Locating sources of sound. In R. F. Thompson & G. F. Bosse (Eds.), Topics in Learning and Performance. New York: Academic Press.

61. Strelow, E. R. (1985). What is needed for a theory of mo-
     bility: Direct perception and cognitive maps - Some lessons
     from the blind. Psychological Review, 92, 226-248.

62. Suterko, S. (1973). Life adjustment. In B. Lowenfeld (Ed.),
     The Visually Handicapped Child in School. New York: John
     Day Co.

63. Tobler, W. (1976). The geometry of mental maps. In R. G.
     Golledge & G. Rushton (Eds.), Spatial Choice and Spatial
     Behavior: Geographic Essays on the Analysis of Preferences
     and Perceptions. Columbus: OH: Ohio State University Press.

64. Tolman, E. C. (1948). Cognitive maps in rats and men. Psy-
     chological Review, 55, 189-208.

65. Wallach, H. (1940). The role of head movements and vestib-
     ular cues in sound localization. Journal of Experimental
     Psychology, 40, 339-368.

ISSUES IN TRAVEL AID DESIGN

Emerson Foulke

University of Louisville

I wish to comment on several basic issues of design for
mobility aids for the blind pedestrian. It may be constructive,
to begin with, to consider a nonelectronic travel aid, the long
cane. The long cane is, by far, the best inanimate travel aid
we know anything about. What could be the reason for the success of a tool as simple as the cane? I propose that, although
the cane's field of view is limited, and although it does not
afford enough perceptual anticipation (1), it does examine the
surface over which the pedestrian will soon walk, and that
pedestrians who have advance notice of surface features have
a substantial portion of the information they need for safe
travel. In other words, the cane works in part because it looks
where the information is. This, then, should be a guiding
principle in travel aid design.

The Nature of the Display

The designer who believes that it is possible, by an appropriate transduction, to present information about the spatial
extension of things to the auditory system, and who considers
the ease of building a device that displays acoustic signals
to the ears and the difficulty of building a device that displays spatially extended patterns to the skin, will probably
design an ETA with an auditory display. Most of the ETAs that
have been built to date have had auditory displays. Although
some blind pedestrians have been able, after considerable practice, to obtain some useful information about space from such
displays, the results have been generally disappointing. As
matters presently stand, we are in the situation of having to

recommend an ETA, which may cost as much as three or four thousand dollars, as an adjunct to the ten dollar cane.

In view of this experience, it may be instructive to consider the results of an experiment reported by Collins, Scadden, and Alden (2). In this experiment, they used a matrix of electrodes to present patterns of electrical stimulation to the abdomen. The electrodes were activated selectively by a camera, mounted on the head, and fitted with a wide-angle lens, which looked down and ahead of the subject. This apparatus was an experimental travel aid. In order to test it, the subject walked through a cluttered room full of furniture and was able, even on the first trial, to avoid the obstacles in his path. That was an impressive performance, as was his report that the display was immediately interpretable. It made sense. He was not confronted with an initially enigmatic display of the type presented by the binaural sensory aid, and he did not have to spend weeks, months, or years in training in order to make sense out of the display. On the first trial, he knew what it meant. Could it be that spatially distributed information was being presented to a perceptual system which is, by design, suited for the acquisition of spatially distributed information?*

The cane provides another example of the same kind. As already mentioned, the cane's field of view is small, and the perceptual anticipation it affords is insufficient, but blind pedestrians easily learn to use their canes to acquire accurate information about the spatial layout of things within its reach. The cane is an extension of the haptic/proprioceptive system, a spatial system, and it presents spatially distributed information to that system.

An Alternative to Transducers

Most travel aids, with the exception of the long cane, are transducers. They receive patterns of energy, which contain spatial information, in a form that cannot be directly sensed by their users, and display analogous patterns in a form that can be sensed by the perceptual system they stimulate. However, the interpretation of the transduced patterns of energy remains the task of the blind pedestrians who use the ETAs.

---

* For perspective, it should be noted that although this was this subject's first experience with this aid, he had considerable experience with similar devices which presented spatially distributed patterns of stimulation to the skin. --(Eds.)

An alternative possibility is to engage the abstract symbol system called language, a system that humans use with remarkable facility. As a result of developments in the large-scale integration of electronic components, signal processing, and the like, it has become practical to consider ETAs which, by preprocessing the patterns of energy they receive instead of simply transducing them, acquire the information they contain, and display that information by means of the symbols of spoken language. The Kurzweil Reading Machine (KRM) (3), though not an ETA, affords a clear analogy. Unlike the Optacon, which senses the patterns on the printed page and displays their tactual analogs, the KRM senses and identifies the characters on the printed page and displays the spoken words they specify. The ETA now under development by Collins and Deering (see Deering, this volume) exemplifies this preprocessing approach. It identifies things in the space through which its user is moving and reports its findings to the user in a language that is already known and easily understood. To put the matter simply, it tells its user what things are in space, and where those things are.

REFERENCES

1. Barth, J. L. & Foulke, E. (1979) Preview: A neglected variable in orientation and mobility. Journal of Visual Impairment & Blindness, 73, 41-48.

2. Collins, C. C., Scadden, L. A., & Alden, A. B. (1977) Mobility studies with a tactile imaging device. Paper presented at the Fourth Annual Conference of Systems and Devices for the Disabled, Seattle, WA.

3. Fender, O. H. (1983) Reading machines for blind people. Journal of Visual Impairment & Blindness, 77, 75-85.

MACHINE VISUAL GUIDANCE FOR THE BLIND

I. Pollack

University of Michigan

I would like to report some informal observations on the usefulness of a technologically advanced visual guidance system. This system can recognize landmarks, can calculate potential hazards of both stationary and moving obstacles, and can instruct the user directly with highly understandable speech.

I did not have direct access to a technologically advanced machine vision system. I only had access to an intelligent dedicated human guide (Leslie Kay). I visited Kay's laboratory full of American enthusiasm for technological aids for the blind. I had believed that, if one could analyze major informational requirements of the blind, such as landmark recognition, obstacle guidance, etc., then one could construct technological solutions to match the specific requirements.

Kay proposed an "existence proof" of my technological system. Instead of constructing such a system, we simulated an advanced machine guidance system with a human observer. This human observer would announce landmarks, would provide a running path commentary, would warn of potential obstacles, and do (almost) everything we might expect of an intelligent machine guidance system.

I tried to walk under a blindfold along Christchurch streets. Despite Leslie Kay's expert guidance and many years of experience in the guidance field, my gait was hesitant, and I felt unsure in moving about. Doubtlessly, I would have improved with practice under Leslie's expert guidance. The informal tests, however, suggested that such a guidance system would be less successful than I had originally thought. By contrast, I navigated reasonably well with Kay's ultrasonic aid.

What is to be learned from this brief "existence proof"? It would be easy to conclude that a sophisticated machine guidance system will be a failure. But I think that is the wrong conclusion. Rather, to succeed, we must incorporate features which were omitted from our simulation. The success that many blind observers have with human or guide-dog guidance in strange environments suggests that continuous tactual guidance may be helpful. The partial success with the ultrasonic aid suggests that the user must be closely coupled with the system, rather than being a consumer of information about the environment.

Perhaps the major lesson to be learned from the simulation was Kay's admonition to me. He, an electrical engineer, had to remind me, a psychologist, "Don't overlook the possibility of utilizing the intelligence of the human brain. If we, as designers, can provide a good well-engineered description of the environment, the human brain will learn to utilize it."

MOBILITY AND ORIENTATION PROCESSES OF THE BLIND

Michael Brambring

University of Bielefeld

The mobility and orientation of the human adult, i.e. the capacity for independent, safe, and goal-directed locomotion in the street, is rarely analyzed in scientific research. In contrast, a voluminous literature exists regarding the development of gross motor behavior of children. Problems of mobility and orientation seem to generate research interest only if certain aspects of athletics, of neurology-psychiatry, or of rehabilitation are concerned.

One exception is found in the theory by Gibson (10,11), in which features of the mobility of adults are analyzed, particularly with regard to the importance of visual information for locomotion. Unfortunately, this theory allows at best only restricted conclusions about mobility problems of the blind, because the mobility of the blind is necessarily based on non-visual information (16).

The present paper examines theoretically the problems of the blind walking in the street. Then, descriptions of routes familiar to the blind are analyzed and compared with descriptions by people who can see. The comparative nature of the investigation is intended first to ascertain whether blind and sighted persons' route descriptions differ with respect to the quantity of information used to communicate particular routes, and second to estimate those informational aspects the blind may need for successfully being oriented in, and navigating through, their spatial environment.

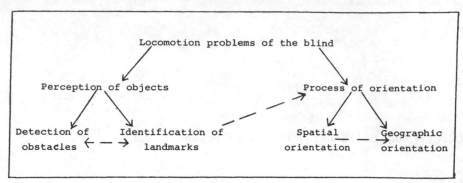

Figure 1.   General locomotion problems of blind persons.

LOCOMOTION OF THE BLIND

There are two main problems in street locomotion for the blind: (a) reliable perception of objects, and (b) adequate orientation (9,19). Each of these problems can be seen as having at least two aspects (Figure 1). The perception of objects includes the detection of obstacles and the identification of landmarks. The orientation process includes spatial and geographical orientation.

These aspects characterize not only the locomotion of the blind, but also that of sighted people. But because of reduced or absent vision, the solution of these problems, especially the first three, is much more difficult for blind than sighted persons. Even the group of the blind is not a homogeneous one: There is a wide range of mobility capacity depending on biographical variables, such as age, age at onset, degree and duration of blindness, education, additional handicaps, and psychological variables such as motivation or personality (4,18,19).

Obstacle Detection

The functional detection of obstacles means that physical objects in the environment that can become dangerous for the blind have to be perceived in time to avoid them. The most dangerous objects are down-steps and low-lying or fast-moving objects.

Only when the long cane, in connection with systematic mobility training, was introduced after the Second World War (12) was the problem of reliable detection of such obstacles by the blind solved satisfactorily. The guide dog, also suitable for this task, is only acceptable to a small percentage of blind people (17,20). By use of the long cane, reliable detection of some of the most dangerous obstacles, such as down-steps or low-lying objects, is possible. The long cane does not solve the problem of detecting objects at the height of the head. In order to solve this problem, as well as to extend both the range and the accuracy of detecting obstacles, technological aids have been developed. These are the so-called obstacle detectors or clear path indicators (e.g. Mowat Sensor, Sicopilot, Nottingham Obstacle Detector, Laser Cane). They deliver only the very simple information whether there is or is not an object there.

Aside from the technological and manual aids, the ear is the primary alternative for perceiving physical objects, by means of perception of sound, sound shadow, and sound reflection by ambient as well as self-generated noise.

The reliable detection of obstacles is a necessary condition, but not a sufficient one with respect to the independent locomotion of the blind. The mastery of this problem is not enough for goal-directed locomotion from a starting point to the destination of the route. Identification of landmarks and spatial and geographic orientation are essential to the adequate solution of this task.

Landmark Identification

In order to identify landmarks, the blind person has to perceive the quality or pattern of the objects and has to determine their location with respect to the specific points of the route. Landmarks may be primarily physical objects, but they may also be odors, changes of temperature, or changes of sound conditions. The ear, the tactual sense through the feet, and the long cane as the extended arm give essential information for the identification of landmarks. Also, some prostheses, such as the TVSS (1) and auditory aids like the Sonicguide, try to solve this problem, but thus far only in a limited manner.

To be effective, landmarks must be stationary and easy to identify under a variety of environmental conditions, such as changes of ambient noise or of weather conditions.

Physical objects, such as trees, parking meters, and steps, may be obstacles as well as landmarks. One can even expect that most of the obstacles will become landmarks after the person has walked a route several times.

The identification of landmarks probably possesses the highest importance with regard to the independent locomotion of the blind: Goal-directed mobility requires the ability to go from one landmark to the next. Further, the blind person seems to require

a great many landmarks to learn a new route, but the distance between the landmarks can be greater once the person has increased
familiarity with or anticipation of the route. The same will
happen if competence increases (2,15).

Spatial Orientation

Spatial orientation means the ability of a person to estimate his own position with regard to the immediate surroundings,
such as the estimation of distances as well as direction of his
own body with respect to the directly perceivable environment.
The most difficult problems regarding spatial orientation are, on
the one hand, the optimal position of the blind person in the
middle of the sidewalk and, on the other hand, the ability to
walk without veering off course. The solution to these problems
does not create too much difficulty if there is a clearly
perceivable inner shoreline, such as houses or bushes, or a
continuous traffic noise at the outer shoreline, by means of
which the blind person can maintain a straight walking direction.

Audition is the most important sense modality for these
tasks, but tactual information through the feet or by the extended arm via the long cane may add to the solution of these
problems. Beyond these natural senses, some prostheses such as
the so-called environmental sensors (Sonicguide, Siemens-Brille,
i.e. Siemens-Glasses) aid in reducing mobility problems.

Geographic orientation, in contrast, is the ability to classify one's position with reference to the topographic space
(8,13), the space that is not directly perceivable. Geographic
orientation may be illustrated by success in finding one's way
around in an unfamiliar terrain, or being able to describe or
draw one's topographic surroundings.

Because of the absence of long distance vision, one may
describe the blind person's mobility situation as a geographic
orientation task, more so than for sighted persons. In addition
to perceptual information, certain cognitive processes such as
memory or mental representation of the environment are essential
for the geographic orientation task. Fortunately, the redundancy
of street situations and the construction of cities supports
the blind person's acquisition of a cognitive picture of his
environment (9). This argument is more valid for the relatively
rectilinear cites in the U.S.A. than for the medieval cities in
Europe. Tactual maps (3,7) have been constructed to improve the
understanding of the topographic surroundings for the blind.

EMPIRICAL WORK

Descriptions of Routes

In two investigations, blind persons were asked for relevant information about their known routes, on the reasonable assumption that those who are most immediately involved should be able to give the most valid answers.

In the first study, four blind students were asked, on several occasions, to describe their daily route from their dormitory to the bus stop. In the second study, nine sighted and nine blind subjects, matched on various criteria, each described two different routes.

Both sets of data were evaluated with regard to their relevant functional implications, with respect to the above-mentioned problems of locomation of the blind. In the second study, a further, differentiated evaluation of the language used was carried out, based on linguistic analyses of interaction sequences involving the requesting and giving of street directions (14).

Study 1: Route Descriptions Given by Blind Persons

Our first study analyzed verbal information which the blind give for a route which they knew well. Here, we were interested in the kind and amount of information provided, as well as the relationship between this information and positions or places along the route in question. Moreover, we wished to examine the extent of agreement among various blind subjects with respect to route information.

Four blind students in their mid-twenties participated in the experiment. All of them traveled without sighted guide. On four different days, each subject was asked to describe the route of approximately 400 meters from his dormitory to the nearest bus stop. The tape recordings were transcribed and evaluated for content with respect to the general problems of locomotion of the blind (see above). The evaluation of the 16 descriptions was carried out by independent judges. The objectivity of all these evaluations, however, was not separately tested.

The catalog of descriptive designations developed included the following four general categories (5):

(1) Data on distances were designated if distance information was expressed either directly, e.g., "about 6-8 meters from the next corner," or indirectly, e.g., "I go straight ahead, as far as the corner."

		Percentage of unique and shared references			
				Shared by	
Information type	Number of distinct items	Unique	2 speakers	3 speakers	4 speakers
Data on distances	15	46.7	26.7	20.0	6.7
Data on directions	13	30.8	23.1	15.4	30.8
Data on landmarks	69	37.7	17.4	21.7	23.2
Data on obstacles	19	68.4	15.8	10.5	5.3

The total frequencies are based on data from four subjects over four trials.

Table 1.   Geographic information given by the blind in route descriptions (dormitory to bus stop).

(2) Data on directions were recorded if the information expressed on actual change, e.g., "I make a 90 degree turn," or an actual change in direction, e.g., "I take two steps to the right,"

(3) Data on landmarks were designated if objects served an orienting purpose and were not mentioned as something to be avoided, e.g., "the irregularities in the sidewalk are especially noticeable here."

(4) Data on obstacles were designated if objects were mentioned by the subjects as something to be avoided, e.g., "here, I have to go more to the left, in order not to bump into the parking meters."

A given sentence could contain more than one of these types of information, but only one category was used to code each partial statement of the sentence.

The results of this analysis are presented in Table 1. As can be seen from Table 1, the four subjects produced 116 distinct items of information during their four walks, i.e., approximately seven items per route per person, or the equivalent of one item about every 60 meters. It can be seen from the table that landmarks were by far the most frequently named items. The verbal descriptions given are in relatively high agreement with respect to directional information, whereas the data on obstacles, on the other hand, appear to be more idiosyncratic and limited to particular individuals.

The results point to the special importance of landmarks for the blind during street locomotion. This conclusion is further underlined by the distribution of landmarks mentioned in relation

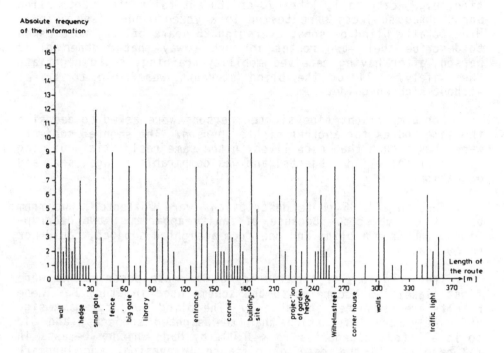

Figure 2. Distribution of information regarding specific landmarks in relation to the route described. The abscissa shows
distances in 30 metre intervals, the ordinate frequency of mention
(total possible = 4 subjects x 4 trails).

to the route. Figure 2 shows that the number of landmarks mentioned in individual sections of the route varied considerably.
They were frequent between 0 and 30 meters, between 150 and 180
meters, and between 240 and 270 meters. These three sections
have in common that at these points of the route, the blind
person had to change direction or cross a street. From this,
it can be inferred that the blind especially need orientation
information about such nodal points if they are to travel safely.
This fact should be given due consideration in describing routes
to blind persons, and in the construction of maps for the blind.

Study 2: A Comparison of Route Descriptions by Blind and Sighted
Persons

In the second study the aim of the research was extended.
The task of the participants was to describe two different

routes, 500-1000 meters long, beginning at the place where they live and having well-known places in the city as their destination, e.g., city hall, library, or student cafeteria. Both blind and sighted subjects were tested in a yoked manner (see below). Nine totally blind persons, averaging 25 years of age, were asked to describe their two routes in such a way that another blind person, after having received mobility training, could negotiate them safely. All of the blind students were able to travel without sighted guide.

For comparison, nine sighted persons were asked to describe the same routes for another sighted person. The sighted subjects were chosen such that each lived in the same residential building as one of the blind subjects, and was comparable in age, sex, and education.

Thus in all 36 route descriptions were collected, two from each of 18 subjects. Because of faulty apparatus, two descriptions, one from a blind and one from a sighted subject, could not be evaluated.

Transcriptions of the remaining 34 route descriptions were first classified according to the scheme used in Study 1. These results are presented in Table 2. The blind subjects gave significantly more information than the sighted subjects, and did so in all four categories ($p < 0.001$ by Mann-Whitney U-tests in all cases). In the case of distance, direction, and landmark information, the blind mentioned nearly three times as many orientation points per route. For the sighted subjects, data on obstacles are almost entirely absent: one subject mentioned one obstacle on one route.

The results suggest that the blind may require considerably more information for locomotion than the sighted. Thus two problems arise. First, the process of acquiring the necessary

Information type	Blind		Sighted	
	Median	Range	Median	Range
Data on distance	26.7	15.0-48.5	8.7	5.0-15.5
Data on directions	14.0	8.0-27.0	5.5	2.0- 7.5
Data on landmarks	46.5	16.5-74.5	18.5	9.5-26.0
Data on obstacles	4.0	0.0-22.5	0.1	0.0- 0.5

Based on nine subjects per group. Group median based on mean per subject over the two routes. Range based on averaged sum of information per subject for the two routes.

Table 2. Geographic information given by blind and sighted subjects in describing two routes each.

information will consume more time, and second, committing the
information to memory will require a greater mnemonic effort by
the blind.

Linguistic units of route description. The second step in
evaluating the results of Study 2 was an analysis of data collected in accordance with a more detailed linguistic scheme based
on a classification system given by Klein (14).

There were two phases in this part of the analysis. In the
first phase, we examined whether the total route described could
be divided into delimitable sections by individual judges. In
the second phase, each section of the route descriptions was
classified in terms of five linguistic categories.

In the task of route subdivisions, the judges were to divide
the overall route description into as many small sections as
possible, in such a way that each section formed a meaningful
unit with clear boundaries. Such a section was considered to be
delimitable if a break was made at these points in describing the
route.

The route subdivisions were marked by six advanced psychology students serving as judges. To determine the reliability of
these judgments, each route description was scored by at least
two different persons. Inter-judge agreement averaged 86%, and
ranged for pairs of judges from 75% to 94%. These figures indicate that the independent judges used were in quite close
agreement on the subdivisions needed. Using this scheme, there
were 129 subdivisions in the 17 descriptions produced by the
sighted persons and 283 subdivisions for the blind subjects,
about 8 segments per route per person for the sighted, on the
average, and about 17 segments for the blind. The average overall length of the routes was about 690 meters, meaning that for
the sighted subjects, one subdivision corresponded to about 90
meters, and for the blind subjects, to about 40 meters.

The length of the subdivisions of the blind was shorter
in the second than in the first study (40 versus 60 meters).
This difference may be due to several factors. First, the blind
subjects had to walk in the first study, whereas they had to
describe the routes from memory in the second. Second, the
blind subjects were probably more familiar with the route in the
first than in the second study. Third, the routes were longer
in the second than in the first study.

In the second phase of the analysis of Study 2, the route
descriptions were classified in terms of five linguistic categories, as follows (6):

(1) Designation of points of departure: Points of departure can be defined by naming a particular object, or by implicitly describing the new point of departure by means of spatial and temporal deixis.

(2) Designation of directions: Statements are designated as data on directions if they either give a direction explicitly, or if the direction can be deduced from the given position.

(3) Designation of distances: Statements are designated as data on distances if they contain information on some number of meters or steps, or length of time.

(4) Designation of destinations: Destinations can be designated by naming objects, analogous to points of departure. If no object is named, it is impossible to define the destination.

(5) Comments: Statements are designated as comments if they consist of an evaluation or of an additional, redundant explanation of the first four categories.

Judgment by means of this more elaborate classification scheme was again made by the six independent judges, with each transcription again scored separately by at least two persons, with the subdivisions in it already marked. For each subdivi-

	Group			
	Sighted		Blind	
Determination of departure by means of	Frequency	Percentage	Frequency	Percentage
(1) Naming of objects				
(a) Explicitly named object, assumed as known	7	5.4	8	2.8
(b) Pointing to an object	0	0.0	0	0.0
(c) Dependent on previous section of route	8	6.2	16	5.7
(d) Independent of previous section of route	9	7.0	20	7.1
Sum	24	18.6	44	15.6
(2) Naming no objects				
(a) Spatial deixis	21	16.3	38	13.4
(b) Temporal deixis	19	14.7	86	30.4
(c) Enumeration	65	50.4	115	40.6
Sum	105	81.4	239	84.4
Total sum	129	100.0	283	100.0

The data are based on nine subjects for each group.

Table 3. Points of departure given in the route descriptions collected.

Type of data	Sighted		Blind	
	Frequency	Percentage	Frequency	Percentage
(1) Explicit data on directions				
(a) Based on previous direction	75	58.1	142	50.2
(b) Based on body rotation	0	0.0	16	5.6
Sum	75	58.1	158	55.8
(2) Implicit data on directions based on particular locality	54	41.9	125	44.2
Total sum	129	100.0	283	100.0
(1) Precise or approximate data on distances				
(a) Precise statements on metres, steps, or time	0	0.0	30	10.6
(b) Approximate statements on metres, steps, or time	2	1.6	29	10.3
Sum	2	1.6	59	20.9
(2) Vague or lacking data on distances				
(a) Vague statements on distances	16	12.4	25	8.8
(b) No statements on distances	111	86.1	199	70.3
Sum	127	98.5	224	79.1
Total sum	129	100.0	283	100.0

The data are based on nine subjects for each group.

Table 4. Distances and directions given in the route descriptions.

sion, a judge decided whether it could be designated as belonging to any of the five categories, and if so, to which. The average percent agreement was 87%, with a range from 72% to 95%.

Tables 3-6 present the results of this frequency analysis for both groups of subjects. For points of departure, the relevant data are shown in Table 3. Both blind and sighted subjects described points of departure mainly without naming any concrete object. This difference was significant in both groups separately ($p < 0.01$ by Wilcoxon tests).

In the category 'naming of objects' sighted persons more frequently assumed objects to be known than the blind did, although the difference was not statistically reliable for the present sample.

Determination of goal points by means of	Group			
	Sighted		Blind	
	Frequency	Percentage	Frequency	Percentage
(1) Naming of objects				
(a) Explicitly named object, assumed as known	21	16.3	24	8.5
(b) Pointing to an object	0	0.0	0	0.0
(c) Dependent on previous section of route	22	17.1	32	11.3
(d) Independent of previous section of route	44	34.1	87	30.7
Sum	87	67.5	143	50.5
(2) No determination of goal points by objects	42	32.5	140	49.5
Total sum	129	100.0	283	100.0

The data are based on nine subjects for each group.

Table 5. Determination of goal points in the route descriptions.

Type of comment	Group			
	Sighted		Blind	
	Frequency	Percentage	Frequency	Percentage
(1) Evaluative	1	0.8	25	8.7
(2) Redundant	40	31.3	134	47.5

The data are based on nine subjects for each group.

Table 6. Evaluative and redundant comments in the route descriptions.

In the category 'no naming of objects', the sighted subjects defined points of departure proportionally more frequently by means of spatial terms, such as 'here' or 'there' and enumeration, whereas the blind more frequently used temporal terms, such as 'then', 'first', or 'afterwards'. However, only the more frequent use of temporal adverbs by the blind was statistically reliable (p < 0.01 by matched pairs sign test by subjects).

The designations of statements on direction as well as distance are summarized in Table 4. The two groups of subjects used direct and indirect statements about direction with approximately equal frequencies. It is striking that the blind subjects, but not the sighted ones, used instructions involving body rotation, such as "turn 90 degrees to the right and then start walking" ($p < 0.05$, matched pair sign test by subjects).

Table 4 shows that almost without exception, the seeing subjects had no precise or approximate information in their statements on distance, while blind persons did so about one time in five ($p < 0.01$, sign test). Even among the blind, such information was consistently less frequent than vague information, or no information about distance ($p < 0.01$, sign test).

Table 5 presents the data with respect to destinations. Table 5 reveals a tendency for the sighted subjects, more regularly than the blind, to choose an object in defining a destination ($p < 0.01$ by matched pairs sign test). Within the subcategory of 'naming of objects', however, there were no significant differences between the two groups.

Finally, Table 6 shows the use of evaluative and redundant comments by subjects in the two groups. An example of an evaluative comment is "It's not hard to find," or, "there you have to pay close attention." An example of a redundant comment is "then you go past [hesitation], and then the next street is the Biegenstreet" (which is redundant). It is evident from Table 6 that the blind subjects used more comments of both kinds combined ($p < 0.05$ for both types summed together by sign test). Separately, however, only the difference for evaluative comments was significant ($p < 0.01$). The sighted subjects injected commentary into about one-third of the subdivisions they produced, whereas the blind injected commentary into more than half of the subdivisions.

CONCLUSIONS

The linguistic analysis of route descriptions given by blind persons reveals that they use less information from the environment and more information relating to their person. This interpretation is suggested by the way in which points of departure and destinations were determined for the individual sections of the route. Blind persons less frequently name objects in defining such points, probably because they cannot test this kind of information visually, and it is thus unreliable for them. They tend to use more temporal and fewer spatial terms in defining new points of departure. It is particularly characteristic that they make explicit statements about distances more frequently than sighted persons, whereas the sighted obviously can do without such information, since it is implied in the description of characteristic features of the surroundings. The blind, on the other hand, obviously make greater use of egocentric information. This is shown by the precise statements made about distances, which permit correct estimates independently of the environment, and also by the information involving body rotation, to which sighted persons never refer.

The difference between route descriptions given by blind and by sighted persons can be cautiously characterized thus: sighted persons give environment-oriented descriptions, whereas the blind tend to use person-oriented descriptions. In other words, sighted persons make more use of external characteristics for locomotion, and the blind tend to rely more on internal characteristics.

In regard to the amount of information given in describing a route, there is a major difference between sighted and blind persons. The latter provide more than twice as much information as the former, and their subdivisions of routes are correspondingly more than twice as detailed. This implies that blind persons may need far more fixed points in such descriptions.

The additional comments apparently serve partly as further verification, and possibly help the listener to construct the more fine-grained plan of the route which is being offered. Evaluative comments also appear to have a verifying function and have, as we have seen, mainly to do with warning against possible dangers. As was shown in the functional classification scheme, information about obstacles is extremely rare in the sighted persons' descriptions of walking routes, but is fairly frequent in those of the blind.

In summary, the findings of these two studies provide insight into the problems of the blind in comparison with sighted persons in regard to street locomotion.

REFERENCES

1. Bach-y-Rita, P., Collins, C. C., Saunders, F., White, B. & Scadden, L. (1969). Vision substitution by tactile image projection. Nature, 221, 963-964.

2. Barth, J. & Foulke, F. (1979). Preview: A neglected variable in orientation and mobility. Journal of Visual Impairment & Blindness, 73, 41-48.

3. Bentzen, B. B. (1980). Orientation aids. In R. L. Welsh & B. B. Blasch (Eds.): Foundations of Orientation and Mobility. New York: American Foundation for the Blind, 291-355.

4. Blasch, B. B. & Welsh, R. L. (1980). Training for persons with functional mobility limitations. In R. L. Welsh & B. B. Blasch (Eds.): Foundations of Orientation and Mobility. New York: American Foundation for the Blind, 461-476.

5. Brambring, M. (1977). Geographische Informationen für Blinde. Zeitschrift für Experimentelle & Angewandte Psychologie, 24, 1-20.

6. Brambring, M. (1982). Language and geographic orientation for the blind. In R. J. Jarvella & W. Klein (Eds.): Speech, Place, and Action. New York: Wiley, 203-218.

7. Brambring, M. & Laufenberg, W. (1979). Construction and complexity of tactual maps for the blind. Psychological Research, 40, 315-327.

8. Downs, R. M. & Stea, D. (1977). Maps in Minds. New York: Harper & Row.

9. Foulke, E. (1971). The perceptual basis for mobility. American Foundation for the Blind: Research Bulletin, 23, 1-8.

10. Gibson, J. J. (1958). Visually controlled locomotion and visual orientation in animals. British Journal of Psychology, 49, 182-194.

11. Gibson, J. J. (1979). The Ecological Approach to Visual Perception. Boston: Houghton-Mifflin.

12. Hoover, R. E. (1950). The cane as a travel aid. In P. A. Zahl (Ed.): Blindness: Modern Approaches to the Unseen Environment. New York: Hafner.

13. Howard, I. P. (1982). Human Visual Orientation. Chichester: Wiley.

14. Klein, W. (1978). Wegauskünfte. In W. Klein (Ed.): Sprache und Kontext. Göttingen: Vandenhöck & Ruprecht.

15. Shingledecker, C. A. (1978). The effect of anticipation on performance and processing load in blind mobility. Ergonomics, 5, 355-371.

16. Strelow, E. R. (1985). What is needed for a theory of mobility--Direct perception and cognitive maps: lessons from the blind. Psychological Review, 92, 226-248.

17. Warnath, C. & Seyfarth, G. J. (1982). Guide dogs--mobility tool and social bridge to the sighted world. Journal of Rehabilitation, 48, 58-61.

18. Welsh, R. L. (1980). Psychosocial dimensions. In R. L. Welsh & B. B. Blasch (Eds.): Foundations of Orientation and Mobility. New York: American Foundation for the Blind, 225-264.

19. Welsh, R. L. & Blasch, B. B. (Eds.) (1980). Foundations of Orientation and Mobility. New York: American Foundation for the Blind.

20. Whitstock, R. H. (1980). Dog guides. In R. L. Welsh & and B. B. Blasch (Eds.): Foundations of Orientation and Mobility. New York: American Foundation for the Blind, 565-580.

FINAL COMMENTARY

The careful reader of the papers in this volume will realize
that there are a multitude of issues in this field: further,
various direct and oblique references in many papers indicate
that there are different viewpoints on many of the most important
issues and that opinions are often very strongly held. We can
not resolve these issues in a short commentary: The issues are
simply too large to be dealt with summarily. However, since most
of these issues are at least potentially amenable to empirical
research, our goal should more properly be to assist the formula-
tion of research questions. Thus, in this final section, we will
draw attention to several of the issues which we feel either are
especially important or which have not been brought out to sufficient extent in the preceding papers.

Technology and Behavioral Research

Our background as experimental psychologists makes us most
able to deal with the behaviorally-oriented issues. If we are
criticized for this bias, it will at least represent a change in a
field which has been more generally criticized as being dominated
by issues of technology. To the present time, the designs that
we have for spatial sensors have come more from a process of technological transfer in which a technology, designed for purposes
other than use by the blind, is adapted to serve as a spatial
sensor. This process has been criticized on the grounds that the
human requirements are being neglected. In some respects this
criticism is valid: The design and use of sensory aids raises
many issues in behavioral science and rehabilitation which require
solution. However, as may be evident from preceding sections,
the behavioral problems associated with sensory aids raise many
fundamental questions which we are currently far from being able
to answer. It would not help the blind to expect the technologist
to wait until these questions are fully understood before attempting the design process.

The process of providing a technological "solution" for a
human problem, prior to substantial basic research, is not unique

to the field of sensory aids. The general pattern of technological innovation in our society is that it is first necessary to demonstrate that a technology is feasible to serve a particular need before the wider prospects and problems raised by the implementation of the technology will be considered, and before the technology will become fully refined.

Given the many imponderables in predicting the success of new technologies, it is not easy to guide technological development by non-technological considerations. As an example, computer vision seems to hold great promise for future development within the area of spatial sensory aids. However, it is impossible to know at this time whether this considerable promise will actually materialize. The situation in regard to behavioral issues is almost as difficult since so many of the questions raised by the use of sensory prostheses tax our current capabilities to conduct scientific studies or even formulate appropriate research questions. However, we feel that the field of spatial sensors has matured to the point where the initial fascination with the technology of artificial sensing is giving way to the realization that the further development of this field will require more sophisticated understanding of these behavioral issues.

Information for Spatial Behavior

In this process of realignment, the behavioral and technological approaches have interests in common. For example, a key issue in both technological and behavioral research is: What environmental stimuli inform the observer about spatial events in the environment? This is important both to the potential blind aid user as well as to the designer of machines such as self-guided vehicles or robots, since both man and machine can potentially use the same information for spatial tasks.

There are several levels within this general question: What environmental information controls spatial activities; what control information can be registered by a spatial sensor; what information can be displayed to a non-visual modality; and, what information can be detected by a user and responded to appropriately? Failure of an electronic prosthesis device could result from difficulty at any of these levels. On the other hand, success requires some measure of success at each level. If there is any single message from the current collection of papers on spatial prostheses, it is that we have managed the task of presenting useful spatial information to a measurable level of success.

Evaluation and Training

Although we can claim some success in presenting useful spatial information, this is not the end of the problem. One of the major stumbling blocks to further progress in this field has been the problem of coming to terms with the behavioral issues of the use of electronic spatial prostheses. Neither in the research laboratory nor in the field have we been conspicuously successful in analyzing the important elements of spatial behavior, such as mobility and locomotor control, or even identifying the types of artificial or natural information which control these processes. The skill of mobility shows many paradoxes. It is apparently controlled by complex visual processes, yet it can still be performed at a useful level of skill by totally blind persons. It can involve several degrees of success and several forms of strategy, and one device or assessment technique may not tap the entire process. Similarly, it can at times be very forgiving of errors and at other times require great precision.

We have made progress on some aspects of the problem of assessing street travel. We now have means for deciding if the street travel of blind users is improved in several key categories by electronic travel aids (ETAs). These procedures have not been given wide use with more than a few sensory aids and a few subjects, who have generally been blind persons with above average travel skills even prior to the use of sensors. That even some number of such a sampling of the blind has been shown to be aided by a number of devices, though, gives some significance to this research area.

However, it must be born in mind that a behavioral assessment of an electronic spatial sensor is not simply an assessment of the technology. It is also an assessment of all the assumptions that we make about the nature of the processes by which we train a person to use this technology. Training users of spatial sensors is not a simple problem. Not only must the blind user learn the correspondences between device signals and spatial structure, but in many cases the potential user must learn more about the environment itself because he or she may have a poor understanding of the spatial environment. This spatial understanding problem may prove to be more difficult than the perceptual learning problem.

We wish to stress that the use of electronic spatial sensors can not be considered in isolation from several other important general issues. The blind user of a spatial aid is not the proverbial scientific black box. He or she is a human being with a wide variability of fundamental spatial skills, and an intellectual and emotional reaction to spatial activity. We need to know not just that travel aids, for example, do or do not help in some global fashion on the street, but also at what level of perceptual, cognitive or emotional functioning this help is occurring or failing to help.

Perceptual Aspects of the Use of Electronic Sensors

The general purpose of an electronic spatial sensor is to present information about the spatial environment, that would ordinarily be processed by vision, to an alternative perceptual system. The "substitute" perceptual system, though, must be able to process the information in an effective way. It does no good to present information that a perceptual system cannot process effectively. The determination of whether the sensory dimensions of a display are detectable is a comparatively straightforward psychophysical problem, and there has been a considerable amount of research on this problem, particularly centering on tactile displays.

However, it is more difficult to decide the type of environmental information to provide in the display, how to code it, or indeed, whether to code it. One general strategy is to try to model features of the visual system in a sensory prosthesis. We know that the visual system performs an excellent job of controlling spatial behavior, and it seems likely that it has evolved around the use of the most effective stimuli. However, it may or may not be the case that present technology would be capable of extracting these cues effectively. An alternative strategy is to employ the best form of spatial sensing, regardless of whether it is modelled on the visual system.

Coding and Preprocessing

Even if aspects of environmental information, such as the stimuli for the control of locomotion, could be extracted, it may not prove possible to preprocess and code them for effective use. This problem becomes very evident as one attempts to present a great deal of information about the spatial world, in order to approach the richness of visual experience.

One extreme answer to this problem is contained in the philosophy of the obstacle detector for mobility, where spatial information is reduced to little more than the indication of whether or not the path ahead is clear. Another alternative also largely avoids the perceptual coding problem by attempting to present at least some of the information about the environment in a verbal form after extensive processing by computer vision programs. This approach holds considerable promise. However, aside from the question of just how far one can go in providing useful verbal descriptions of the environment in real time, this approach would obviously be unsuitable for young, preverbal blind infants.

Several of the papers from both designers and psychologists have argued, alternatively, that there may be little point in attempting to optimize the display of information along some "ideal" of visual simulation, but rather that devices should present a rich and complex stimulation out of which the user can extract, through processes of perceptual learning and differentiation, the most useful information. It may be that devices that make heavy use of preprocessing will prove to be very effective aids to mobility, whereas the goal of understanding environmental structure will be better served by devices that present a richer array of stimulation.

Regardless of the position one takes on the issues of the amount and form of environmental information to present, it should be clear that the ultimate criterion must be the effectiveness of device use and that much research must be done on these issues before any alternative should be discarded.

Interference

Travel by the blind requires the acquisition and use of perceptual information by several sense modalities. The acquisition and use of such information must not be significantly impeded by the demands of a sensor: it is unlikely that any device will be able to substitute completely for the information that comes naturally to other sensory modalities, thus the traveler must continue to rely to some extent on those other modalities.

The question of such interference was not substantially addressed in any of the current papers, and it deserves more mention here. Most criticisms of devices have been directed to designs of mobility aids which use auditory displays, because of their potential interference with the natural hearing or use of echo cues, both used extensively in mobility by the blind. However, there are some characteristics of the use of sensory aids in travel which make this a lesser problem than it first appears. If the sensing range is comparatively short (e.g. less than 8 m), as it now is on most devices, then the presence of signals indicates that potential obstacles are present; information about these should probably have prominence. When no objects are present, no signal need be registered, as is the case with the

Nottingham devices, and there is no interference with normal hearing. The Kay sonars generate some extraneous noise at a low level even when no targets are present. The commercial Sonicguide has more background noise in the absence of obstacles because it detects the ground ahead of the traveler.

Still there is a potential problem of interference for all auditory displays when obstacles are present. One means to reduce the interference between the use of an auditory display and the simultaneous use of natural hearing has been the use of automatic level controllers for the displays. This involves monitoring ambient noise levels and adjusting the output of the auditory display to keep it only loud enough to be detected. Thus two objectives are served at once: The auditory display is not masked by very loud background sounds, and the display is kept to a level where the interference with hearing other natural sounds is kept minimal.

Information Overload

The problem of interference does not just arise with auditory displays. Any psychological task can potentially interfere with another task being performed simultaneously. For the sighted person, some aspects of locomotor control, such as remaining on a well defined travel path, apparently require very little attention and take place with a minimum of interference from other mental activities. Whether this is true for the blind is less clear. However, as the cognitive demands of the travel task become more complex, the issue of information overload may become critical. It is not known whether performance can become largely automatic in these circumstances. The relationship between the cognitive demands of travel and the perceptual demands of the processing of the information provided by a mobility aid is a critical one which needs research.

Developmental Research

A surprisingly strong theme of current research with spatial prostheses is work with blind children and infants. Most of this work has been done with Kay-type devices. One reason for this is that the richness of the display of these devices makes them of interest for the study of the processes of perceptual learning. By comparison, the obstacle detector which indicates only the presence of a clear path is of very little interest in relation to the developing non-mobile infant. On the practical side, the Kay devices are comparatively compact; even with batteries, complete systems weighs no more than .6 kg, and the animal research versions require that only 36 gm of apparatus be worn on the head. These devices have also proved reliable in operation even in the very demanding continuous use situation where the Trisensor is worn by an infant monkey. However, probably the major research attraction of these devices has simply been their availability, either in the commercial Sonicguide form or in the various research designs provided by Kay to several laboratories around the world. While there is no shortage of research questions to be formulated around the Kay technology, information is also needed about other forms of sensory substitution in the developmental research context.

The issue of intensive use is especially important. Such use is very difficult to achieve with human infants and children, and most of our research conclusions to date are based on studies in which few users have experienced more than several hours a week of sensor use. Primate models allow this question to be addressed without the attendant possibility of risk to the human subject. We should not underestimate the difficulty of assessing the perceptual-motor skills of young animals, or the pitfalls in contrasting animal with human use. However, against these concerns, we think that the advantages of intensive use, the savings in research time (most animals reach perceptual and motor maturity more rapidly than humans), and the possibilities for more thorough environmental control are quite significant and recommend the use of animal research models on these issues.

Summary

There has been much progress in technological developments applied to sensory aids for the blind in recent decades, and the promise of the application of newer technologies, particularly in spatial sensing, is great. We are impressed by the potential for advances in computer technology for application to these problems. All those who are involved recognize the need for an ever-closer interaction among engineers, rehabilitation professionals, and behavioral scientists. The degree of such interaction represented in several of the papers in this volume is encouraging. It is also encouraging to see the emerging involvement of perceptual and cognitive psychologists with roots in the more basic research areas, since this signals a recognition that the issues of spatial behavior of the blind are not circumscribed or unrelated to the larger questions of psychology. Indeed, the application of traditional psychological issues and methodologies to issues of spatial behavior and the use of electronic sensors by the blind may have as great an impact on the traditional questions of psychology as on the specific issues relating to the blind.

However, it is by no means the case that the overall field is ready to deal with the problem of designing the ideal spatial sensor. There are many issues of technological design that must be addressed. Perhaps more importantly, there are many questions about spatial interaction that must be actively addressed by both behavioral and engineering research so that both may be better informed by their answers. Although we have advanced a great deal, the path ahead is still a long one.

The Editors

SUBJECT INDEX

Far space and near space   20, 50, 51, 162, 188-189, 219-220, 240
    259-267, 270-272, 281-282
Feature detection   69, 70, 151, 438
Feedback   212-214, 231, 327, 338
Field of view   37, 48, 61, 75, 77, 380
Figural features   41, 176-178

Gait   5, 194, 281, 315, 491
Generalization of performance, aid benefits 205-210, 241-253, 300
Genetic factors   325, 326, 329
Goal direction   22, 388, 404, 464, 493, 495
Governmental policy in science and rehabilitation   377, 378, 385
Ground information   47, 48, 51, 53, 74, 78, 86, 112, 405, 431,
    433, 434, 468, 479, 487
Guide dogs   15, 41, 83, 371, 378, 415, 492, 494

Iconic   65, 423
Imagery   245, 369, 423
Independence   13, 191
Infants   189-190, 287-295, 299, 324, 514-515
Information overload   20, 37, 54, 135, 162, 165, 398
Interactive control   49, 51, 59, 175
Interdisciplinary cooperation   9, 22, 366, 381-385, 415, 509,
    515-516

Kinetic Depth Effect   180-183

Landmarks   17, 22, 37, 41, 51, 225, 231, 379, 390, 467, 472,
    491, 495, 502
Layout   17, 32, 225, 389, 398, 431-459
    Cognitive   5, 299, 388, 389, 398, 433-439, 457, 458
    Perceptual   5, 389, 431-459, 472
Localization   205-214, 219-331, 241-252, 301-319
Locomotor control   5, 18-20, 305, 388, 404-409, 431
Long cane   13, 15, 41, 51, 74, 83, 94, 125, 126, 193, 371, 378,
    398, 399, 487, 488, 494, 495

Manufacturing   4, 127, 134, 375
Marketing   6, 15, 17, 22, 125, 133, 375, 376, 382, 384
Masking   473, 475
    Auditory   16, 54, 135, 513-514
    Tactile   39
Mental manipulation   177, 184, 243-253
Microprocessor   41, 88, 161, 163, 164, 169, 184
Modelling Tasks   243-253, 259-267, 270-272, 444-445, 456
Molyneux's Question   7, 8, 30, 179, 180, 203, 426
Motivation   274, 277, 278, 316, 383
Multiple object detection   39, 132, 133, 136, 147, 151, 165,
    166, 168, 147
Multiple handicaps   375